Handbook on
Ethical Issues
in Aging

HANDBOOK ON ETHICAL ISSUES IN AGING

Edited by
Tanya Fusco Johnson

174.2 H191j

Handbook on ethical issues
in aging

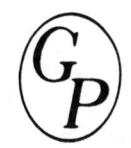

Greenwood Press
Westport, Connecticut • London

Library of Congress Cataloging-in-Publication Data

Handbook on ethical issues in aging / edited by Tanya Fusco Johnson.
   p. cm.
Includes bibliographical references and index.
ISBN 0-313-28726-0 (alk. paper)
1. Aged—Care—Moral and ethical aspects. 2. Aging—Moral and ethical aspects. I. Johnson, Tanya F.
HV1451.H35   1999
174'.2—dc21   98-8235

British Library Cataloguing in Publication Data is available.

Copyright © 1999 by Tanya Fusco Johnson

All rights reserved. No portion of this book may be reproduced, by any process or technique, without the express written consent of the publisher.

Library of Congress Catalog Card Number: 98-8235
ISBN: 0-313-28726-0

First published in 1999

Greenwood Press, 88 Post Road West, Westport, CT 06881
An imprint of Greenwood Publishing Group, Inc.
www.greenwood.com

Printed in the United States of America

∞

The paper used in this book complies with the Permanent Paper Standard issued by the National Information Standards Organization (Z39.48-1984).

10 9 8 7 6 5 4 3 2 1

This book is dedicated to my parents, Edna Dulany Fusco and Jack Quido Fusco, who have been my models and mentors for nearly six decades. Now, at the ages of 85 and 88, they continue to hold to what is good and right and to show the way to their children, grandchildren, and great-grandchildren. Without their nurturing in my young life and beyond, I could not have contributed this work. Happily, this book provides a way to carry on their legacy of ethical behavior for generations to come.

Contents

Preface		ix
1.	Ethical Issues: In Whose Best Interest? *Tanya Fusco Johnson*	1
2.	Ethical Issues in a Subculturally Diverse Society *Anthony J. Cortese*	24
3.	Ethical Issues in a Religiously Diverse Society *Cromwell Crawford*	59
4.	Ethical Issues in Spiritual Care *Patricia Suggs*	78
5.	Ethical Issues in Medical Care *Anthony Back and Robert Pearlman*	94
6.	Ethical Issues in the Quality of Care *Kathy A. Marquis and Bette A. Ide*	114
7.	Ethical Issues in Terminal Care *Dallas M. High*	125
8.	Ethical Issues in the Care of the Judgment Impaired *Lawrence Heintz*	150
9.	Ethical Issues in Mental Health Care *Martha Holstein and David McCurdy*	165
10.	Ethical Issues in Personal Safety *Georgia J. Anetzberger*	187

11.	Ethical Issues in Nonfamily Care *Phyllis B. Mitzen and Arlene Gruber*	220
12.	Ethical Issues in Family Care *Jennifer Crew Solomon*	239
13.	Ethical Issues in Legal Care *Marshall B. Kapp*	261
14.	Ethical Issues in a High-Tech Society *Gari Lesnoff-Caravaglia*	271
15.	Ethical Issues in Research on Aging *Beth A. Virnig, Robert O. Morgan, and Carolee A. DeVito*	289
16.	Ethical Issues in Long-Term Care *Laurence B. McCullough, Nancy L. Wilson, Jill A. Rhymes, and Thomas A. Teasdale*	305
17.	Ethical Issues in Decision Making: A Balanced Interest Perspective *Tanya Fusco Johnson*	326
18.	Ethical Issues in Aging: Synthesis and Prospects for the Twenty-first Century *W. Andrew Achenbaum*	340
References		351
Author Index		393
Subject Index		405
About the Editor and Contributors		415

Preface

The *Handbook on Ethical Issues in Aging* has afforded me a rare privilege to explore what I consider the most important element of all human relationships—ethical behavior—and to share in this learning with a number of able and committed colleagues. I wanted to produce a handbook about specific ethical issues adults may encounter as they grow older. Therefore, not only did I look for colleagues knowledgeable about ethics and aging, but I also approached specialists with particular expertise in the areas of ethical issues in a culturally and religiously diverse society, spiritual care, medical care, quality of health care, terminal care, care of the judgment-impaired, mental health care, personal safety with an emphasis on elder mistreatment, home health care, family care, technological care with emphasis on assistive devices to prolong life or compensate for health limitations, legal care, boundaries and possibilities for aging research, and long-term care. Consequently, a number of disciplines are represented in the handbook. These include sociology, anthropology, theology, medicine, philosophy, humanities, social work, law, social policy, public health, and history. The professional focuses of these contributors range from teaching to research to policy making to human services practice. This array of subjects, disciplines, and professions has led to a comprehensive volume and a richness of meaning for the theme of ethical issues in aging.

The contributors to the handbook have made a concerted effort to present the state of the art in ethical issues in aging by examining how specific topics have been and are currently being perceived and implemented in practice. In addition to previous and contemporary thinking in the respective subjects mentioned above, the handbook contributors have posed new questions and proposed thoughtful solutions for ethical practice in aging in the future. Several contributors have used case studies, both actual and hypothetical, to describe ethical issues and evaluate solutions. In some chapters, the contributors have advocated specific ideologies, and some have developed their own approaches to ethical decision making. The result is not only a handbook based on careful scholarship but also spirited arguments about what we ought to "do" and "be" as older adults, family, friends, paraprofessionals, and professionals. In other words, the contributors have not been content merely to review the literature. Rather, they have also presented a thorough analysis and substantive recommendations for improvements in ethical practice. In some chapters, the authors propose concrete approaches for ethical decision making. In particular, Dallas M. High in chapter 7, Georgia Anetzberger in chapter 10, Laurence B. McCullough, Nancy L. Wilson, Jill A. Rhymes, and Thomas A. Teasdale in chapter 16, and I in chapter 17 have developed more systematic guidelines for ethical evaluation and decision making.

The handbook contains 18 chapters. Chapter 1 introduces the nature and scope of ethical issues in aging, lays the groundwork for the meaning of terms in ethics and aging, and guides the reader to relevant chapters where these concepts are discussed. Chapters 2 through 4 center on cultural and religious contexts. In chapter 2, Anthony Cortese describes how various ethnic groups, especially minority ethnics, define ethical issues, and he notes how the human services delivery system has responded to the needs of different ethnic groups. Cromwell Crawford compares the ethical underpinnings for the religions of Judaism, Christianity, Islam, Confucianism, Buddhism, and Hinduism in chapter 3. In chapter 4, Patricia Suggs focuses on the spiritual dimension of people's lives and notes the ways it may impact their overall health and well-being.

Chapters 5 through 9 focus on physical and mental health issues. Anthony Back and Robert Pearlman describe changing ethical practices in medical care because of technology, costs, and the policies dictating new structures in health delivery in chapter 5. In chapter 6, Kathy A. Marquis and Bette A. Ide discuss the factors that enhance or limit the quality of health care delivery and quality assurance and describe the challenges for ethical practice. Dallas M. High looks at the ethical issues those with terminal illnesses are likely to face and presents systematic guidelines for the resolution of dilemmas in chapter 7. In chapter 8, Lawrence Heintz describes the dilemmas and decision-making responses when older adults lack the mental capacity to make decisions for themselves. Martha Holstein and David McCurdy look at the problems in mental health in general in chapter 9 and describe a number of system barriers to treatment, including the reticence of this particular age cohort to seek treatment for mental problems.

In chapters 10 through 13, the contributors focus on environmental-psychosocial-legal care needs. Georgia J. Anetzberger in chapter 10 explores issues related to personal safety. Contexts include abuse, neglect and crime, and risks for harm in the home and in institutional settings. In addition, she introduces her hierarchy of principles for adult protective services workers. In chapter 11, Phyllis B. Mitzen and Arlene Gruber examine professional and paraprofessional in-home support for older adults who are able to remain in the community because of a variety of compensatory services. Jennifer Crew Solomon takes up those issues related to the family role in elder care in chapter 12. In particular, she examines the limits of responsibility as well as the impact of differential family structures on ethical responses to elder care. In chapter 13, Marshall B. Kapp addresses the special domain called Elder Law which has evolved because, in some ways, older adults are a unique group of legal consumers. The chapter focuses on entitlements, competence, guardianship, and the role service providers play in promoting legal autonomy.

In chapters 14 and 15, the contributors look at technological advances and research in ethics and aging. Gari Lesnoff-Caravaglia describes technological applications in medicine, institutions, home, and person-oriented technologies such as organ transplants in chapter 14. Beth A. Vernig, Robert O. Morgan, and Carolee A. DeVito discuss ethics in research with the elderly in chapter 15. The authors note the benefits of research for the well-being of older adults now and, increasingly so, in the future. However, they describe the types of research activities that spawn ethical dilemmas and caution those engaged in this enterprise to use greater care in research methodology to prevent these dilemmas.

Chapters 16 and 17 center on ethical decision making. In chapter 16, Laurence B. McCullough, Nancy L. Wilson, Jill A. Rhymes, and Thomas A. Teasdale point out the ethical issues in long-term care and present a model for preventive ethics designed to avoid many of the inevitable issues that arise in this type of care. In chapter 17, I describe the "balanced perspective" for managing ethical issues in the applied setting and demonstrate this point of view by drawing on Jürgen Habermas's notion of "communication ethics" in developing a model for ethical decision making. W. Andrew Achenbaum summarizes the major ethical themes in the handbook in the final chapter, chapter 18. He compares the contributors' conclusions to those of a wide range of ethical thinkers in the past and present, and offers a critique of gaps in the literature that need to be addressed in the future, such as gender differences and comparative ethics in other countries.

The twenty-first century will most certainly give rise to ethical issues other than those raised here in the handbook. This reference volume anticipates the need to explore these new horizons and to work toward a consensus on how older adults, their social and service networks, and members of the society in general should advocate for and enforce ethical conduct. At this juncture, the handbook is a benchmark of how far we have come in protecting the well-being of our older citizens, but, more important, it serves to point the way to new directions in ethical policy and practice. I would like to take this opportunity to thank all of the contributors for playing this critical role in shaping the nature and destiny of ethical issues in aging for the next century.

I would also like to thank all of our colleagues who have reviewed our work and, in so doing, have helped us chart a clearer course for our understanding of ethical issues in aging. Further, my thanks are extended to Greenwood Publishing Group, to George Butler, a former social science editor, who conceptualized the handbook and extended the invitation to me to write it, to Nita Romer, the present social science editor, for her encouragement and continuing support, and to Charles Eberline for the most responsible copyediting effort I have ever encountered. Closer to home, I would like to express my gratitude to my student assistants at the University of Hawaii at Hilo who have helped to bring the book into its final stages—Pearl Moore, Serene Silverman, Debbie Agbayani, Ethel Wensler, and Pua Evans. Even closer to home, my thanks also to my husband, Ron Johnson, and our son, Joel Johnson, and daughter-in-law, Deb Johnson, for their expertise in the more advanced areas in word processing. Their skills were essential in putting the 18 chapters into a uniform format and compiling a master reference list from the respective chapters in the handbook. Finally, on behalf of all the contributors, I would like to thank you the reader for being our audience and for giving us this opportunity to share our current understanding of ethical issues in aging and our hope for greater wisdom in ethical practice with older adults in the future.

1

Ethical Issues: In Whose Best Interest?

Tanya Fusco Johnson

> It is precisely because life so often fails our expectations that we need one another. It is precisely because moral demands to give of self can be so outrageous, so utterly devastating, that we need to know others are prepared to do the same for us. . . . Vulnerability is understood to be part of the human condition, some being visited with greater needs than others, but others being blessed with greater strength. . . . A good society is one that finds ways to match needs and strengths, one that cares for not only public injustice visited on minority and other weak groups, but also for private injustices that nature and life visit upon individual people.
> —Daniel Callahan, in Nancy Jecker, *Aging and Ethics*, pp. 167–169

ETHICS IN AGING

This handbook follows a growing number of writings on ethics in aging, and we are indebted to their authors for the breadth of ethical issues they have addressed and their insights in charting a course for resolution. Many writers, including those who have contributed to this volume, have moved this field of ethics in aging to a higher level of understanding, and we wish to acknowledge their pioneering efforts, especially those of the many who are unnamed. Illustrative of the more well-known works, but certainly not exhaustive, are Jecker, 1991; R. A. Kane and Caplan, 1990, 1993; Kapp, Pies, and Doudera, 1985; Lesnoff-Caravaglia, 1985; McCullough and Wilson, 1995; Moody, 1992; and G. P. Smith, 1996. This reference volume has built upon these works and has attempted to develop and expand upon the ethical issues they address.

Aging as a Catalyst in the Growth of Ethics

Aging and ethics have more than a casual link. Aging has played a significant role in moving ethics into the forefront in decision making. One reason it has been a magnet for ethics is the sheer increase in the numbers of older adults, which has led to the greater visibility of aging issues. In chapter 7, Dallas High cites Gardner and Hudson's (1996) statistics that at the turn of the century the average life expectancy was 47, while currently it is over 75. With the increase in aging has come a new generation, one that we were not prepared for in some ways. John Bond (1993) has declared that this new generation of aging is a triumph of the twentieth century, as indeed it is. Although this observation was primarily for a British audience, it certainly spans continents.

We do find several arenas in which the society has responded effectively to this new generation. For example, Gari Lesnoff-Caravaglia in chapter 14 describes the benefits older adults have derived from technology. For some, technology has allowed an "electronic lifestyle" from wheelchairs and hearing aids to Hoyer lifts and lifesaving lifeline communications. These advances have enhanced the older adult's quality of life immeasurably. But technology has also presented us with questions about prolonging life. It has provided life-sustaining devices that may pose problems for those whose body is being kept alive, but whose consciousness has been extinguished. Anthony Cortese in chapter 2 observes that an outcome of modernization is to shift "death" primarily to the older adult population. Here is the major link with ethics. Issues of life and death are fertile ground for ethics. Therefore, aging itself has led to several changes in how all of us see ourselves as individuals in the society. Attendant to this aging enterprise are concerns about (1) disability and who will care for us, (2) long-term care and how we shall pay for it, (3) whether we need to have a rationing of resources, and (4) how we assess quality of life when technological advances can keep us alive. These concerns in aging have compelled us to take a closer look at what is good and right. Ethics in the past has tended to be detached from life events in such a way as to make it a separate phenomenon. However, with changes and challenges in the life course of older adults, ethics has come more and more into a central place as aging issues call for the evaluative perspective that ethics can provide.

With longevity come the likelihood of chronic illness and the possibility of disability and long-term-care needs that, among other costs, are subsequently translated into economic issues for family and professional caregivers. This leads to a question of resource allocation and whether older adults are valued as much as those who are younger. Finally, there is the question of whether human life is worth living if it means that we are merely being kept alive. Is it sufficient just to be alive, or is there something more? This calls to mind a comment a medical colleague once made: "There are worse things in life than death." His intention was to consider how much suffering we can endure for the sake of merely living, along with the socio-emotional costs that are traded off for the benefit. Consequently, we may be called upon to assess the question "Is life *worth* the living of it?" In this regard, the aging process has caused us to go beyond ethical issues based primarily in physical health care to ethical issues of a psychological nature such as self-determination, the social realm of distributive justice, and meaningful participation in the broader community. In chapter 9, Holstein and McCurdy develop this more encompassing view when they discuss mental health. Other events in recent history have demanded that ethics come closer to the center of everyday life. However, aging has certainly played a significant role.

Older Adults as a Subject of Study

As the title indicates, this handbook focuses on older adults. In doing so, the intention is not to isolate age in the life course and hence characterize the ethical issues older adults face as somehow different from those of other age cohorts. The chapter topics in the handbook—ethnicity, religion, spiritual care, medical care, the quality of care, terminal care, judgment impairment, mental health care, personal safety, nonfamily care, family care, legal care, the impact of technology and research on the practice of ethics, and long-term care—span all ages. The issues and dilemmas that arise from these situations are fundamentally the same. Further, we recognize that singling out an age cohort may lead to interpretations so exclusionary of other groups as to unintentionally set up competition and possibly conflict between groups. Even in the face of these important reasons for integrating aging into the life course rather than setting it apart, aging, nevertheless, does have its own special boundaries—biologically, mentally, socially, and culturally. Therefore, until we become what Bernice Neugarten has called an age-irrelevant society, we must, for better or for worse, view aging as a distinctive sphere in the ethics universe while at the same time recognizing that aging is, ultimately, a part of the life course and should not be examined over against it but as very much a part of it. Therefore, we have set aging apart to understand the issues distinctive to it rather than lifting up this stage of life as somehow more important than any other.

Being old creates a different profile as compared with the young and middle-aged. This profile includes (1) the potential for an increase in "losses"—physical, mental, relational, and professional—which are illustrated by Anetzberger in chapter 10 with "Anna's Story"; (2) the likelihood that the circumference of one's circle of life will be drawn smaller, into what Lesnoff-Caravaglia in chapter 14 calls an "encapsulated environment," with the center of our existence lived in the bedroom, kitchen, and bathroom, a smaller surround that Suggs sees as a catalyst for the growth of "spirituality" in chapter 4; (3) the expectation that more attention will be given to one's well-being through a variety of caregiving (Marquis and Ide in chapter 6 note that there will likely be an increase in services as one ages and that the cost of caring for the elderly will be high; of course, cost will be measured by more than just the financial burden); (4) a greater likelihood of long-term aging. For example, in chapter 7, Dallas High notes that "for most of us, death most likely will not be rapid and sudden." The usual pattern will likely be several years of gradual decline.

In spite of our observations of sustained health and fitness for many older adults, images of aging have tended to be negative for most of this century (T. F. Johnson, 1995a). Besides the picture of natural consequences of the aging process being one of decline, there remains an adverse cultural attitude toward aging in some corners. In chapter 9, Holstein and McCurdy discuss the consequence of this denigration by describing aging as a process of "deculturation." This negative image of aging has sometimes been translated by human services providers into discriminatory practice characterized by the concept of "ageism," which Robert Butler has described (1969, 1989), policies of rationing of resources in favor of younger people, and, in some instances, a deepening disregard for older adults who find themselves in a dependent care situation. T. F. Johnson (1991) notes that ageism stretches far beyond laypersons' attitudes to institutional policy and practice areas—societal ageism (antiage legislation), community ageism (programs that exclude the elderly), and professional ageism (treating the elderly like children). In chapter 9, Holstein and McCurdy talk about societal ageism as well. For these and other reasons mentioned by the contributors in the following chapters, ethics does take a somewhat specific turn in its meaning when applied to the elderly.

Some Differences among Older Adults

The study of ethical issues in aging is complicated by the fact that there are individual differences among older adults that come from a number of sources, from peculiarities in personality to culturally rooted behaviors. Some older adults are strong willed and have managed to be in control all their lives. Others may be willingly submissive because they feel overwhelmed by making decisions. Some are decisionally incapacitated and, as a consequence, present condition-specific ethical issues, many of which Heintz discusses in chapter 8. Several of the contributors note that ethical issues become more complex for groups with different religious, ethnic, racial, and social-class starting points. Cortese explores all of these dilemmas in chapter 2. In spite of great strides in our society against sexism, racism, ethnocentrism, and classism, there are still issues that revolve around these demographics.

Sex and gender are good examples. Gilligan (1982) contends that women respond to moral dilemmas differently than men. In chapter 4, Patricia Suggs notes that spirituality may be experienced differently in men and women. Solomon in chapter 12 and McCullough, Wilson, Rhymes, and Teasdale in chapters 12 and 16 observe that women are more likely to be the primary caregivers in dependent care situations. Solomon, more specifically, points out that this identification with the caregiving role could lead to negative gender typing in elder care and subsequent exploitation. Lesnoff-Caravaglia in chapter 14 notes that sex is a factor in the structure of relationships in older age. Older women are less likely to remarry than older men. This presents ethical issues of different kinds. For those older women who do not remarry, the circumference of care diminishes, often causing them to rely on professional assistance. On the other hand, for men, new in-laws pose questions about moral responsibilities for the aging parent-in-law who may be a stranger to younger family members. Nevertheless, as legally constituted family members, without the trappings of socioemotional ties, in-laws may be looked upon as potential caregivers.

With regard to racial and ethnic issues, Marquis and Ide in chapter 6 state that medical decisions may be based on racial considerations. Mitzen and Gruber in chapter 11 note the potential for conflict in situations in which an African American paraprofessional is placed in a non–African American household. It is also the case that the same racial or ethnic-group affiliation between the paraprofessional and the older adult can cause problems. In some cases, loyalties based on these demographic factors may promote an alliance of the two against the agency.

Finally, there is the recognition that political jurisdictions, both small and large, will be different in their management of ethical issues. For example, several of the contributors talk about policies in other countries. In chapter 2, Cortese observes that Canada and Australia train more physicians in primary care than the United States—a fact that could have implications for the "preventive ethics" that McCullough, Wilson, Rhymes, and Teasdale discuss in chapter 16. In chapter 7, Dallas High compares the United States to the Netherlands, where active euthanasia and physician-assisted suicide are permitted for persons with preexisting conditions. National consensus of this type could change the ethical interpretation of life and death, especially the taking of one's own life. Marshall Kapp observes a difference in the orientation to guardianship between the United States and Great Britain in chapter 13. In the United States, there is a heavy emphasis on autonomy, while in Great Britain, the stress is on beneficence. Kapp points out that the pursuit of autonomy for the older adult by trying to prevent guardianship could get in the way of meeting the care needs of the older adult. There is a similar difference between the United States and Great Britain in cases of elder mistreatment. In the United States, elder mistreaters tend to be "criminalized" or approached in an adversarial way. However, in research this author conducted in the United Kingdom in 1991, it seemed that the "criminal" label was replaced by a more "compassionate" posture. In the case of the latter, both the victim and the mistreater were believed to be in need of care and support, much more so than in the United States.

Older Adults in the Community

Having recognized that the needs of older adults are like those of others in many ways and different in other ways, we assume that their participation in the community (their rights and obligations) is not any different from that of other members. Therefore, we would expect them to be much invested in their destiny, to avoid dependence when they can, and to be their own advocates through the life course. At the same time, we would expect them to reciprocate and honor the same circumstances for others. In chapter 9, Holstein and McCurdy note that even "dementia does not remove the sufferer from the ranks of being a person." Older adults' feelings, desires, responsibilities, successes, and failures are a part of the "humanness" they share with others in the community. Except for those who are temporarily or permanently mentally incapacitated, they are accountable just as everyone else is. Jennifer Solomon observes in chapter 12 that care flows back and forth between generations. Therefore, there is a need for sharing rights and duties. In chapter 10, Georgia Anetzberger notes that even in the nursing-home setting, there are not only resident rights but also responsibilities. Older adults should not be treated like children (helpless and dependent), but, rather, competent older adults should be expected to participate in give-and-take relationships like noninstitutionalized adults.

Therefore, when we examine ethical issues in aging, we must view the older adult as a part of a constellation of intergenerational and community relationships—bottom up and top down. The older adult's well-being cannot be assessed apart from the community, nor can those in the community detach themselves from the older adult. Therefore, this book focuses on the individual older adult in the community and the community of which the older adult is a part. Each and every individual in this setting—the older adult, family, friends, neighbors, paraprofessionals, and professionals—is expected to pursue ethical rights as well as duties in a network of reciprocal encounters. Along with times of mutual support and cooperation, we recognize that there are likely to be "clashes" of interests. These are the circumstances under which we raise the questions of in whose "best interest" the ethical decisions are made. While we would hope that there would be consensus among parties, we may expect situations in which decision making is confounded by misunderstanding, a lack of clarity, and real differences. "Complexity, ambiguity, conflict, and stress are, to put it simply, the normal conditions of the moral life" according to McCullough, Wilson, Rhymes, and Teasdale in chapter 16.

When we look at managing different interests, we imagine a puzzle. The goal is to fit the various pieces together so that they form a unified picture. We start with the easiest pieces, the boundaries, and then move toward the center. The closer we move toward the center, the more hard pressed we are to find parts that fit. We must find the best connections between the closed places and the open portions. The task requires repeated attempts with some pieces almost fitting, but not quite. Sometimes we try to force them into place. Eventually, we know that in the end, if we are patient, a complete picture will be constucted. The pieces become linked together into a perfect wholeness. When there are competing interests, we suspect that the process is similar to putting the puzzle together. We are a bit more certain of the boundaries than how things will take shape in the center. We also understand that in order for the pieces to fit together, we must allow the shape of concerns to control the outcome, all the while recognizing that, ultimately, these differing configurations, closed views and open, can fit together into a unified whole.

A Case-based Approach to Ethical Issues

Most of the contributors in this handbook use cases to discuss ethical issues. This method of analysis is found in other works in ethics (Rhodes, 1991; Beauchamp & Childress, 1994; T. F. Johnson, 1995b). Using cases is another way in which ethics can be more centered in actual day-to-day life. Here is an example of how complicated decisions can become when interests are competing.

A Case Study of Best Interest

The social worker and the public health nurse agree that the disabled arthritic 83-year-old older adult must move from the apartment into a nursing home for greater safety and health monitoring. The retarded son, age 45, who lives with the parent and helps with household activities, cannot manage to live on his own. If the parent goes to the nursing home, he will either have to live with his sister, age 50, who is married with two teenagers, or will need to be institutionalized as well. The daughter believes that it is time for the parent to have more competent supervision but is feeling pressure about having the parent and brother live with her. She feels obligated to bring them to live with her. However, she fears that it would greatly disrupt the household, take time away from her husband and children, and require a considerable economic investment that might jeopardize the savings for the children's college education. The parent, who is assessed as a competent adult, refuses to leave and is supported in this decesion by an ombudsman. However, the neighbors tell the landlord that if the parent stays, they are afraid that this person may set the apartment complex on fire in the process of fixing meals on the gas range. The landlord cannot evict without medical certification that the older adult is unable to manage self-care and the care of her son. However, the primary-care physician has attested to the fact that the older adult is perfectly competent and able to perform most of the activities of daily living. For things that the parent cannot do, the son seems able to manage. Each party in this situation has his or her own interests that are quite legitimate but, nevertheless, in competition.

The perspective of this handbook is to consider each interest, neither elevating nor subordinating the older person or others involved in the life of the older adult. Everyone's point of view in the relationship must be acknowledged and addressed if consensus is to take place. More particularly, we will follow the same orientation John Arras (1995) proposes: a *balance* perspective in which best interest favors neither the client nor others in the community. This assertion does not mean that there is a leveling of expectations in which nobody is satisfied, with compromise being the best outcome, or a stalemate or an uneasy alliance. This approach seeks to push toward a win-win perspective that emerges out of information, deliberation, and negotiation so that in the end, the pieces of the puzzle fit to make an integrated whole. In chapter 17, we will examine this "balanced-interest" approach in greater depth in the discussion on ethical decision making presented by this author.

The Presentation of Multiple Perspectives

This handbook includes multiple points of view. The contributors have several starting points: (1) they come from a variety of disciplines that have developed discipline-specific conventions and specialized tools of analysis; (2) their views are drawn from different roles in the practice setting; (3) their work is bound by specific professional codes that have an impact on ethics; and (4) quite understandably, each contributor is likely to be governed by his or her own personal perspective on what is ethical. This mix, far from creating bedlam in the following chapters, makes for a rich rendering of interpretations in their discussion of ethical issues.

The contributors to this volume have necessarily approached aging, ethics, and the subject matter through the eyes of their own disciplines: sociology, religion, medicine, philosophy, social work, law, social policy, public health, and history. Consequently, it is a difficult task to speak the same "ethics language" because starting points are discipline specific. Beauchamp and Childress (1994, p. 37) make this point when they observe that what they call "principles" may be termed "right," "virtues," or "values" by others. Back and Pearlman in chapter 5 refer to what this writer elsewhere (T. F. Johnson, 1995b) has called values as principles, and, conversely, they speak of values using the terminology that this writer has called principles. We note that McCullough, Wilson, Rhymes, and Teasdale in chapter 16 use principles and values similarly. Since we have yet to come to a consensus on terminology, the reader is asked to grasp the issues in the context of the specific ethics language each contributor adopts, a task that is quite easy once it is understood that terms are not necessarily used in the same way.

Various practice settings are represented: research, policy, practice, or a combination. For example, Vernig, Morgan, and DeVito in chapter 15 discuss research issues, Anetzberger provides a formula for doing ethics from an adult-protective-services point of view in chapter 10, and Mitzen and Gruber look at ethical issues from the practice perspective for paraprofessionals in chapter 11. In addition, ethical issues in aging are filtered through the perspective of the contributors' various professional codes. For example, Vernig, Morgan, and DeVito discuss the impact of various codes such as the Nuremberg and Helsinki codes and the Belmont Report in doing research. Each profession tends to have its own code of ethics. Finally, the reader will find that personal positions for an ethical perspective may be seen in the writing of some. For example, Anthony Cortese in chapter 2 and Marshall Kapp in chapter 13 seem to have adopted a "social justice" ideology, while Dallas High in chapter 7 and Jennifer Solomon in chapter 12 emphasize an "ethics of care" approach.

As the reader will see, this diversity may not only mean that there will be different word usage for the same notion, it will also demonstrate that some issues and their resolutions are stressed more than others. In fact, most contributors have not attempted to be encyclopedic. Cortese's chapter that follows is the most comprehensive, focusing on the broad-brush complexities of aging minority subcultures from family relations, transportation, work and retirement, intergenerational relations, gender differences, and health care to attitudes toward death. At the other end of the spectrum, Mitzen and Gruber in chapter 11 on nonfamily social care narrow their discussion primarily to the ethical issues for the home care worker.

It is important to keep the multiple starting points of the contributors in mind as one reads the following chapters. These points of view have necessarily shaped the ethical issues that are most critical to one's competing specialization, whether of medicine, mental health, religious tenets, legal mandates, or social care—whether examined by the professional researcher or the family. As a consequence, the authors demonstrate just how complex ethical issues can be.

Congruence of Meaning on the Subject of Ethical Issues

Given such diverse starting points in the exploration of ethical issues in aging, the reader will find that there is no unified terminological framework. However, it is the intrinsic meanings of the terms that are important in the communication of ideas, not what we in the various professions elect to name them. In this respect, there is considerable congruence. In fact, there is a noticeable uniformity in the identification of ethical issues and the dilemmas the authors pose for the older adult, the family, and the professional. At the end of the twentieth century, we and our colleagues have not achieved consensus in the usage of terms among disciplines or, in some cases, even within them, but this in no way diminishes our concerted attempts to find a common substantive meaning in discussing ethical issues in aging.

At this juncture in our understanding, we have not come as far as we would have liked in our multidisciplinary dialogues. However, when we see how far we have come during this century, we believe that we are where we ought to be in terms of progress toward this goal. This handbook comes at an important time in this process. It is an opportune time to take stock of the state of the art in ethical issues in aging as the next century draws near. As we stand at the threshold of the twenty-first century, there is an atmosphere of renewal, reform, and invention. It is in this vivifying climate that this handbook has been prepared.

PARAMETERS OF ETHICS

Despite differences in labeling ethical phenomena, there are some common notions about ethics that have formed the foundation for this handbook. We shall begin by framing ethics per se and providing a method for mapping meaning. The primary goal here is to demystify ethics, bringing its usage into the everyday world of laypersons as well as professionals. This is not to be confused with our coming to an ultimate recognition of truth or some profound apprehension of reality, but merely, through the limits of our place in history, to operationalize a notion that first and last is essential to promoting our collective survival. Ethics as a subject of study belongs to philosophy. However, the practice of ethics is grounded in our everyday lives, whether personal or professional, public or private. Because of its roots in philosophy, ethics has developed a reputation for being abstract, even esoteric. In some ways, ethics in the past has cast a spell of being incomprehensible over us and has prevented those who were not students of this subject from linking it with daily experiences. Philosophers are not expected to be practitioners, and it would be unusual for practitioners to study philosophical theories to any great length. What is needed is a bridge between these two spheres. This handbook is intended to dispel the belief that ethics is too restricted for nonethicists to grasp. The contributors will show how ethical issues and decisions emerge out of a number of everyday experiences in which older adults find themselves. Overall, our goal is to convince private individuals and professionals that this perspective on our lives is quite embedded in mundane, ordinary existence as well as out-of-the-ordinary crises. Therefore, all of us, including laypersons, need to become moral gatekeepers. Lawrence Heintz in chapter 8 illustrates this point in his discussion of advance directives. Social workers are not prepared for clients to talk back, but they need to be; physicians are not always responsive to advance directives that would permit the patient to be a player in the health outcome, although they should be.

The root of the word "ethics" comes from the Greek term "ethos" or "ethikos," meaning character or moral. Moral, in turn, refers to the Latin word "mores," or cultural rules or customs of the people. Culture or customs do not refer to a specific group of people. Rather, they make reference to a generic script or recipe for living based on what one "ought to do" as contrasted with what one "prefers to do" or "actually does." Mores become loaded with meaning when we develop a specific governing system. As Cortese says in chapter 2, "Morality is socially constructed." In this sense, ethics is a marker that helps us measure how close our actual conduct is to an absolute that is defined in terms of the "ought to." Ethics is a dynamic word that includes a process involving means and ends as well as a field of study. As a field of study, ethics has several branches: *metaethics, descriptive ethics, ideology*, and *applied ethics*. Some call the first two nonnormative ethics (Beauchamp & Childress, 1994), and some consider ideology and applied ethics normative (Singer, 1994). *Metaethics* involves raising questions about various ideologies while not subscribing to a particular one, and *descriptive ethics* refers to the enterprise of characterizing ideologies, also without advocating for a particular ideology. While both are alike in some ways, there is a clear difference in that metaethics is evaluative while descriptive ethics is a matter of mirroring or depicting ideas. *Ideology* is the advocacy of a set or system of beliefs, and *applied ethics* refers to linking an ideological framework with a real-life situation. Since descriptive ethics is more of a journaling endeavor, we will not explore this effort further here. However, more needs to be said about metaethics, ideology, and applied ethics.

ETHICS AS A FIELD OF STUDY

Metaethics

Metaethics centers on raising questions about conceptualizations in the domain of ethics. It is not the goal of metaethics to espouse a particular system, but rather to explore how we decide what is ethical. The works of Mackie (1977) and Hare (1981) are good illustrations of using metaethics. There is a search for meaning, not as an ultimate but as the immediate. Metaethics raises questions about how individuals and groups develop their ethical meaning—the various ways people evaluate life and subsequently how their assessment promotes certain standards. It assumes that there is differential perception, subjectivity, a grounding in time and space—geography, the political context, the social structure, occupational protocols, and, perhaps, different stages in the life course. It is the study of how people create ethics that promotes their best interests. For example, the metaethicist would like to know the process of formulating ethical standards of elder care between the home health aide and the spouse. Why is it that the aide violates ethical standards if she or he acts as an intimate, while the family members violate ethical standards if they do not do so? In Mitzen and Gruber's chapter 11, it is in the best interest of the home health aide to be professionally attached but personally detached in order to be most helpful to the client. On the other hand, the client may wish for a familylike relationship between the aide and himself or herself before trust can really be established. After all, the family would be expected to be personally attached.

Ideology

Ideology, the second branch of ethics, includes the ethical theories that have been systematically constructed to make judgments of right conduct and to explicitly or implicitly state beliefs that are wrong. This branch provides the criteria for a system that analyzes right and wrong. It is divided into two spheres: the secular and the sacred. There are so many books on ethics that it is hard to distill and sort meaning. We have elected to use secondary sources that have done the work of synthesis. There are several, of course, but two will be mentioned here: Newman and Brown (1996) and Beauchamp and Childress (1994). Newman and Brown separate these ideologies into five categories. (1) *Consequence* theory (Bentham, 1970) is a teleological theory assessing right and wrong on the basis of consequences. The goal is the greatest good for the greatest number of people. (2) *Duty* theory (Kant, 1956) is a deontological theory based on obligation as the rationale for right and wrong. (3) *Rights* theory (Feinberg, 1984) is related to deontological theory. This theory focuses on the "rights" of individuals to not have others infringe on their privacy and participation. (4) In *social justice* theory (Rawls, 1971), everyone should be equal, and if not everyone is equal, unequal distribution in favor of the disenfranchised is appropriate to bring them up to the norm. (5) *Ethics of care* theory (Gilligan, 1982) is a feminist reaction to "reason" as the dominant driver in ethics based on relationships and the contextual relationships in which people find themselves rather than abstract, rational notions.

Tom Beauchamp and James Childress (1994) use eight categories. (1) In *utilitarianism* or *consequence-based theory* (Mill, 1969), while happiness and pleasure have been salient in terms of goals, other goals such as friendship, health, and understanding have also been advocated. (2) In *Kantianism or obligation-based theory* (Donegan, 1977), morality springs from reason and is an expectation that the individual meets because every other person is obliged to do the same. Others are treated as ends, not means. (3) In *character ethics or virtue ethics* (Aristotle, 1985), the individual's motivations are taken into account, and conduct is based on the self-development of each individual. (4) In *liberal individualism or rights-based theory* (Dworkin, 1977), individual freedom is the focus. The rights of all, whether private or public, are protected from the intrusion of others. (5) In *communitarianism or community-based theory* (Sandel, 1982), there is a focus on the common goal, social solidarity. The individual is subordinated to the group. Common history and the welfare of the group as a whole take precedence over the individual's needs. (6) In *ethics of care or relationship-based accounts* (Baier, 1985), personal involvement is more important than impartiality, emotions are more critical than reason, and persons who are "unequals" can be in a relational network. (7) In *casuistry or case-based reasoning* (Jonsen & Toulmin, 1988), casuistry means being skeptical of rules and therefore taking an intimate look at a particular situation. This leads to examining similar situations and precedents. Ethics develops out of consensus about a case. (8) *Principle-based or common-morality theories* (Frankena, 1980) are based on rules coming from tradition and common sense that promote universal standards.

In comparing the two classificatory models, we see that Beauchamp and Childress include the five of Newman and Brown, but go beyond this listing to include virtue ethics, case-based ethics, and principle-based ethics. Other typologies have been constructed using other categories. Margaret Rhodes's (1991) classification is an example. However, Beauchamp and Childress have provided a reference that is more than sufficient for this handbook.

A second context for doing ethics is the sacred. The sacred is comprised of religious philosophies that include, primarily, the categories of (1) *theism* (a belief in gods or goddesses), illustrated by Christianity, Islam, Judaism, and Hinduism; (2) *the simple supernatural* (impersonal forces found in animate and inanimate objects that influence human activities), illustrated by mana and Shintoism; (3) *animism* (spirits that can be benevolent or evil and may inhabit persons or objects), illustrated by black magic and voodoo; and (4) *abstract ideals* (a focus on higher levels of thinking and personal conduct based on principles such as truth and justice), illustrated by Buddhism and Confucianism. When one looks for ethical guidelines, one is not required to choose the sacred or the secular. These guidelines can include both. A. D. Hunt, Crotty, and Crotty (1991) point this out when they note, "My everyday culture instructs me. It regulates morality and provides moral directives. Religious culture also instructs me" (p. 8).

Cromwell Crawford describes the different ethical approaches of Judaism, Christianity, Islam, Confucianism, Buddhism, and Hinduism in chapter 3. In chapter 2, Cortese links religious beliefs with various ethnic minorities, demonstrating the union between the sacred and the secular. In particular, he shows the influence of the Far Eastern religions—Buddhism, Shintoism, and Confucianism—on death and dying within the Japanese ethnic group. Patricia Suggs then develops another dimension of the sacred in her discussion of spirituality in chapter 4. Probably all religions have some form of spirituality, but spirituality need not be preceded by a particular religious affiliation. Spirituality tends to be a more personal manifestation of the sacred as opposed to group norms set out in established religions. For this reason, it has less reliance on external systems and standard polities. Therefore, when one includes the sacred in the ethics repertoire, it is important to identify both whether one has the backdrop of an established religion and whether that individual may also have a private interpretation of the sacred as defined by that person's spiritual nature. Holstein and McCurdy in chapter 9 stress the importance of the spiritual as well as the psychosocial in the maintenance of mental health of older adults.

Applied Ethics

The third branch of ethics is called applied ethics. In this form, an ideology is brought to bear on a particular condition in life. Peter Singer (1986) notes that while applied ethics had been discussed in previous centuries, it had very little impact on specific life events until the second half of the twentieth century. A number of events beginning in the 1960s were a springboard: "the American civil rights movement, and then the Vietnam War and the rise of student activism began to draw philosophers into discussions of moral issues: equality, justice, war, and civil disobedience" (Singer, 1986, p. 3). As a sign of the rapid growth of this section of the field of ethics, journals have been established that focus only on applied ethics. Chief among these has been the journal *Philosophy and Public Affairs*, which began publication in 1971. When we think of older adults specifically, topics in applied ethics that come to mind include (1) suicide (including physician-assisted suicide), (2) persons with Alzheimer's disease, (3) rationed care, (4) quality of life, (5) active and passive euthanasia, (6) ageism, (7) sexism, (8) ethnocentrism, (9) the rights and duties of cohabiting partners,

(10) the right to be abused (because the other parts of the relationship are good), (11) the right to die, and (12) the right to lie. In applied ethics, one brings a specific ideology to bear on topics like these. That ideology may arise from private or public expectations—the personal, informal interpretation or the professional, formal one. Given the fact that there is such a wide variety of ideological starting points, it is obvious that there could be different interpretations. The levels of disagreement on ethical ideologies might include differences among laypersons, differences between laypersons and professionals, or differences among professionals, even those in the same occupations.

Most of the contexts described here imply a crisis or a problem, and indeed, most of the chapters in this handbook look at problems in aging. However, we must not lose sight of the fact that ethics is a part of wholeness and wellness in aging and can be applied to prevent crises. To this end, Marquis and Ide in chapter 6, Holstein and McCurdy in chapter 9, and McCullough, Wilson, Rhymes, and Teasdale in chapter 16 discuss the importance of preventive ethics. The intent is to manage conflicts before we ever raise the question of ethics or whether something or someone is right. We shall take a closer look at this notion in chapter 17.

ETHICS AS A PROCESS

The Practice of Ethics

In order to make ethics an applied concept, we must move from the armchair of speculation to the avenues of unpredictable, ever-changing day-to-day encounters. We leave the study of ethics as a conceptual phenomenon and direct our attention to the practice setting. McCullough and Wilson (1995) talk about ethics as a "downward-up" process, that is, one in which we probably do not start with ethics in the practice setting. Rather, we begin with a situation—more specifically, the individual case. If the resolution of an issue or dilemma is complex, and there is not consensus in the decision, then we most likely will move to the stage in which ethics is called to settle differences. In order to get a handle on starting points, we must look at the steps that actually lead to practice, or what Charles J. Fahey has called "doing ethics" (1992, p. 3), the term we shall adopt.

From this writer's point of view, there are four basic steps in the process of doing ethics:

1. The *identification* of key ethical concepts that name attitudes and behavior.
2. The *implications* of these concepts for interpersonal relationships that are articulated in propositions. Among professionals there are codes of ethics.
3. The *interpretation* of the propositions into protocols (specific procedures for action).

4. The *implementation* of the protocols in interaction (decision making among major parties to the ethical issue).

Couched in academic language, the first three steps are primarily homework, and the fourth is bringing what one has learned into the classroom where one will discuss, agree or disagree, and, hopefully, come to some consensus while, at the same time, preserving and even affirming differences. Although the process may look like a clearly marked footpath of identification, implications, interpretation, and implementation, it is not nearly as formulaic in its execution. First of all, we must note that there is a subjective element in each step. Ethics is the paramount recipe for goodness—the ultimate quality aspired to in our human condition, not just for one particular individual, but for all the citizenry. Who among us does not wish to do good and prevent evil? This goal of goodness is probably hoped for even among many who do evil. But having said this, do we really know *what* is good, and then do we know *how to be* good? By whose calculus? What we believe is good may be different from what is good. How do we know what is ethical as private individuals, or as public figures, or as a society as a whole? To our chagrin, the answer is that we probably can never really know. Our human condition that is vulnerable to the ebb and flow of historical events and embedded in cultural prescriptions mires our attempts to translate the pure quintessential principles into practice. We speculate and approximate what would be ethical conduct in our efforts to do what is right, but we tend to only see through the glass darkly. It is a double challenge both to know what is ethical and then to enact the ethical in everyday life—to actually "do" ethics. At the philosophical, abstract level, the nature and scope of the ethical seems much clearer. However, when we try to see how it fits with the unpredictable conditions of everyday life, certainty is challenged. A closer look at the four steps will show why certainty in doing ethics is difficult to achieve.

Ethical Concepts

In order to avoid the confusion in the use of "values" and "principles" mentioned earlier, we will call the single-word notions concepts. Concepts are handles around which we wrap ethical practice. There is a growing consensus in this last quarter of the twentieth century about which concepts are central to ethical practice. Here too, there is disagreement on the usage of terms—whether to have umbrella terms under which related terms are subsumed, or to expand the categories. Beauchamp and Childress (1994) take a conservative approach and include only four (*autonomy, nonmaleficence, beneficence, justice*). They call these four "principlism" and link principlism to the ideology of common-morality or principle-based theory mentioned earlier in the descriptions of types of ideologies. Others include *fidelity* (filial piety) (Sung, 1990; Kitchener, 1984), *confidentiality* (privacy), and *veracity* (accountability). Beauchamp and Childress (1994) consider truth telling, confidentiality, privacy, and fidelity "substantive rules" but not principles.

The contributors to this handbook discuss some or all of seven concepts: *autonomy, privacy, benevolence, justice, nonmaleficence, fidelity*, and *accountability*. In fact, the application of these concepts constitutes the major focus of the following chapters. However, some are emphasized more than others. It is important to mention at this point that the contributors' use of these terms does not imply that they have adopted the principle-based ethics that Beauchamp and Childress have so eloquently developed through four editions of *Principles of Biomedical Ethics*. Rather, these concepts are used simply to name the context in which ethical issues and dilemmas are centered. We must also note that although they imply that elders have the right to have these seven conditions operative, the wish to claim these rights is not universal. It depends on the older adult's orientation. As Solomon points out in chapter 12, there are some older adults who do not want to make decisions or do not want to hear the truth about their condition. Under some circumstances, the desire not to know (the abdication of autonomy) or choosing not to tell (not being accountable) may be beneficent. Therefore, the application of these concepts must be case based, which again does not refer to the ideology mentioned earlier, but simply draws attention to the uniqueness of each ethical situation. Cortese observes in chapter 2 that these concepts may be moderated by one's religion. For example, in the fatalistic notions of the Mexican American, if you are sick and terminal and your time is up, there is nothing you or the doctor can do. In such instances, several of these concepts become irrelevant. Furthermore, deference to the group may supersede one's individual preferences. Therefore, it is important to recognize that while these seven concepts appear to be the major pegs for ethical discussion and debate, we must not presume that all older adults subscribe to them in the same way or to the same degree. They are merely guides, not mandates. A brief description of each follows.

Autonomy

Autonomy refers to self-rule or the right to have control over one's situation as long as others are not harmed, or assigning others to act on the older adult's behalf. This concept is the most frequently cited one among the contributors to this handbook. In addition, some contributors, including Anetzberger in chapter 10 and Kapp in chapter 13, see a hierarchy among the concepts and place autonomy at the top. Achenbaum in chapter 18 implies this in his discussion of power. In chapter 17, this author takes a different perspective and elects to view autonomy and the other six concepts as coequal. Considerable research has been conducted on the notion of autonomy, breaking it down into different types (Collopy, 1988), different forms of consent (Moody, 1988), and different parties in the decision-making process (High, 1989, 1994a). Lesnoff-Caravaglia in chapter 14 points out that technology has greatly enhanced autonomy. Newman and Brown (1996, p. 38) point out that autonomy is not one-sided. It implies responsibilities as well as rights. Thus the elder, the family, other informal caregivers, paraprofessionals, and professionals all have rights and responsibilities in the network of interaction. By extension, the rights of each must be honored by others, and, in so doing, all must be responsive and responsible to each other. Herein lies the basis for competing interests. For this author, rights and duties are also embedded in the other six concepts.

Privacy

This author has chosen to use the term "privacy" rather than confidentiality because the former term is more encompassing. Rosalie Kane (1993b) probes the nuances of this concept in the home care setting. From this writer's point of view, privacy includes more than restricting information. It also encompasses the sphere of where one resides and with whom one chooses to associate. Privacy, along with accountability and fidelity, is discussed least among the contributors. However, this does not make them any less important. It may be that these notions are least developed because they are the hardest to pin down in practice. They are less tangible than the concepts of autonomy, beneficence, justice, and nonmaleficence. Because Beauchamp and Childress have tended to dominate the field of bioethics with the four principles of autonomy, beneficence, justice, and nonmaleficence, it may be that the other three have been either ignored or, as has been done by Beauchamp and Childress, absorbed into these four.

Beneficence

Beneficence is the second most frequently cited concept among contributors to this handbook. The meaning of beneficence is to seek to provide benefit for others (Collopy, 1993). In some ways, this concept is the crux of "best interest." Since benefit implies cost, and since the older adult, family, paraprofessional, or professional may disagree with what is in the older adult's best interest, beneficence is likely to spill over into the issue of autonomy (Abramson, 1989). Doing good, therefore, often resides in the eye of the beholder rather than in the system. As an example of reciprocal beneficence, in chapter 9, Holstein and McCurdy talk about the need for older adults to be drawn out of self-absorption and into contributing to the welfare of others as a preventive to mental illness.

Justice

Justice and nonmaleficence tie for third place among the seven concepts as the most frequently cited by the handbook contributors. Justice refers to fair play. It includes notions of equity for all parties, especially if there is status denigration because of sex, race, ethnicity, or socioeconomic status (Rawls, 1971). It spans the macro as well as the micro levels. At the macro level, it refers to categories of persons such as Native Americans, Italians, Jews, rural elderly, institutionalized elderly, or a patient population. At the micro level, it includes smaller groups such as specific older adults, their families, and their specific paraprofessional or professional care provider. At the macro level, Wetle and Fulmer observe, "Although the primary role of the health care providers involves advocacy for a specific patient, both individual professionals and the organizations in which they work also have responsibilities for *populations* of patients. It is not uncommon that the interests of a single patient are weighed against the interests of other patients" (1995, p. 35). Back and Pearlman in chapter 5 illustrate this dilemma with Case 4, the case of Frances. In this example, not only are Frances's needs compared with others and rationed accordingly, but the physician's needs are also highlighted. It is in his best interest not to pursue her case because of the terms of the physician's contract with the HMO, which favors categories and quotas rather than individual cases.

Nonmaleficence

Beneficence and nonmaleficence are often found together. Certainly one can make a case that they are sides of the same coin. In chapter 13, Kapp simply combines beneficence and nonmaleficence in the notion of *parens patriae*. The specific focus for nonmaleficence is on doing no harm. In the extreme, when elder mistreatment occurs, this author has referred to this elsewhere as "unnecessary suffering" (T. F. Johnson, 1991). In this respect, Anetzberger points out in chapter 10 that when no help is available to protect older adults from mistreatment, exposing the situation may do more harm, and so one must question whether to report abuse. Unnecessary suffering could be used in the broader context of doing no harm as well. That is, some degree of suffering may be necessary when the care of the older adult requires extraordinary measures. For example, there is the older adult who does not want to go to the nursing home, but must go because of care needs; there is another who becomes weak and dizzy through overmedication in order to control a life-threatening condition. Therefore, besides those situations in which pain can be prevented, one must also recognize that sometimes it is necessary to experience pain to prevent more severe pain.

Fidelity

Fidelity refers to the commitment of persons to one another, whether they are older adults, family, informal caregivers, paraprofessionals, or professionals. It is the promise to be faithful—to follow through with a commitment to be of help to the older adult (Sung, 1990). While some use the term "filial piety," this seems to be a limited conceptualization. It is not just family members who are included in fidelity, but also friends, paraprofessionals, and professionals. When paraprofessionals or professionals have agreed to the care of the older adult and the process of care, they will be expected to honor their contract of care—to not abandon the older adult and his or her family unless there are circumstances outside their control such as illness, a job change, moving away, or death.

Accountability

Accountability is often called veracity. It refers to being responsible for accurate information, not misrepresenting the situation or practicing deception, whether one is an older adult, family member, paraprofessional, or professional. McCullough, Wilson, Rhymes, and Teasdale in chapter 16, Back and Pearlman in chapter 5, and High in chapter 7 talk about the professional's role in helping family members process information and make decisions: "nondirective counseling," the "deliberative approach," and the professional's responsibility to make sure family members communicate with one another even if there is hostility among them. Each of these modes requires some degree of paraprofessional as well as professional accountability. Mitzen and Gruber in chapter 11 illustrate the issues surrounding accountability when the paraprofessional takes time off from work illegitimately. Holstein and McCurdy in chapter 9 discuss the need for older adults to be accountable for their mental illness when it is self-inflicted, as in the case of alcoholism.

Propositions

Propositions do not settle disagreements, nor do they facilitate decision making. What they do is develop the intrinsic meaning of the concepts included in the previous section. To "do ethics," the implications of these concepts must be converted into propositions. Propositions lead us in the direction of action, but they are not prescriptions. They suggest a means to an end. They are "ought to" statements intended to direct us to what is good. While older adults may not have systematic principles, they nevertheless may have a clear notion of what is implied for them with regard to autonomy, privacy, beneficence, justice, nonmaleficence, fidelity, and accountability. This is also true for professionals. Most professions, at the very least the helping professions, set up their own codes of ethics or standards of conduct that advance the process of "doing ethics."

Protocols

Propositions are interpreted into protocols (procedures) in the applied setting. These may be profession specific and most likely agency specific. There is considerable latitude in usage, and often the procedures are dictated by a particular political jurisdiction. These systems then reflect the agency or institutional limitations and possibilities for services. Ethics must be filtered through administrative policy. At the theological level, Crawford points out in chapter 3 that according to Christianity, human needs must be given priority over institutions (Mark 2:27). However, Back and Pearlman in chapter 5 observe that in medical practice it is sometimes the case that the institution takes precedence over the patient, illustrated by their case study of Frances and the preferred-provider organization. Institutions may tie workers down as the Lilliputians did Gulliver. For example, Margaret Rhodes (1991) observes, "They discourage workers from questioning rules, goals, methods of evaluation.... The professional role of discretion, then, instead of serving clients' best interests, serves more often to mask bureaucratic features" (p. 144). Mitzen and Gruber in chapter 11 point out this dilemma when agency protocol conflicts with the needs of the client. The client expects the paraprofessional to be an intimate, while the service agency expects him or her to be detached. Marshall Kapp in chapter 13 is also concerned about the impact of agency protocols on human services with regard to guardianship. He fears that agencies spend too much time and money on the guardianship process. These resources could be better used in the care of the elderly.

Older adults also have protocols—plans for action in everyday life. Suggs in chapter 4 notes the importance of discerning the "spiritual" beliefs of clients before a care plan is developed. Those persons in residential care are likely to have routines established in preinstitutionalized times, and as long as they do not cause harm to others, they should be permitted to maintain these familiar and customary ways of doing things. As we read the following chapters, we will find several examples of professional and individual procedures that play a major role in either promoting ethical decision making or undermining it.

Decision Making

Ethical concepts, propositions, and protocols are the foundations for decision making. Ethical decisions in the practice area are most likely the consequence of much discussion and debate among individuals who attempt to do what is good in the face of limited material and human resources. It would be rare to find any two people, even two people in the same occupation, approaching a situation in the same way. The decision making may vary, but not the goal. John Hospers makes this point: "Ethics not merely describes moral ideals held by human beings, but asks which ideal is better than others.... Two people might agree on the empirical facts of the case and yet disagree about what course of action to follow in view of the facts" (1961, pp. 6–7). The following illustrates differential perceptions in decision making: A social work student recently interviewed for a position in a local nursing home where there are three social workers on staff. When the student asked the director of social work whom among the social workers he should approach about patient care questions, the director observed that any of them would be fine. They were all qualified and highly skilled, but she believed that there would be three different opinions about the best plan to achieve a common outcome because each worker had different gifts, experiences, and perceptions. Therefore, each decision would be valid and valuable. She believed that each colleague should use her own gifts in problem solving. However, there was no disagreement about the goal of beneficence. Each social worker had the preservation of the well-being of the client in mind.

Several contributors discuss the merits of ethics committees as well as their cost, especially Heintz in chapter 8 and Anetzberger in chapter 10. Anetzberger also highlights the development of "residents' councils" in nursing homes in order to demonstrate that the patients are very much partners in the decision-making plan. In their discussion of "preventive ethics" in chapter 16, McCullough, Wilson, Rhymes, and Teasdale observe that this prospective approach presumes that the plan of care will be open to review and renegotiation as the situations in one's life change. What may be a good ethical decision for today may not be how things look tomorrow. Therefore, decision making is at best tentative.

While some would place the "communicative ethics" of Jürgen Habermas in the category of an ethical ideology, Anthony Cortese included, to this author it seems to be more of an ethical process. Preventive ethics would seem to fit into this context as well. In particular, both are decision-making systems. McCullough, Wilson, Rhymes, and Teasdale develop their model in chapter 16, and this writer builds upon Habermas's communicative ethics in chapter 17.

ETHICAL ISSUES AND DILEMMAS

Ethical Issues

Before we conclude this introduction to the handbook, there are a few more terms to define. These include *ethical issues, ethical dilemmas*, and *nonethical issues*. Ethical practice can be clear-cut, but there may be questions. Joan C. Callahan (1988, p. 6) defines issues as "questions" arising from a single ethical concept, and dilemmas as "questions" that emerge because two or more concepts are in conflict. For example, in the case of autonomy, should grandma be allowed to seek quackery medicine when all else has failed? Relative to distributive justice, does the son owe something to himself when he is consumed by his mother's care?

Ethical issues usually arise from questions about one of the seven concepts—autonomy, privacy, beneficence, justice, nonmaleficence, fidelity, and accountability. A good illustration of an ethical issue in the context of autonomy is the advance directive that Back and Pearlman, High, and Heintz discuss. In different ways, these contributors raise questions such as the following: (1) What if the physician does not comply? (2) What if the patient's preferences change? (3) How can the patient know his or her preference when that person has never been in this situation before? (4) How will we know if the patient and the physician have the same interpretation of such conditions as "incapacity" and "extraordinary measures"? (5) What if the doctor and the patient are reluctant to discuss the conditions set out in the advance directive?

Ethical Dilemmas

On the other hand, ethical dilemmas typically emerge when there are conflicts within, between, and among the seven concepts. The contributors provide several illustrations. Chief among them is the dilemma between physician-assisted suicide (autonomy) and preventing death (nonmaleficence). There are cases in which terminal illness can create a dilemma between telling the patient (accountability) and preventing emotional harm (nonmaleficence). Back and Pearlman in chapter 5 offer the particularly disturbing case of Frances, mentioned earlier, and the discovery of the breast mass. The physician seeks to preserve his own welfare through a commitment to the institutional rules (beneficence) but places his patient in a potentially life-threatening situation by not telling her about the breast mass (accountability). Vernig, Morgan, and DeVito in chapter 15 describe a dilemma in a nursing home where a family refuses to take part in a study (autonomy) that could be beneficial to the residents, including their relative (beneficence).

Nonethical Issues

How do we distinguish between ethical issues and nonethical issues? Daily living most likely does not consist of moving from one ethical decision to the next. There is much that is nonethical. The nonethical refers to our preferences as long as those preferences do no harm. McCullough, Wilson, Rhymes, and Teasdale in chapter 16 talk about Mrs. G's decision to go to a nursing home. There are a number of decisions she must make with reference to this. These include (1) whether to sell her home, (2) what personal possessions to take to the nursing home, (3) whether to ask for a single or double room, (4) what activities she will engage in while there, and (5) with whom she will form relationships. Each of these decisions is based on personal preference, and as long as one's preference does not violate the rights of others, it is not defined as a part of the ethical realm. However, we see in this case that the daughter has objections. She believes that her mother's plans are not in her mother's best interest. If disagreement ensues, then ethics comes into the picture. Therefore, ethics is not an absolute criterion that we use to sort attitudes and behaviors. It is an interpretive response to a situation as a consequence of a conflict of interest as to what is right either within the individual or between or among individuals no matter what their status. Therefore, we may expect that such conflicts will trigger the need for ethics. On the other hand, consensus precludes the need for ethical decision making. McCullough, Wilson, Rhymes, and Teasdale speak to this separation between conditions for nonethical decisions and ethical decisions in chapter 16.

CONCLUSION

In this chapter, we have laid the groundwork for what is to follow by introducing the overall goals for this handbook and by providing a terminological framework with which to approach the chapters that follow. However, while each contributor is "in the same church," each is not necessarily "in the same pew." The contributors have been free to address their subjects as they chose, like the social workers in the nursing home noted earlier—with their own gifts, experiences, and perceptions. As a consequence, they have launched their ideas about their topics in the context of ethics in aging with a sense of urgency, immediacy, and uncompromising honesty. As the reader will see, the results have been thought-provoking and provocative. For their determination to be candid, prodding, and especially pioneering, this writer is most grateful.

2

Ethical Issues in a Subculturally Diverse Society

Anthony J. Cortese

The major objective of this chapter is to provide a comparative reference on ethical issues that emerge for subculturally diverse older adults within the following contexts:

(1) The broader sociocultural environment
(2) Particular subcultural constructions of
   (a) attitudes about the elderly, and
   (b) interaction rituals involving older adults, including beliefs about death and dying
(3) Health and health care delivery

There is a focus on subcultural ethical practices, moral principles of conduct, and ideology. I examine the following racial/ethnic categories: African Americans, Latinos, Japanese Americans, Native Americans, and whites. There are case studies on most of these categories. Comparisons and contrasts between the dominant culture and the particular subculture are made, as well as comparisons between subcultures.

This chapter explores ethical issues in a subculturally diverse society, including moral aspects of care for elderly of color. There is a particular focus on ethnicity, race, age, and sex. Wherever possible, data are broken down and presented by race or ethnicity. Finally, implications for social policy are offered.

The proportion of the population that is elderly is growing increasingly larger. This will have an important impact on health care delivery systems. Disproportionately high birth rates for ethnic minorities and near-record rates of immigration from Mexico, Latin America, the Caribbean, and Asia have significantly altered demographics in U.S. society. These changes in the ethnic composition of the U.S. society have affected (and will continue to affect) the sociocultural system, including social mores and ethical decision making.

In 1980, over 2.5 million persons, or 10% of all persons aged 65 years or over, were nonwhite (U.S. Department of Health and Human Services, 1990a). Racial and ethnic-minority elderly have been increasing at a faster rate than white elderly in recent years. This tendency is anticipated to continue in the next century, with tremendous implications for public and educational policy for the training of physicians, sociologists, nurses, social workers, dentists, pharmacists, psychologists, occupational and physical therapists, and nursing aides. Between 1985 and 2030, the white elderly will grow by 97%, compared to 265% for older African Americans and other races and an amazing 530% for Latino elderly (U.S. Department of Health and Human Services, 1990a, p. vi). Demographers predict that in the next century, the minority part of the elderly population will swell rapidly from 13% in 1985 to 21% in 2020 and 30% in 2050.

The social responsibility of applied ethics requires us to examine how the increase of culturally diverse elderly directly or residually affects the larger society. Issues include unequal access to and unequal quality of health care, housing, transportation, affordability of health care, racism, and sexism. Since the 1930s, the remarkable development of gerontology, geriatrics, and social gerontology has taken place without adequate attention to ethnic background and minority status (Markides & Mindel, 1987). It was not until the 1960s that important studies of the African American elderly were published. Concentration on Latino elderly came even later, during the 1970s. Even so, there has been little research on Latino elderly except for Mexican Americans in California and southwest Texas. More recently, gerontologists have begun to study elderly Native Americans and Asian Americans.

From these studies, we know that ethnic-minority elderly have the following problems:

1. A generally lower life expectancy than their white counterparts
2. Linguistic and cultural barriers that hinder access to social, legal, and health care services and to public transportation
3. Less education than their white counterparts
4. Lower-paying blue-collar jobs (many without Social Security or retirement benefits)
5. Inadequate income
6. Poor housing conditions
7. Poor access to health care, social services, and preventive health services
8. Inadequate representation in policy and legislative bodies
9. Emotional attachment to their ethnic communities
10. Underutilization of long-term-care and mental health services

The ethnic-minority elderly also have many strengths, including the following:

a. Strong kinship bonds, family unity, loyalty, and interfamily cooperation (ability to provide for the physical, emotional, and spiritual needs of the family)
b. Strong work and achievement orientation (ability for self-help and mutual help)
c. Adaptability of family roles (ability to perform family roles flexibly)
d. Strong religious orientation (ability to discern spiritually)

MORAL PLURALISM VERSUS UNIVERSALISTIC MORALITY

Justice is an essential theme in social life. The notion of justice as fairness underscores the claims of legitimacy by a society's social and political institutions (Greenberg & Cohen, 1982). When such claims start to lose their legitimacy, social change usually occurs. At the same time, the issue of social justice in everyday life is pervasive. However, the definition of justice and its implications or guidelines for rules of ethical conduct may vary considerably between subcultural groups. This raises the important issue: Is a universal justice possible? Within the context of this chapter, is there "fair treatment" in the arena of health care for subculturally diverse older people? Is there "fair play" in decision making involving the ethnic-minority elderly?

Minority groups have a culture of their own—a *subculture*, with a distinct set of values (Meyers, 1984). Each ethnic-minority group has its own unique *ethical ideology*—systematic belief systems about what one ought to do or who one ought to be. The negation of subcultural values and the related ethical ideology places *majority groups* in the elitist position of asserting that they know what is good for a people even though those in question may not want it (Henshel, 1990). *Cultural relativism* (see Herskovits, 1972) observes the validity and equality of all cultures and, therefore, the right to cultural self-determination. The problem with cultural relativism is that it implies nonintervention or a laissez-faire approach to social problems. If all values are relative, there are no objective criteria in moral reasoning.

Any discussion of human rights, however, implies *universalistic ethics*, applicable to all people regardless of ethnicity, culture, social class, or gender. If one assumes a position of cultural relativism, nevertheless, ethical criteria become intuitive and insufficient. Thus a tension emerges from the attempt to reconcile universal ethics or human rights with *pluralistic ethics* or moral relativism.

It is clear that just, good, or acceptable behavior varies tremendously across cultures (and even between and within subcultures within a more general culture) and time. Happiness is achieved in exceedingly diverse ways that are fluid and subjective (Moore, 1970). Yet a considerable degree of consensus or accord exists among the ways subcultures characterize extreme misery, torment, or suffering. This type of discourse allows one to move beyond cultural relativism by focusing on conditions of extreme misery, conditions on which there is substantial agreement. Such analyses can be gainfully applied to ethical issues in a subculturally diverse society.

DISTRIBUTIVE JUSTICE

Distributive justice is a major ethical issue in a subculturally diverse society. On what basis do we distribute resources for the elderly? Given that the need for medical services and products is greater than what is available, who should receive an artificial heart or a lung transplant? What is the fairest way to assess need? "First-come, first-served"?

There is a great deal of inequality in health care. The case can be made that too much of the medical profession's attention, effort, research, technology, and financial resources is geared toward costly cures for the rich at the expense of basic, preventive health care for the poor, working, and middle classes. Medical schools train too many specialists and not enough primary-care physicians. Australian medical schools instruct three-fourths of their students in primary care, those in Canada, half, but those in the United States, only a third. Growth in specialization has also resulted in an overabundance of hospitals and physicians concentrated in the affluent suburbs. Consequently, inner-city communities and rural areas are stranded, with unsuitable access to health care delivery.

The problem of distributive justice also emerges at a more basic level: How should society distribute resources that develop particular types of new procedures at the expense of others or that acquire new knowledge in some areas while ignoring others? "Personnel and facilities for medical research and treatment are scarce resources. Is the development of a new technology the best use of the limited resources given current circumstances?" (Kass, 1985, p. 26). We must consider that the resources used in medicine and biology are also needed to reduce gender and ethnic discrimination, urban decay, environmental pollution, and poverty and to improve the quality of education.

American society is experiencing an internal "brain drain" that squeezes our brightest youths into rigid careers focused on the search for biochemical defeats in rare genetic diseases while the much more fundamental issues of social and economic inequality are chiefly ignored. These judgments are usually made within a framework of conflict between competing interests. The sociolegal system in the United States is based on a complex that is inherently power and conflict oriented. Institutional arrangements are grounded on the balance of power and checks and balances. The question starts as "How should X be justly distributed?" However, it ends up "Who will decide how to distribute X?" Consequently, a moral issue is often turned into a power play.

Some people, with knowledge of medicine as their instrument, exercise power over others. It is the marriage of science and politics that makes this possible. Science and politics combine to decide the limits of population growth. Fertility control is typically coercive, including brute force as well as the imposition of forceful sanctions. During the Nixon administration, a high-level psychologist-advisor called for the psychological testing of all 6-year-olds to detect future criminals and misfits. The suggestion was rejected because current tests lacked the required predictability. What would have occurred had reliable tests been available?

The most fundamental social problems regarding health care are ultimately issues of power and justice. Technologically induced dehumanization, the abuse of power, and the distribution of scarce resources are topics that provide a window for defining and implementing an ethically based health program. Technology has increasingly come to be the primary rationale for scientific inquiry. Science has come to be associated with power, and less with knowledge. We hold the power to manipulate most of the unfavorable consequences of technology, yet we lack the ethical decision making to decide what technology should be developed in the first place.

The delivery of effective health care depends on scientifically reliable ways for improving the quality of life and decreasing unnecessary death and premature death. As medical technology hastily advances, the amount of cases for which potential public health activity might be taken on is proliferating quickly. Moreover, various innovative strategies are used to implement new and existing technology. Since resources are always finite, it is crucial that distributive justice be implemented to ensure equitable distribution of scarce resources among the various segments of our population.

HEALTH AND HEALTH CARE

Elderly ethnic minorities generally have greater health problems than their white counterparts. Moreover, minorities tend to have chronic disability at an earlier age than nonminorities (Hawkins & Kildee, 1990). Forty-one percent of elderly Latinos viewed themselves to be in poor or fair health, compared with 29.9% of all elderly (C. Lopez & Aguilera, 1991). Elderly Latinos also have disproportionately higher rates of disability than non-Latinos. Elderly minorities of color face serious problems in the arena of health care delivery. Many begin working at a very early age (often as young as 5 years of age) and are often employed in hard labor (factory work, farm work, or manufacturing) that leaves them with an assortment of work-related illnesses or disabilities. Access to the health care system (e.g., transportation, cost of care, communication) is another problem. Without adequate transportation, many Latino elderly have problems getting to their doctor's office, hospitals, or clinics. When they do arrive, they rarely discover bilingual staff to assist them.

Thirty-one percent of elderly Latinos had been bedridden for 1 to 30 days in the previous year, compared to 22% of elderly whites and 27% of elderly African Americans. In addition, elderly African Americans had an average of 43 "restricted activity days" during that same period, compared to 31 days for whites and 37 days for Latinos (C. Lopez & Aguilera, 1991). Latino elderly are less likely to visit a physician when having a health problem (8 visits annually, compared to 9.1 visits for white elderly and 9 for African Americans) (U.S. House Select Committee on Aging, 1989, pp. 9–10).

Even with Medicare, the elderly must put more than 15% of their income toward health care (Ehrenreich, 1990). Latinos are more underinsured for health care than any other racial or ethnic group and suffer disproportionately from disability or illness. Latino elderly are more likely to depend on Medicare to pay for health care; the general elderly population is more likely to have a private source of health insurance. Nevertheless, only 82% of Latino elderly were covered by Medicare, compared to 96% of all elderly (Andrews, 1989, p. 38). Eight percent of Latino elderly have no health insurance, compared to only 1% of all elderly (Andrews, 1989, pp. 37–39).

Data on personal care activities are not always consistent. For example, census data report that a higher proportion of Latino elderly have obstacles to personal care activities and tasks of household management than the overall elderly population (U.S. Bureau of the Census, 1990c, p. 4). A robust indicator of poor health is the need for assistance with activities of daily living (personal care, preparing meals, doing housework, getting around outside, basic finance keeping). However, in another study, it was discovered that nearly 23% of African American elderly need help with one or more of these activities, compared with 15% for whites and 19% for Latinos (C. Lopez & Aguilera, 1991).

In another study by the Commonwealth Fund, ethnic minorities were more likely to have problems with the most basic activities of daily living (eating, toileting, dressing, bathing, and transferring to bed or chair). Forty percent of Latino elderly had such problems, compared with 23% of all elderly. (Transferring was the most troublesome activity for Latinos.) Moreover, 54% of Latino elderly had problems with at least one instrumental activity (money management, telephone use, meal preparation, shopping, and light to heavy housework), compared with 27% of all elderly. Most burdensome for Latinos was heavy housework (Andrews, 1989, pp. 40–43).

Latino elderly rely on their families (typically a spouse or child) more than on other relatives and nonrelatives for assistance with the activities of daily living. Among Latino elderly living with others, more than 60% receive help from a child in the household with the most basic activities of daily living (Westat, 1989). Most Latino elderly do not pay for this family-based support. They live with others because they need such assistance and cannot pay for it (Westat, 1989, tables 2–30, 2–34). Following is an illustration of health and health care delivery problems for an elderly Latino. This story is based on fact. (The name has been changed to protect confidentiality.)

Case Study 1: Latinos

Eighty-three-year-old Samuele Perales, of Mexican descent, has fallen through the cracks of the American Dream. He is one of the countless people whom census takers cannot even find. Samuele is not very sick, but he feels weak and looks pale. He had tried to obtain medical treatment a couple of years ago by hitching a ride early one morning from outside the housing project where he stays with relatives who do not really want him. When he finally arrived at the outpatient clinic, he waited 14 hours without being seen by a physician or a nurse, then returned home. In the weeks that followed, Samuele did not return to the clinic.

Samuele did not, however, disappear completely. Most of the time, he could be seen in the basement cafeteria of an elderly day-care facility located near the center of the barrio and run by a religious agency. It is a nice place for the elderly poor to chat with friends, play cards, listen to music, watch television, eat a hot meal or two, and be safe for a while from the haunting visions of loneliness and the trauma of urban violence. Late one afternoon, volunteer workers at the center noticed that Samuele seemed listless and pale. After asking some questions of him, they communicated his symptoms to a member of the clinic's staff.

The clinic serves a predominantly Latino community, but pamphlets about high blood pressure, smoking, and breast cancer now come in Kurdish, Vietnamese, and Cambodian as well as in Spanish and English. The faces of the outpatients reflect the cultural diversity of the area—and often the hesitation of people for whom the very idea of going to the physician remains foreign. (Once a small group of Kurdish women from Iraq refused to get off the bus at the clinic because they were not sick; they were pregnant but inexperienced with prenatal care.)

The physician ordered some blood tests for Samuele; results indicated anemia. Further tests revealed that Samuele cannot digest vitamin B-12. The nausea and illness the old man has been experiencing for untold years is a simple problem, with a simple solution—a B-12 injection once a month. All Samuele had to do was show up for his appointment. Today Samuele is keeping his end of the agreement.

The clinic is a community-oriented primary-care (COPC) system where patients do not just get rushed in and out. The physician also noticed that Samuele was short of breath and wanted to know why. Samuele admitted that he was not sleeping well. Why not? He said that he was not getting along with the relatives he has been staying with. Why not? Because he was old and forgetful. The physician continued to pry. But why did this adversely affect his sleep? Finally, Samuele revealed that his relatives had kicked him out of the tiny apartment. Then where was he staying? "With friends at night." The physician knew that this signified that Samuele was very close to living on the street. Dignified, polite, and proud, the old man would not come out and say it.

While the physician prescribed a sedative to help with sleep, the clinic nurse took notes on Samuele's condition to pass on to a social worker who, hopefully, would be able to find Samuele a safe place to sleep at night. As they talked, the physician asked Samuele to remove his tattered straw cowboy hat. It was obvious why he always wore it. An oval growth—benign—bulged from the right side of his head. The physician measured the growth to discover whether it had enlarged. It had—a little—but perhaps that was a side effect of the B-12 injections. The physician told Samuele to return in two weeks, partly to continue monitoring his condition, and partly just to make sure that he was still around.

This case study illustrates possible subcultural responses to aging, the role of the elderly in Latino culture, and the need for and right to maximum support and care by others (the moral value of beneficence). Samuele's poverty and his poor health have clearly made him dependent on family and other caregivers. He has a right to have his personal welfare and physical well-being restored and maintained. His family and other caregivers are obligated to him in this regard. Moreover, members of Samuele's family are obliged to offer the highest standards of care of which they are capable in order to prevent any further adverse consequences for him (the moral value of nonmaleficence).

Samuele's professional caregivers are expected to offer preventive care in order to preserve his health and well-being (once again, the moral value of nonmaleficence). Samuele also has the right of continued assistance as long as he needs it (the moral value of fidelity). Since Samuele obviously needs help, his family is obligated to either offer help itself or recruit the services of others. They should not abandon him. In the case study, recall that the health care staff referred Samuele to a local social worker; the moral value of fidelity requires this.

At the macro level, this is an ethical issue of *distributive justice*. Society has a commitment to share material and/or human resources without regard to ethnicity, race, gender, social class, or subcultural differences. This discussion has offered *moral principles*—rules of moral conduct—that key on Samuele's health care needs and how he and his family and professional caregivers should respond in light of relevant ethical values and the subcultural context.

Latino elderly are among the most unprotected yet least conspicuous parts of the Latino community; they are unprotected from violent and property crime, health care risks in the environment, and financial liability. Since Latinos, in general, are a young population and among the most poverty-stricken segments of the U.S. population, the needs of Latino elderly tend to be ignored (C. Lopez & Aguilera, 1991). The rapid growth of the Latino elderly population has significant implications for the Latino community as well as for ethical issues of social responsibility and distributive justice, since this elderly population is among the neediest in the nation (Macionis, 1996).

Health care is unquestionably very expensive and therefore, for this reason alone, not equally accessible to all. The limits of biomedical technology are also being questioned (Beauchamp & Childress, 1994). The medical profession and some of those satisfied with the current health care delivery system work to avoid government intervention and regulation. Yet some of the most critical problems involving culturally diverse populations have not received adequate attention.

The following section addresses how subcultures construct their own ethical systems, with a focus on how these systems compare and contrast with the ethical system of the dominant culture. This involves discussion of how conflicts between the two systems are managed.

ETHNIC ETHICS

Human social and cognitive development is largely an outcome of the child-rearing practices of the cultural subgroups that compose a modern complex society (Havighurst, 1976, p. 56). *Ethnic groups* are people who have a common history and generally share ways of life, including language, religion, and social identity. They affect individuals through family activity, peer group, linguistic concepts, common literature, work in formal associations, in-group marriage, and residential and work segregation. *Social classes*, too, are pervasive and powerful in their influence on individuals (Macionis, 1996; Gordon, 1964, p. 52; Havighurst, 1976, p. 56). Ethnic groups, however, are also effective, more so at the lower- and working-class levels than at the middle- and upper-middle-class levels.

Sociologists use the term *subculture* to refer to the cultural patterns of any type of subgroup within the national society (Gordon, 1964, pp. 38–39). Each ethnic group is a subculture with its own set of behaviors and attitudes (Havighurst, 1976, p. 56). Subcultures, nevertheless, do not exist in isolation. They affect and are affected by the general culture as well as other subcultures. One may speak of the subculture of a neighborhood, a factory, a hospital, a university campus, or even a gang. A. Cohen's (1955) study of the cultural patterns of a delinquent gang uses this notion of subculture.

Recent research guided by a critical approach to cognitive-development theory offers insights into the humanizing effects of the ethnic and cultural sources of moral values (Cortese, 1990). Morality is socially constructed, not based on rational principles of individuals (Cortese, 1989a). This alternative theory conflicts with the universal theories of morality and societal development as formulated by Immanuel Kant (1949), Jean Piaget (1965), Lawrence Kohlberg (1969, 1981, 1984), John Rawls (1971), Jürgen Habermas (1984), and J. C. Harsanyi (1982).

Critical analyses of ethnicity and moral judgment combine two controversial and central areas: morality and race relations (Cortese, 1989a, 1989b). Critiquing the cognitive-developmental model, Cortese (1980, 1982a, 1982b, 1984b) examines social class, gender, and ethnic differences in moral judgment. This argument (Cortese, 1990) is situated in relation to both Kohlbergian theory and the feminist critique thereof (Gilligan, 1982). The major thesis is that "moral judgment reflects the structure of social relations, not the structure of human cognition" (Cortese 1990, p. 4). The agenda is to (1) explore the impact of ethnicity, culture, and language on moral development (Cortese & Mestrovic, 1990), (2) elucidate conceptual problems linked to justice and objectivistic-subjectivistic tensions (Cortese & Mestrovic, 1990), (3) identify methodological problems in the study of moral judgment (Cortese, 1984b, 1987, 1989c), and (4) clarify the relationship between Kohlberg's (1984) approach and sociological theory (Cortese, 1985). This critique of Kohlberg (Cortese, 1986a) also constitutes a challenge to the moral theory of Jürgen Habermas (1984).

Moral reasoning and behavior are determined largely by social factors—role demands, class interests, national policies, and ethnic antagonisms. One cannot be moral in an immoral social role, whatever one's childhood socialization, psychological predispositions, or commitment to abstract rational principles

(Cortese, 1990, p. 2). Social forces and individual cognition interact to shape moral judgment (Cortese, 1985). A purely sociostructural framework cannot totally account for the wide range in moral reasoning among people in similar social roles. Yet it is important to focus on the ethnic origins of moral reasoning. Latinos and African Americans typically base their moral judgments on principles of responsibility, fidelity, and caring rather than abstract principles of justice (Cortese, 1984a). Any universal theory of ethics must account for epistemological relativism.

Kohlberg's work borrows from Piaget's (1965) theory of cognitive moral development, Kant's (1949, 1950, 1963) philosophy of science, Rawls's (1971) theory of justice, and Émile Durkheim's (1961) concept of morality and has been criticized by adopting Karl Mannheim's (1971) sociology of knowledge (Cortese, 1990). Habermas makes extensive use of Kohlberg's ideas in his theory of communicative ethics. Habermas recognized that the implicit social evolutionary model in Kohlberg's stage theory fits nicely with his own developmental theory of communicative ethics and instrumental rationality.

The pivotal issue in examining ethical issues and minority elderly is the alleged universal generalizability Kohlberg attached to his six-stage developmental model. Kohlberg postulated that as individuals mature, they move from simplistic forms of moral reasoning to the use of more complex moral principles, although most never achieve the higher stages. Kohlberg's theory has spawned considerable research and controversy (Cortese, 1986b; Gilligan, 1982; Simpson, 1974).

The central argument is that Kohlberg's theory is, at best, a heuristic model and, at worst, false, because it ignores the fact that ethnic and cultural factors shape the moral development of individuals in ways that would make any universalized model of moral development fail when comparative testing was used (Cortese, 1990). While Kohlberg's hypothetical moral dilemmas were designed to test the ability to comprehend and implement more highly complicated forms of "justice," real-life decisions are complex and go beyond abstract questions of justice. Kohlberg's moral dilemmas can be criticized as unrealistic and depicting situations as having rigid either/or choices and consequences (Cortese, 1984b). In particular, Latino and African American responses to moral questions frequently differ significantly from the responses of whites. Moreover, women's responses differ from those of men, indicating gender-specific socialization regarding moral reasoning (Gilligan, 1982). For example, in the now-famous Heinz Dilemma (a destitute man is faced with the choice of stealing lifesaving drugs for his wife from a pharmacy or allowing her to die), women focused on Heinz's care, responsibility, and love for his wife, not justice or rights, the intended focus of the question.

American ethnic minorities and those raised in non-Western cultures sometimes gave responses that indicated alternative forms of moral reasoning. Labeling these alternate forms of reasoning as indicating lower levels of moral development makes Kohlberg's work subject to criticisms of ethnocentrism. The

Standard Issue Scoring system tends to favor complex reasoning and abstract dialogue; thus alternate types of solutions are typically scored at the lower stages. In addition, Kohlberg's (1984) presumption that individuals move as they mature from lower, less sophisticated stages to higher, more complex ones makes his theory open to the criticisms of various forms of evolutionary theories and related forms of developmental thought. What Kohlberg has done is to create ideal types of discrete forms of moral reasoning and presume an inevitable sequence of development, much as nineteenth-century anthropologists presumed that they had uncovered the inevitable sequence of social change that led from savagery to civilization. The fact that Habermas (1984) chose to transform Kohlberg's individual stages of moral growth into stages of increasingly rational societal communication demonstrates that developmentalism is inherent in both theories. Developmentalism is acknowledged as an important dimension of human nature and social order.

MINORITY AGING AND HEALTH PROBLEMS: ETHNIC COMPARISONS

While people in the United States are living longer, life expectancy remains lower for ethnic minorities (C. Lopez & Aguilera, 1991; U.S. Department of Health and Human Services, 1990a). Life expectancy for the general U.S. population increased from 69.7 years in 1960 to 74.9 years in 1988 and is projected to increase to 77.0 years in 2000 (U.S. Bureau of the Census, 1990d, p. 72).

Ethnic-minority families place remarkable priority on caring for their elderly; this puts distinct moral responsibilities on the family. Latino elderly are more likely to rely on their families for care and assistance than other elderly. This represents the ethical value of fidelity, under which loyalty in times of need is manifested in assistance. Latino elderly are also less likely to be institutionalized than both white and African American elderly. Besides elders' reliance on frequent familial support, Latino families must also face heavy economic hurdles. (One out of every four Latino families are poor.)

COMPARATIVE LIFE EXPECTANCY

Although data are collected by race and ethnicity, the National Center for Health Statistics does not publish life-expectancy tables for Latinos or Latino subgroup populations. Data, nonetheless, suggest that life expectancy for ethnic-minority groups (71.3 years) is less than for all races (75.0 years). The life-expectancy rate for African Americans (69.4 years) is substantially less (a difference of 6.2 years) than for whites (75.6 years) and, perhaps even more disturbing, has been steadily declining since at least 1984 (69.7 years in 1984, 69.5 years in 1985, 69.4 years in 1986, 69.2 years in 1990) (National Center for Health Statistics, 1997).

Latinos are less likely to reach the age of 85 (or over) than non-Latinos (U.S.

Bureau of the Census, 1990a). Ethnic minorities comprise a smaller portion of the over-75 elderly population than they do of the elderly over 60 years of age (Hawkins & Kildee, 1990, p. 7). At age 55 and later, mortality rates of Latinos are somewhat lower than those of non-Latinos (Markides & Mindel, 1987, p. 79).

RACIAL MORTALITY CROSSOVER PHENOMENON

There is a notable exception to lower life expectancy for African Americans compared to whites: 75 to 80 years of age. At this point, a convergence occurs whereby African Americans have more expected years remaining than whites (Wing, Manton, Stallard, Harnes, & Tyroler, 1985; Manton, 1980). We call this the *racial mortality crossover phenomenon*. There are also racial crossover patterns in death from heart disease and certain types of cancer (National Center for Health Statistics, 1980).

Racial mortality crossover suggests that whites and African Americans age physiologically at various speeds. This calls into question the validity of chronological age as a measure of aging when African Americans and whites are compared (Jackson, 1985; Markides & Machalek, 1984). This is but one example of how ethnic background may play an increasingly larger role in the distribution of health care services, the scientific investigation of the elderly, and the strategies of health behavior intervention. The crossover phenomenon, at about age 75, appears to suggest that the relative health and environmental position of the disadvantaged African American has improved. However, the overall situation of African Americans relative to whites has not improved substantially (Sullivan, 1989).

The crossover phenomenon exists also for American Indians. There are 1.4 million American Indians and Alaska Natives who identify themselves as Indians. Life expectancy of American Indians and Alaska Natives was 50 in 1940 and approximately 70 in 1980. Once they reach their 55th birthday, however, they die at a slower rate than all other U.S. ethnic groups. Almost half of the Indian elderly living alone live in poverty (U.S. Department of Health and Human Services, 1990a). Among those 75 and older, 61% live in poverty.

Latino men show minimal crossover when compared to their white counterparts after the age of 45. This pattern may be due, in part, to a somewhat higher mortality rate among Latinos at younger ages.

MINORITY ELDERLY DATA INADEQUACIES

There is a lack of sufficient research data on minorities of color. We do not know enough about their perceptions about their own health, how often they are bedridden or otherwise restrictively limited, or the financial influence on such limitations. Most epidemiological studies of minority elderly focus on broad racial comparisons instead of actual ethnic, ecological, or social factors that may affect the health or the delivery of health care of the minority elderly (e.g., the relationship of obesity to diabetes, the effects of inner-city population density and crime on restrictions in the activities of daily living, or out-of-pocket expenses for the elderly poor).

As stated earlier, many Latinos have problems getting to their doctor's office or health care clinic. Despite these research findings, there are still insufficient data on how access and transportation to health care facilities and wellness clinics, living arrangements, marital status, employment and employability, occupation, income, and education are distributed by ethnicity, gender, and age. Moreover, there are deficiencies in census data that have important implications for estimating the extent of poverty as well as for public policy (Passel & Robinson, 1984).

RETIREMENT

Ethnic-minority elderly face serious financial problems. Since most have worked at relatively low-paying jobs or are forced to exit the work force before retirement age for health reasons, they are likely to receive minimum or near-minimum benefits when they retire. This results in high rates of poverty and near poverty. Many elderly minorities have incomes so low that they cannot survive without assistance from families and friends.

Latino elderly have typically worked hard throughout their lives. Many suffer physical disabilities due to a lifetime of manual labor, often since childhood. Nevertheless, most Latino elderly are not financially secure at the time of their retirement. While most elderly in the United States receive Social Security, Latinos are less likely than whites to receive this type of benefit. Despite great need, Latino elderly are less likely to receive Social Security than the rest of the eligible population. Nearly 1 in 4 (23%) Latino elderly receive no Social Security, compared to about 1 in 8 African Americans (11%) and 1 in 12 whites (7%) (C. Lopez & Aguilera, 1991). Latinos are also less likely than whites to receive private pensions and to have income from interest and other assets.

Latinos are likely to depend on earnings and public assistance to survive retirement because of high rates of poverty and low rates of participation in Social Security and other retirement plans (C. Lopez & Aguilera, 1991). The median income for Latino elderly is only slightly above the poverty threshold for an individual 65 or over; older Latinos are more than twice as likely to be poor as white elderly. Although the poverty rate for Latino elderly decreased from 30.8% in 1980 to 20.6% in 1989, the total number of Latinos 65 or over in poverty has steadily increased, from about 179,000 in 1980 to approximately 211,000 in 1989.

LATINO ELDERLY HEALTH CARE DELIVERY

Latino elderly have low rates of health insurance coverage. Most of the jobs Latino elderly have had are unlikely to include health benefits; thus access to health care is limited even for employed Latinos. About one out of three Latinos of all ages have no health insurance coverage. Latino elderly have a much lower rate of Medicare coverage than non-Latino elderly. This is likely a reflection of the lower rate of receiving Social Security. Latino elderly, consequently, are more dependent on Medicaid. Latinos, moreover, are more likely not to have any health insurance than the general elderly population. Private supplemental insurance (Medigap coverage) is also less common among elderly Latinos than among all elderly. The lack of supplemental insurance leaves elderly not covered by Medicaid vulnerable to costly medical expenses—premiums, deductibles, cost-sharing requirements, and services not paid for by Medicare.

Latino elderly not only have greater unmet acute-care needs, but seem to have greater long-term-care needs as well. A higher percentage of elderly have difficulties with self-care activities and household management tasks than white elderly. Unable to care for themselves or manage their affairs, these elderly are dependent on others, usually family members, for assistance. As Latino elderly live longer, and Latino families need greater financial and political support in caring for their elderly, Latino community-based agencies are being called upon more frequently to provide services to homebound Latino elderly.

Accessibility and affordability of transportation have become central issues in serving the poor Latino elderly. Even agencies that offer their own transportation services to clients cannot begin to transport all the elderly who wish to participate in their programs. Where agencies do not have their own transportation for clients, the elderly must depend on public transportation, other private sources (for example, Dial-a-Ride), or family members. Most staff and elderly describe public transportation systems, when they are available at all, as very inadequate. Local buses sometimes run infrequently, are not convenient to places of residence, or do not accommodate the needs of the especially frail elderly. Private services, requiring elderly clients to call in advance to reserve a ride, often have neither bilingual staff people to handle calls from Spanish-speaking elderly nor bilingual drivers to understand them once they are on the bus or van; many have inflexible schedules.

Decent affordable housing is a major need for the Latino elderly, especially as the Latino family structure shifts away from the traditional multigenerational model. Latino elderly will need housing that will allow them to stay in their communities and maintain an independent living status while receiving necessary support services. Families who want to have their elderly members continue to live with them will need housing assistance—now available only if the elderly members live in their own apartments.

There is a misconception that because Latino families take care of their elderly, older Latinos have little need for services and programs. Caring for an elderly relative imposes a financial as well as an emotional strain on families, particularly those with limited resources. Furthermore, as the growth of the elderly Latino population outpaces the growth of younger generations, families face greater difficulties in meeting elderly needs. Social services and programs that can supplement family care and, consequently, ease the burden of caregiving are critical for Latinos.

ELDERLY LIVING ARRANGEMENTS: ETHNIC COMPARISONS

Latino elderly are more likely to live in the community and less likely to be institutionalized than white elderly. In a recent National Nursing Home Survey, out of a total of 1.5 million elderly cared for in nursing homes, 2.7% were Latino, 7.8% were African American, and 89.5% were white. In addition, Latino elderly are less likely to live in homes for the aged than white and African American elderly (Cubillos & Prieto, 1987). For example, the ratio of white females 75 or over (12.4%) cared for in nursing homes was more than twice as great as the proportion of Latinos the same age (5.4%).

Latinos are less likely to live alone and more likely to live with family members than white and African American elderly. Over three-fourths (76.6%) of Latino elderly lived with family, compared with two-thirds (67.5%) of white elderly and approximately 6 out of 10 African American elderly (63.1%) (U.S. Bureau of the Census, 1990b). About 2 out of 10 elderly Latinos (22.0%) lived alone, compared to 3 out of 10 white elderly (30.6%), and one-third of African American elderly (33.4%) (U.S. Bureau of the Census, 1990b).

Latino elderly are more likely than other elderly to live in a multigenerational family where the child is the householder. In 1989, Latino elderly were less likely to be householders (60.2%) than white (70.7%) and African American (68.1%) elderly. Moreover, a larger percentage of elderly Latinos (38.7%) were nonhouseholders living with family members than white (30.7%) or African American (27.5%) elderly (U.S. Bureau of the Census, 1990b).

Latino elderly are less likely than other senior citizens to own their homes. In 1987, three out of four senior citizens owned their homes, but a disproportionate percentage of homeowners were white. More than three-fourths of white elderly owned homes (77%), while a little more than half of Latino elderly (56%) and more than three-fifths of African American (62%) were homeowners (U.S. Bureau of the Census & Department of Housing and Urban Development, 1989).

A 1988 survey (Westat, 1989) found that 22.4% of elderly Latinos lived alone, 48.7% lived with their spouse, and 28.9% lived with others. Respondents living with their spouse were more likely to own homes (65%) than those living alone (44%) or with others (34%). Respondents living alone were most likely to rent (52%), compared to those living with a spouse (31%) or with others (40%). A comparison of housing occupied by Latino elderly shows that those living with their spouse were more likely to live in a house (75%) than those living with others (71%) or living alone (48%). Latino elderly living alone were most likely to live in an apartment (48%), compared to those living with a spouse (22%) or those living with others (28%) (Westat, 1989, table 2-6).

ETHNIC DIFFERENCES IN DEATH AND DYING

Rituals and belief systems surrounding death have developed universally in societies to help individuals deal with fears and anxieties provoked by death as well as to help them deal with the loss of loved ones (Mandelbaum, 1959; Palgi & Abramovitch, 1984).

Industrialization and modernization have resulted in remarkable declines in death rates and substantial increases in life expectancy through improvements in food production, public health, and medical care. These improvements have primarily affected infants, who, in premodern times, were the most vulnerable to malnutrition and widespread disease (Goldscheider, 1971). Such progress in life expectancy is mainly the result of reductions in infant and childhood mortality.

One of the major effects of modernization has been to shift much of the occurrence of death to old age (Kalish, 1985). Despite homicides, accidents, and AIDS, it is increasingly old people who die. One consequence of the transformation in mortality to the older years is to make death more predictable, more controllable, and therefore less socially disruptive, leading to diminished importance of elaborate rituals (Ward, 1979; Blauner, 1966, p. 386).

There are ethnic differences in such beliefs and practices within the United States. There are several reasons why it is important to understand how groups of various ethnic backgrounds conceptualize death. By exposure to alternative views of death, we may learn more ethical ways of life and better ethical treatment of the dying and their loved ones. We can gain considerably from learning how the ethnic elderly view death.

African Americans

The attitudes toward the elderly, death, and death-related rituals/practices in the African American community can be traced to lower socioeconomic status, general American culture, a previous history of slavery, and African culture (Kalish & Reynolds, 1976; Herskovits, 1941; Wylie, 1971). In my comparative research on moral reasoning in Mexican Americans, African Americans, and whites (Cortese, 1990), some African Americans expressed deep respect for their elderly. This veneration for older people, as well as the practice of ancestor deference, has been credited to West African values, specifically, the authority and prestige of the elderly within the family and village community. I did not find this same pattern of respect for the elderly in individuals of other ethnic groups within the semiclinical moral-judgment interview setting from which the data were gathered (Cortese, 1990).

Despite the survival of some African values in the African American community, the experience of African Americans is distinct and qualitatively diverse from African culture. In terms of social theory, this issue is highly significant. *Ethnogenesis* refers to people from the same or similar geographical origins (e.g., West Africa) who blend to form a new ethnic group within a different society. Accordingly, African American culture in the United States represents exactly this.

This process may occur initially because the members of a group share certain historical and cultural characteristics, but from this perspective, the importance of these shared characteristics derives from the common experiences of the group's members in the new society, most notably for African Americans, slavery, discrimination, oppression, and rejection by the dominant group. This common experience, in turn, provides a basis for a transformed ethnicity, one that is not a simple derivative of the society from which the immigrants or refugees come. Immigrant communities usually are not communities when they come (slavery is an extreme example); their ethnic identities are, to a surprising extent, constructed in the United States.

The effects of slavery on the experience of death began early and often, during capture and the journey to the Western Hemisphere (Markides & Mindel, 1987). Millions of Africans never finished the trip to America: "victims of starvation, suffocation, drowning, suicide, disease, and the whippings, beatings, mutilation, and direct killing by those who held them in bondage" (Jackson, 1985, p. 203). The death-causing social structures of oppression and institutional discrimination continued during slavery (Weld, 1969) and afterwards, during segregation. Today death is common in ghettos in the United States. Within a context of deprivation, some African Americans have considered death as a covert form of desire for freedom (in spirituals, for example) (Markides & Mindel, 1987). Nevertheless, the spiritual image of African Americans has been misinterpreted (Jackson, 1972; S. A. Brown, 1958; M. M. Fischer, 1969). The significance of the African American church and religious beliefs lies not in its sacredness, but in its ability to address itself to everyday problems of human existence and survival, as well as providing rituals of social solidarity or communal bonding.

A review of African American history and literature shows that death (often in a violent manner) is sometimes a central theme. Scant empirical findings from the social sciences corroborate what has been termed a *preoccupation* (see Markides & Mindel, 1987, p. 152) with death. A preoccupation with violent death has been linked to negative self-image, frustration, and anger that eventually view violent death as more honorable than passive death, the symbol of acquiescence to the structures of white political authority.

Attitudes toward Life, Death, and Suicide Behavior

Case Study 2: African Americans

The only lights in the large hall of the worn but colorful community center were coming from the bright flames on the tops of the candles on a very large birthday cake. Too numerous to count, each candle represented one of the first hundred years in the life of Henry Hughes. Henry smiled while he listened to a roughly harmonized version of "Happy Birthday" and was deeply touched by an explosion of spirited shouts and applause that followed. The dozens of guests included five generations of family members, numerous friends, members of the local media, and some health care professionals. Henry was frail, reflecting a lifetime of heavy physical labor, but seemed in good spirits. One of the local television news reporters curiously asked, "Mr. Hughes, to what do you attribute your long life?"

Henry thought for a couple of seconds and replied, "Complete faith in God, a good attitude toward life, a never-ending quest for learning, and an occasional glass of red wine." He smiled as the crowd broke into laughter. "I've tried to live a simple life. All I've ever needed was a clever accountant, a forgiving minister, and a passionate wife." Henry added. Henry had outlived each of his three wives, and rumor had it that he was courting a possible fourth.

The reporter then asked, "Do you have any goals at this point in your life?" Without hesitation, Henry retorted, "I want to live to be 110." Everyone knew that Henry was serious by the conviction in his tone.

Henry had worked as a sharecropper in rural Mississippi and had lived his entire life in abject poverty. He had suffered continuous discrimination from a racially stratified social structure with a long history of demanding and enforcing pervasive public segregation. Despite his hard life, Henry was grateful and upbeat.

"The Chinese have a beautiful saying: 'As calm as the sea . . . and as long-lasting as the mountains.' In other words—happiness and a long life. And I thank God that I've had both of them. Just because life is often painful and you're real old—that don't give you the right to check out early—Dr. Kevorkian style. You just make do with the opportunities that God gives you."

This case study illustrates African American subcultural scripts on aging and mortality. The ethical value of accountability discourages elderly suicide even in the event of terminal illness. There is subcultural resistance to autonomy that supports freedom to make decisions about ending one's own life. The ethical value of privacy is demonstrated by subcultural cues to pursue activities of daily living in any way one chooses as long as it does not cause harm to others. The African saying "It takes a village to raise a child" is consistent with the moral value of beneficence. Everyone is involved in the welfare of the individual and the community.

Despite the relatively short life expectancy of African Americans or their alleged preoccupation with death, African Americans expect to and wish to live longer than whites, Mexican Americans, and Japanese Americans (Bengston, Cuellar, & Ragan, 1977; Kalish & Reynolds, 1976; Reynolds & Kalish, 1974). Given the economic pressures, prejudice, and discrimination that African Americans endure, this seems to reflect optimism, hope, resiliency, an appreciation of life, and religious faith. Life seems to take on greater significance and appreciation in the wake of requiring so much energy, endurance, resourcefulness, and suffering. This clearly is an example of *virtue ethics*, with a focus on how adverse living conditions develop the character of the individual.

Older African Americans are much more likely than older whites to believe that one should live as long as one can and that pain and suffering do not justify dying (R. Koenig, Goldner, Kresojevich, & Lockwood, 1971) (death with dignity). More African Americans than whites are opposed to allowing people who wish to die to do so (Kalish & Reynolds, 1976, p. 100). This speaks highly of their self-determination even in the context of terminal illness.

The finding of greater expectations and desires for longevity by African Americans is consistent with the generally lower suicide rate among older African Americans (Seiden, 1981; Markides & Machalek, 1984). This is indicative of a high degree of integration into the community (Durkheim, 1951). While the suicide rate increases with age among whites, it declines with age for African Americans (Markides & Mindel, 1987). Low suicide rates among older African Americans, as well as high expectations and desires for a longer life, hint toward a high degree of acceptance of life. Given the relative inequalities of life that African Americans experience vis-à-vis whites, this is somewhat paradoxical. Perhaps recent gains by African Americans have exceeded the expectations of older African Americans. Meanwhile, they have not met the heightened expectations of young African Americans who display their frustration and hopelessness through increasing suicide (Seiden, 1970) and homicide rates. In addition, the low survival rate of African Americans may lead to a relatively robust group of those who attain old age and are much less disposed to commit suicide (Markides & Machalek, 1984; Seiden, 1981).

Funerals and the Church

African Americans and whites depend less on family support during death and dying than Mexican and Japanese Americans (Kalish & Reynolds, 1976). Church-related support, as surrogate family, in the African American community compensates for less traditional family emphasis. Lewis's (1971, pp. 103–104) narrative of funeral customs in a small southern town underlines the importance of the church in African American funerals. The funeral affirms self-worth and status (Markides & Mindel, 1987) and functions as an opportunity for social gathering (McDonald, 1973). Most important, funerals serve the purpose of facilitating grief. African American funerals engender emotional release, catharsis, and interaction and confrontation with the deceased through music that is appreciably rhythmic. The eulogy confirms significant respect for the deceased by focusing exclusively on positive attributes. Ostensibly, one can leave African American funerals with the belief that the deceased was saintlike.

Mexican Americans

While the effect of African values on the attitudes and behavior of African Americans is questionable, the influence of Mexican culture on Mexican Americans is undeniable. In contrast to Anglo conceptions of death, "the Mexican . . . is familiar with [it], jokes about it, caresses it, sleeps with it, celebrates it, it is one of his favorite toys and his most steadfast love" (Paz, 1961, p. 58). Although evidence does not suggest less fear of death, Mexican Americans do seem to take a matter-of-fact attitude about it, refusing to hide it away. Mexicans and Mexican Americans even celebrate a Day of the Dead on November 2 (an equivalent to All Souls Day in the Catholic church).

There is great diversity within the Mexican American community regarding traditional rituals and beliefs about death (Markides & Mindel, 1987). Typical Day of the Dead activities include taking flowers to the graves of their loved ones or lighting candles in church (Kalish & Reynolds, 1976). This is not very different from what Catholics, in general, do (e.g., Memorial Day visits to cemeteries).

The intensity with which Mexican Americans deal with death is not unlike what is found in Mexico. Regular concern and absorption with death result from the amalgamation of Indian and Spanish culture as evidenced in Mexican literature, art, poetry, folk music, and folk proverbs (Perez-Tamayo, 1977). Outsiders do well to avoid the ethnocentric view that such occupation may appear morbid and disturbing. Mexican American culture supports more open overflowing of emotional responses to death by a larger network of kin than is found with the other groups.

Attitudes toward Life and Death

Mexican Americans expect to and wish to live fewer years than whites, African Americans, or Japanese Americans (Kalish & Reynolds, 1976). This appears inconsistent with the notion that Mexican American elderly occupy a reputable position within the family unless one considers a modernization approach (discussed later). The expectations and wishes of Mexican American elderly are fairly good matches to actual predictions of their life expectancies. One hypothesis is that Mexican Americans have greater acceptance of death than other racial/ethnic categories: "the elderly Mexican American accepts death as a valued experience, a thing of beauty, and an entrance into another world that is real. For him, death is an inevitable event that takes place in the presence of his entire family" (Madsen, 1969, p. 233). This hypothesis, as yet, has not received conclusive support. At any rate, death themes are abundant in Mexican cultural symbols, arts, and ceremonies (Markides & Mindel, 1987).

If we frame the discussion as an ethical dilemma between two moral values, autonomy versus beneficence (or nonmaleficence), we are better able to clarify the more important ethical issues that need to be addressed. What if preserving the autonomy of the individual conflicts with providing maximum support and care by others, including the highest standards of caregiver ability and training? If an elderly Latino has a terminal illness, subcultural scripts would point us in the direction of honoring an individual's autonomy over beneficence or nonmaleficence. However, if an elderly Latino is considering suicide, subcultural scripts would perhaps signal us to devalue autonomy and to provide the maximum support and care available with the highest standards of ability and training (beneficence or nonmaleficence).

Death Issues and Suicide Rates

Mexican Americans and African Americans, more than whites or Japanese Americans, have "experienced or felt the presence of someone after he had died" (Kalish & Reynolds, 1976, p. 158). Such encounters tended to be pleasant or, at least, positive. Mexican Americans, nevertheless, varied from African Americans in that fewer reported knowing anyone who had died during the previous two years, and fewer knew eight or more persons who had died during this period. Mexican Americans were similar to whites on these two items. While nearly all Mexican Americans (96%) who knew someone who had died during the previous two years said that at least one of these deaths was the result of natural causes, 34% knew persons who had died in accidents, 10% in war, 5% by suicide, and 4% who were victims of homicide (Kalish & Reynolds, 1976, p. 164).

The self-reported knowledge of homicide victims was consistent with official homicide rates for the ethnic group—lower among Anglos, Mexican Americans, and Japanese Americans, and much higher among African Americans. However, knowledge of suicide victims by Mexican Americans was much higher than would be expected from the very low reported suicide rate for Mexican Americans. In response to the question "Has anyone you have known well ever committed suicide?" almost one-third of the Mexican Americans responded affirmatively, a proportion slightly higher than that among whites, but considerably higher than that among African Americans and Japanese Americans (Reynolds, Kalish, & Farberow, 1975). This unusually high level of knowledge about suicides among Mexican Americans raises doubts about the validity of official rates. Mexican Americans may be more likely than others to conceal suicide due to its religious implications. The Catholic church views suicide as a mortal sin against the fifth commandment, "Thou shalt not kill." Suicide victims are not eligible for funeral masses or consecrative burials.

Theories of lower suicide rates among Mexican Americans have focused primarily on their Catholic background (the same reason that contributes to underreporting) and high integration into the family (Hoppe & Martin, 1978). Like African American suicide rates, but in contrast to the pattern displayed by whites, Mexican American suicide rates decline with age (Anatore & Loya, 1973; Hatcher & Hatcher, 1975). While older Mexican Americans are better integrated into the family and community than younger ones, recent increases in suicide rates among younger Mexican Americans may reflect greater acculturation into mainstream society or an increasing frustration with a lack of access to social mobility.

Religion, Family, and Acceptance of Death

Mexican Americans are more likely than African Americans, whites, and Japanese Americans to prefer to die in a hospital; fewer (except for African Americans) wish to die at home (Kalish & Reynolds, 1976). Proportionately fewer

Mexican Americans than whites actually do die at home (Richardson, Solis, & Hisserich, 1984). Considering the powerful bonding of Mexican American families, this is somewhat unexpected. Perhaps the elderly exhibit such attitudes and practices for altruistic reasons. Ill or dying elderly realize that their presence at home places a great deal of moral responsibility on the family and major demands upon available space. The strong emphasis that Mexican American culture places on familism translates into additional importance of the moral values of fidelity and beneficence where ill or dying elderly are concerned.

Contrary to the notion that Mexican Americans are more accepting of death than others, there is some indication that Mexican Americans desire to conceal death from the elderly family member, including her or his own. More Mexican Americans than members of other groups feel that dying persons should not be told that they will die; significantly fewer Mexican Americans feel capable of telling someone that she or he is about to die; and more said that they would not want young children to attend their funeral (Kalish & Reynolds, 1976, p. 166).

These data suggest potential ethical dilemmas for Mexican American families that pit the values of accountability and fidelity against the value of autonomy. The ethical value of accountability calls into question the issues of deception and withholding important information. Accountability means that everyone should be responsible for the truth and for his or her actions. Consequently, a dying person has the obligation to tell the truth about his or her condition. Moreover, the family and health professionals also have an obligation to be truthful with a dying individual about his or her circumstances. The ethical value of autonomy involves the individual's right to decide to exclude children from those who are to be told about the elderly's imminent death.

Fidelity requires everyone to show loyalty to one another and to offer assistance in times of need. An elderly person who is dying has the right to expect others to help him or her if he or she becomes dependent in any way. The family members are expected to offer help. The ethical value of autonomy gives the dying individual the right to make choices about one's health and well-being as long as he or she is competent and causes no harm to anyone else in the process. The family has an obligation to act on behalf of the client.

This leads us to the notion of *best interest*. Sometimes family members are authorized to make decisions regarding the welfare of an ill or dying family member. Decisions are based on what would be best for the family elder, but from the perspective of the broader Mexican American cultural system of values rather than what the family elder might personally wish. Thus subcultural beliefs that knowledge of impending death should not be revealed to a family member may take precedence over the individual's desire to know.

The notion of best interest may be contrasted with the concept of *substituted judgment*, which is an effort by someone to make ethical decisions for the dying family elder that are most congruent with what one believes the older person would wish. Best interest differs from *paternalism* because in the case of the latter someone preempts the individual's decision-making right because one feels that his or her judgment is better than that of the client.

There are two very different ways of interpreting such data. First, Mexican Americans attempt to "protect people from openly acknowledging the personal encounter with their own death or with that of a close relative" (Kalish & Reynolds, 1976, p. 170). Conversely, there may be greater resistance within Mexican American culture to accepting death. Clearly, there is ritualistic and symbolic acceptance of death on the cultural or macro level. Empirical data at the individual or micro level, however, suggest greater difficulty adjusting to death, whether a person's own or that of a loved one (Kalish & Reynolds, 1976). Ritualistic and symbolic preoccupation with death in ceremony, art, music, and literature does not necessarily imply acceptance of death by individuals.

Despite empirical refutation of the traditional stereotype that Mexican Americans are generally fatalistic (Farris & Glenn, 1976), it still may hold in the area of facing death. Proportionately more Mexican Americans than other ethnic groups believe that people cannot hasten or slow their own death through a *will to live* or a *will to die* (Kalish & Reynolds, 1976, p. 174). This represents a belief in an external versus an internal locus of control. More of them opposed the idea that people should be allowed to die if they wish. More Mexican Americans than other groups believed that "accidental" deaths indicate the power of God working among people. From this perspective, life and death contain a deeply spiritual or mysterious element.

If Mexican American immigrants do experience greater difficulty in accepting death, what is the cause? Perhaps greater fears and anxieties about death are found in persons socialized in traditional rural Mexican culture with pervasive symbolism and ritual regarding death who then migrate to urban areas in the United States, where this ritualistic support is considerably diminished. This is a question for future research.

Japanese Americans

The attitudes and practices surrounding death of Japanese Americans cover a wide range depending on the degree of assimilation into mainstream culture.

Japanese Ethical Systems

In order to evaluate how Japanese moral and religious frameworks affect attitudes and behavior about death in Japanese Americans, it is important to make an artificial, yet heuristically useful, distinction between individual and social ethics. This entails a brief sociohistorical examination of the major ethical and religious traditions in Japan (Confucianism, Shinto, and Buddhism; see Cortese, 1996) in order to sense why issues of social ethics (e.g., social justice and social equality) are not central to them. Rather, Japanese concerns focus on social aesthetics; a harmonious and orderly society without overt conflict and with minimal envy is beautiful. (See chapter 3 in this volume for a more detailed discussion of ethical principles in Far Eastern religions.)

Shintoism

Shinto, "the way of the gods," is the name given to the faith possessed by the ancient Japanese. It is often considered to be the "soul" of Japan. While Confucianism had been imported from China, and Buddhism from India (through China and Korea), Shinto is native to Japan. Shinto is a system of nature (the physical world) and ancestor deference. Unlike Christianity, Judaism, Islam, Hinduism, and other theistic religions that include the belief in one or more supreme beings, Shinto is an animistic religion. It rejects the notion of a supreme being; instead, it empowers nature with supernatural power. Shinto has no particular teachings or dogma, but allows each person his or her own meaning. Perhaps its label as a religion is inappropriate. Shinto is merely a belief in the power of human spirits and in the natural elements.

Kami is the name given to spiritual power and may include one's ancestors or all of the dead. It is also possessed by natural phenomena such as trees, rocks, rain, wind, mountains, and the sun. *Kami* is benevolent to those who pay homage, but when it is neglected, it becomes indignant and may be provoked to wrath and possible calamity. Therefore, it is always prudent to respect *kami*. In short, Shinto provides a very simple basis for faith. As in other animistic religions, Shintoists appease the spirits in objects and ancestors by honoring them and by taking care of them. Lacking any real ethical system or meaningful concept of an afterlife, Shinto is a folk faith whose essentially austere nature is suggested by the fact that its word for god—*kami*—is associated with the homonym *kami*, meaning up, on top, or paper.

What has incorrectly been called *ancestor worship* by outsiders who study Japanese culture can be more accurately viewed as a system of symbolic communication with deceased relatives. This may entail keeping a family altar with offerings of food and drink (Yamamoto, Okonogi, Iwasaki, & Yoshimura, 1969). Those who adhere to the traditional beliefs and practices of so-called ancestor worship have less difficulty adapting to the loss of family members. Shintoism provides direct implications for resolving ethical issues concerning the terminal illness or potential suicide of a Japanese older person. It leans toward autonomy and a right-to-die position on the issue of euthanasia. Shintoism also carries the moral values of fidelity and beneficence one step further than most other sacred or secular ethical ideologies. While fidelity requires us to show loyalty to one another and to not abandon someone, Shintoism urges continued loyalty, support, and nonabandonment even after the death of a family member. Consequently, the death of a loved one may not be viewed as a sorrowful catastrophe.

Ancestor deference symbolizes the need of the deceased for continued assistance from living relatives. This may also be viewed as an extension of beneficence: Everyone has a right to maximum support and care by others in the maintenance or enhancement of his or her well-being. Well-being has numerous dimensions: physical, psychological, social, legal, and spiritual. Shintoism may suggest that a family provide continuous reverence for dead family members. Consequently, the ritual of ancestor deference plays a role in ethical issues, but it does not represent a life-after-death ideology.

Buddhism

Shinto was inadequate to meet the spiritual needs of the increasingly sophisticated society that Prince Shotoku and his successors created in Japan. That void was filled by the arrival of Buddhism from China, with its concern for individual salvation and its complex philosophical overtones. Carrying with it a dynamic impact on architecture, the arts and literature, technology, and philosophical thought, Buddhism spread rapidly in the upper classes of Japan. From the ninth century on, it pervaded the intellectual and political life of the elite.

Buddhism has often been viewed as the road to enlightenment and was the first systematic method of thought brought to Japan. Buddhist teachings focus on how to resolve and persevere in the problems of life and death; perpetual change (also a feature of most North American Indian spiritual systems) is another dominant theme.

Buddha, a sixth-century B.C. Indian, believed that through meditation, one can escape suffering by liberating the self from all desires. Meditation involves stilling the mind in order to grasp universal truth. This is an ideal condition called nirvana. Zen Buddhism has traditionally contributed toward self-understanding and a deeper sense of one's place in the universe. Consequently, this challenges one to learn to live harmoniously within oneself, with one another, and with the earth that sustains us. In the pursuit of truth, Zen's most basic principle is not to rely on words. Since truth goes beyond the boundaries of rational thought, one must grasp truth directly through meditation. Buddhism assumes that humans possess a latent intuitive power. The goal of meditation is to ignite intuitive insight through unconscious, involuntary processes. The meditative and silent emphasis of Japanese culture is compatible with Zen.

In following the rules for harmonious social relations, self-affirmation or affirmation from others is difficult. It might lead to ostracism or create envy. Consequently, many Japanese often feel that they can only let their inner self show when they are alone or alone in nature. One's inner self is never socially affirmed; it has no social reality. Zen seems to make a positive attribute of this social arrangement (i.e., the selfless individual). Perhaps it is Zen that contributes to outsider complaints that the Japanese are difficult to understand or illogical.

According to Buddhism (Japan's dominant religion), life does not end with death; it is merely transformed and continues in a different form. Buddhism promotes and, in fact, ultimately requires acceptance of death. Death takes precedence over human desire. Since death may occur at any time without warning, recognition of the unpredictable, transitory, and trivial nature of life in the finite world must finally result in a weaning from action taken to satisfy desire. The ultimate is to detach oneself from pleasure and desire. Having accomplished this, the enlightened individual is free from hope, anxiety, ambition, and frustration (Long, 1975). The most effective way to detach oneself from desire is meditation that channels the unconscious toward the impermanence of life and the inevitability of death. In short, one conquers death by accepting it. Accepting death, for a Buddhist, is eased by the belief that it leads to a new life, which, depending on one's actions in the present life, may be preferred to the present one.

Confucianism

A considerable share of the world's population, especially India and East Asia, have religions that concentrate more on sets of ideal principles than on the supernatural power of gods, objects, or animals. The most major of these religions are Buddhism, Confucianism, and Taoism. Such religions tend to focus on how people can achieve a better life on earth. Confucianism has a long history in Japan; it has provided a practical ethic to guide individuals in their daily lives. Confucianism prevails in human relationships and has provided the normative grounding for the vertical structure of Japanese society.

Confucius, a sixth-century B.C. contemporary of Buddha, believed that salvation was based on acting according to correct manners and respecting those of higher social rank. The objective of a Confucianist is to always act in a manner whereby one can mesh harmoniously with one's environment, relationships, and circumstances. Salvation, for a Confucianist, is oriented to the present life; it is harmonious living according to the ideas of an orchestrated universe. Confucianism emphasizes respect for others and goodness and love as the means of attaining harmony with the universe. It also stresses respect for and subservience toward family elders and those in higher social classes. Confucian thought plays into the ethical value of autonomy. Is the individual ever free to make decisions about his or her life or death?

Confucianism demands support for maintaining the status quo of the existing social system as the means for ethical decision making. Because of this conservative stance, it can be criticized as deterministic and resistant to social change. Confucian ideology goes against the central notion of autonomy: Everyone has the right to make choices (as long as he or she is competent). Confucianism, meanwhile, strongly values fidelity—the expectation that everyone is expected to show loyalty to one another.

Essentially an ethical system rather than a religious faith, Confucianism, with its emphasis on loyalty, personal relationships, and etiquette and with the high value that it places on education and hard work, is ideally suited to the pragmatic Japanese character. Today Confucian values still permeate the Japanese and Japanese American populations. Those impressed by the seeming discipline of the Japanese Americans and the efficiency of Japanese society emphasize the authority of the group over the attitudes and behavior of the individual and the accountability of the individual to the group. This authority of the group over the individual flies in the face of the ethical value of autonomy. Accountability, however, is a moral value that is central to Confucian doctrine; the individual is responsible to the group for one's actions and for the truth.

Japanese American Attitudes toward Death

Case Study 3: Japanese Americans

Ichiro Hajime is an elderly Japanese American dying from stomach cancer. He has just suffered a third major relapse and is in the intensive-care unit of a public hospital. The prognosis is not good; physicians tell the family that Ichiro is not likely to live another month. His family plans to conceal the bad news from Ichiro. Ichiro, however, seems to realize that he is dying and has made peace with himself and his family.

As the days go by, Ichiro is removed from intensive care and placed in a private room. He begins to frequently complain to his family about the total lack of privacy; Ichiro is constantly being monitored by hospital staff. He feels very uncomfortable with the seemingly increasing frequency of interruptions by hospital staff and with the curt manner in which people approach and handle him.

Soon Ichiro tells his family that he wants to return to his own home to die. The medicine, radiation, and chemotherapies have not been able to improve his condition. The impersonal living conditions have also taken a heavy toll. Ichiro has become severely depressed. Family members, nevertheless, argue that Ichiro should remain in the hospital where his condition can be carefully monitored. Furthermore, family members will not always be able to stay and care for him at his home.

After an intense open dialogue and debate, a consensus is reached (communicative ethics). The family agrees that Ichiro should return home and hires a private nurse to assist in Ichiro's daily activity needs. Ichiro insists that for their own emotional well-being, his grandchildren are not to be told about the severity of his condition; the family concurs.

The ethical decision not to disclose the impending death of an elder relative to grandchildren is justified by the subcultural belief that it is in their best interest not to know. First-generation Japanese Americans (*issei*) demonstrate controlled acceptance of grieving and death, an attitude based in Buddhism (Kalish & Reynolds, 1976, p. 131). Third-generation Japanese Americans (*sansei*) are more likely to have a Western attitude toward death, involving understanding and control of the external world rather than acceptance of it. *Sansei* tend to fear and avoid thoughts of death, since it is a topic that does not comfortably fit in a rational worldview.

It is not clear whether Japanese Americans are very accepting of death. Fewer Japanese Americans than African Americans and whites (but not Mexican Americans) feel that a dying person should be told that he or she is dying (Kalish & Reynolds, 1976, p. 136). This shows the high degree of sensitivity Japanese Americans have regarding the feelings of others. Even fewer think about their own death. Sometimes dying patients in nursing homes are kept in separate rooms away from other patients. Such data may be interpreted as indicating difficulties in accepting death. Moreover, Japanese Americans (like Mexican Americans) are considerably more likely to express fear of death (Kalish & Reynolds, 1976, p. 145). The overwhelming majority of Japanese Americans, unlike Mexican Americans, reported that they wanted to die at home.

Japanese interaction rituals, in general, and Japanese American attitudes about death and dying, in particular, support a high degree of individual privacy. Accordingly, everyone has the right to maintain his or her privacy even within the context of information about himself or herself concerning a terminal illness or impending death. Data indicating that Japanese Americans prefer to die in the seclusion of their own homes or, at least, in private hospital rooms demonstrate the importance of privacy as an ethical value. Privacy includes the right to live and die wherever one chooses without interference so long as it does not infringe upon the rights of others.

Japanese Americans are not likely to believe in life after death, suggesting that they are not particularly religious in terms of traditional Christian and Buddhist teachings and practices (the two most common religious backgrounds). Perhaps devout Buddhists prefer nirvana (a state of bliss) to life after death. Nirvana represents an escape from the continuous cycle of reincarnations (Long, 1975). Japanese American elderly, who hold traditional Buddhist beliefs, may prefer death to life in an institution, since death may result in a better afterlife or possibly even nirvana. An alternate view is that the high degree of willingness to die among Japanese American elderly is linked to the strong cultural work ethic. Many elderly would rather die than be unproductive or a burden on others (Kalish & Reynolds, 1976). Either way, it would appear that death is viewed positively.

These Buddhist beliefs about death and dying potentially create a conflict between nonmaleficence and autonomy. The family and others in the informal support role are obliged to preserve the safety of the older family member. This includes providing the highest standards of care of which they are capable in order to prevent any adverse consequences for the older person. However, the optimistic nature of Buddhist reincarnation ideology (i.e., the possibility of a better afterlife or nirvana) slants ethical decision making toward an emphasis on autonomy. This gives the individual a right to make choices, even about one's death, as long as one is competent and causes no harm to anyone else in the process. Autonomy clearly conflicts with nonmaleficence in this context, setting up an ethical dilemma.

Acceptance of death is characteristic mainly in Japanese American elderly (Kiefer, 1974a). The younger generation has greater difficulty dealing with death. Buddhist tradition proposes that death is natural, and thus fear of death means fear of nature. Moreover, the elderly who are healthy have a clear notion of their obligations to the world, a notion that helps them achieve a sense of the completeness and wholeness of their lives (Kiefer, 1974b). Although familism is strong in the Japanese family, elderly Japanese Americans who lack the support and gratitude of family or followers may feel overwhelmed by the significance of the end of their lives. Social isolation is especially unfortunate for them.

Suicide

It is sometimes difficult to know how deeply the roots of an ethnic group in the United States can be traced to its geographical origin. Japan has one of the highest suicide rates in the world (Markides & Mindel, 1987). This had been blamed on belief that suicide is an honorable way out of an intolerable situation, a rigid and hierarchical social structure, extreme emphasis placed on individual success, and the dysfunctions of rapid modernization (Iga & Tatai, 1975). Belief that suicide is a fair way out of a crushing predicament can be traced to the Buddhist notion that life is negative and death should be embraced.

The Japanese operate carefully on the basis of social rules. While these rules do not claim to be absolute, at times they may be rigid, incredibly autocratic, and capricious. These rules aim mainly to regulate individual behavior within the group. This points to a very coercive element of Japanese dynamics. Suicide may be viewed as the only reasonable alternative. This has significant ethical implications since a moral system based on constraint cannot satisfy a prerequisite of individual choice and cooperation.

Despite the high suicide rate for Japan, Japanese Americans have relatively low (Kalish, 1968; Yamamoto, 1976) to intermediate (Reynolds et al., 1975) rates. Perhaps the strong cohesiveness of the Japanese American community prevents many potential suicides. Conceivably, low suicide rates for Japanese Americans may also represent successful assimilation into U.S. society. This implies that their adjustment patterns would be more similar to those of Americans than to those of Japanese (in Japan) (Dunham, 1976). This, however, does not explain why the official Japanese American suicide rate is lower than the white rate. There is evidence that the reported suicide rate of Japanese Americans is artificially low (Kalish & Reynolds, 1976, p. 138). More Japanese Americans than other groups know of a suicide that has been concealed. Suicides, like many other potentially embarrassing events, are often concealed by Japanese American families who are greatly influenced by what others think of them (Kalish & Reynolds, 1976). This sets the stage for an ethical dilemma between autonomy and accountability. Autonomy is suggested by data that show that Japanese American suicide rates, like those of whites, increase with age (McIntosh & Santos, 1981b). Similar patterns have also been observed among Filipino and Chinese Americans. A deemphasis on accountability is the trade-off that comes from choosing autonomy. Accountability would include exposing the deception of concealing a suicide in the family.

Funerals

Japanese Americans, more than any other racial/ethnic group, prefer simple funerals attended only by relatives and a few especially close friends (the moral value of privacy) (Kalish & Reynolds, 1976, p. 143). Social etiquette in the

Japanese American community, however, obliges representatives from the community to attend and financially contribute (*koden*) to the high cost of a funeral (the moral value of fidelity). This drives attendance up, which, in turn, drives the cost further up.

The majority of Japanese Americans wish to be cremated; one-third choose burial (Kalish & Reynolds, 1976). A small percentage (11%) want their remains sent to Japan. The majority of those desiring cremation have no travel plans for their remains. This makes sense because grave visiting is very important in the Japanese American community. It is not surprising that most Japanese Americans would prefer that their remains be near their relatives (Kalish & Reynolds, 1976, p. 153).

Besides visiting graves more often than other racial/ethnic groups, Japanese Americans attend more funerals than others. Kalish and Reynolds (1976) found that 84% of their sample had attended at least one funeral in the previous two years. It is not unanticipated that older Japanese Americans have higher rates of attendance than the younger generations (Kalish & Reynolds, 1976, p. 153). Few Japanese Americans make arrangements for their own funeral, suggesting communal responsibility for funerals and other matters of the deceased (the moral value of fidelity).

Native Americans

There is tremendous intertribal diversity regarding death-related beliefs and practices among Native Americans. Older people in such tribes as the Apache have relatively little fear and anxiety facing their own death (Opler, 1946). The Navajos, conversely, have an especially great fear of death and the dead (Markides & Mindel, 1987). Avoidance of the dead and related matters can be traced to belief in and intense fear of spirits (Kluckhohn, 1962). Traditional Navajos bury their dead quickly and unceremoniously away from the village since they are believed to have harmful effects on the living. This pattern was also common in Europe in the Middle Ages. Since people were ignorant about the spread of viruses and disease, they believed that the dead caused death. When workers quickly burned diseased infected bodies, rates of illness decreased. This fostered greater avoidance and fear of the dead.

Such apprehension about death was ingeniously captured, shaped, and expanded by Gothic writers like Bram Stoker. They created a most powerfully evil yet mysteriously enamoring cultural icon: the vampire. The simultaneous, rapid, and deadly spread of tuberculosis also helped to fuel fear of vampires. Victims of tuberculosis displayed the same symptoms that opportunistic writers characterized as vampirish: spitting up blood, rapid physical weakening, pale complexion, and difficulty breathing at night. Native American fear of death carries over into persons with terminal illness, who are often kept in shelters away from home (Markides & Mindel, 1987). Today terminally ill Navajos spend their last few days of life in a hospital. Indian Health Services or religious workers usually take care of funerals. This allows family members to avoid any contact with the corpse (Kunitz & Levy, 1981, p. 384).

Pueblo cultural beliefs about death help the dying neutralize fear that may arise at the time of death or a dangerous crisis (Markides & Mindel, 1987). When these cultural beliefs (e.g., the continuation of life, ancestral prayers for healthy crops) are internalized, as they seem to be here, death is calmly accepted.

Increasingly high suicide rates for Native Americans (McIntosh & Santos, 1981b) have received considerable attention from social scientists. Although the overall rate is high, there is a great deal of variance among tribes. Thus one should avoid the stereotype that Native Americans are suicidal.

Native American suicide rates are higher among younger persons than among the elderly (Markides & Mindel, 1987). Low rates for the elderly are possibly due to the high status they receive within their community. Moreover, since few Native Americans survive to old age, those who do are the hardiest and, presumably, would be less likely to have suicidal tendencies (McIntosh & Santos, 1981a). Finally, elderly Native Americans are less likely to undergo the stress of cultural assimilation (Ogden, Spector, & Hill, 1970).

CONCLUSIONS ON DEATH, DYING, AND ETHNICITY

Death, as part of the life process, affects every individual and culture. It produces anxiety and is disruptive to social dynamics. Each culture has its own beliefs, norms, and rituals about death and dying. Funerals function to provide people an outlet to commiserate and grieve together. This seems necessary in order to get on with life and alleviate the disruption caused by the departure of a group member.

There is a general attitude in the dominant culture to deny and avoid the topic of death and dying. The open examination of death appears to be nearly taboo in the United States. Nevertheless, there has been recent interest by the media, professionals, students, and those most directly affected—the dying and their caretakers and family. For example, support groups aim to enable persons with AIDS to die with dignity and purpose.

There are both significant interethnic (between two or more ethnic groups) and intraethnic (within a single ethnic group) differences in beliefs and behavior related to death. Attitudes toward death are sometimes more personal than other cultural attitudes and more predictable by individual experiences rather than macrolevel characteristics (Bengtson et al., 1977). Although there are subcultural scripts, a member of the subculture is ultimately free to adhere to or reject them.

This analysis, hopefully, has not only shown the richness and diversity of approaches to death and dying by U.S. ethnic groups, but has also raised ethical issues (tied to values) that each of us face regarding our own death or the death of a loved one. Contemporary medical ethics must be sensitive to the ethnic background of the elderly or terminally ill patients. When a patient is elderly, terminally ill, and embedded in ethnic tradition, it is especially challenging to avoid stereotyping him or her (Kastenbaum, 1977) and to honor ethnic ethics (Cortese, 1990).

A MODERNIZATION APPROACH TO AGING AND ETHNICITY

Immigration during the latter half of the nineteenth century and the early twentieth century consisted largely of people from societies that were less industrialized and less modernized than the United States (Italians, Mexicans, Puerto Ricans, Polish, and Irish). While it is true that in some cases, the country of origin was in the process of urbanizing and industrializing, most immigrants came from the agricultural peasant regions of these countries (Markides & Mindel, 1987). Most Italian immigrants to the United States, for example, came from Sicily and the less developed rural South (C. L. Johnson, 1985).

We can gainfully compare the experience of immigrants moving from agricultural to urban-industrial environments to analysis of modernized societies and less modernized ones or the modernization of one society over time. If modernization weakens the extended family and subsequent status of the elderly, likewise, the transplantation of a group from a traditional society to a modern one can be expected to have similar consequences (Markides & Mindel, 1987). Conversely, one could argue that immigrant enclaves are more tightly knit than the communities from which they emigrated because of their minority status. (Recall the notion of ethnogenesis introduced earlier.) Accordingly, immigrants would have strong family ties and commitment to ethnic heritage because of their isolation, subjective feelings of being a cultural outsider, the foreign environment, and the need to reinforce the familiar. Modernization theory aids us in understanding the experiences of the Mexican American elderly (Maldonado, 1975; Korte, 1981). Rapid social change since World War II has significantly changed the role of the elderly in the Mexican American family. Members of the older generation, typically raised in rural society, now find themselves in large and hostile complex urban areas. In another sense, modernization theory has hindered, more than helped, a better understanding of minority elderly. The notion that modernized families are less supportive of elderly members than traditional families has not always been supported by research (Rosenthal, 1983, 1986). Rather, a more dynamic view of ethnicity and culture is fruitful: "Ethnic culture [is] a pool of meanings from which people may draw as they wish [or] need according to their situations. Ethnicity may change its salience to people at different periods in the life course" (Rosenthal, 1983, p. 11).

While the minority status of the elderly minority is certainly important, it is not the whole story. The sweeping idea of ethnicity, as well as cultural disparity between groups, needs special consideration. The focus on minority aging is related to an increasing emphasis on minority groups that began with the civil rights movement. As ethnic minorities became politically empowered, older people too began to view themselves and began to be viewed by others as a political base with which to be reckoned. Gray power piggybacked on the success of the civil rights, Chicano, and feminist movements. It is not surprising that the exploding field of gerontology during the 1970s placed great emphasis on minority status. However, the deemphasis of cultural diversity in aging among Euro-American scholars and policymakers reflects our society's assimilationist ideology that defines all people as having similar traits, aspirations, and problems.

CONCLUSION: POLICY RECOMMENDATION

"Social intervention is any act, planned or unplanned, that alters the characteristics of another individual or the pattern of relationships between individuals" (Kelman & Warwick, 1978, p. 3). This includes such macrolevel phenomena as public policy, national planning, military intervention in the affairs of other nations, and technical assistance. It also covers microlevel phenomena such as psychotherapy, neighborhood security watch programs, sensitivity training, and experiments done with human research participants.

There are four aspects of any social intervention that are likely to raise ethical issues:

1. The choice of goals to which the change effort is directed
2. The definition of the point of the change
3. The choice of means used to implement the intervention
4. The assessment of the results of the intervention

At each of these steps, the ethical issues that arise may involve conflicting ethical values, that is, questions about what values are to be maximized at the expense of what other values.

Ethical values in the human service professions in the United States (e.g., autonomy, privacy, fidelity, and accountability) determine the choice of goals to which a change effort is directed. Intervention is clearly designed to maximize a particular set of values and minimize the loss of specific other values. These "at-risk" values, consequently, serve as examples of acceptable costs in a given intervention.

For example, rapid demographic growth in ethnic-minority populations, limited resources, and the sharply rising cost of health care have forced the government to set financial limits on various types of health care delivery. Such public policy ostensibly benefits the common welfare. At the same time, policymakers should be concerned about the effects of this program on the ethical values of beneficence (maximum support and care by others in the maintenance or enhancement of one's well-being) and distributive justice (sharing material and/or human resources without regard to ethnicity, gender, social class, religion, or other subcultural differences). These ethical values should be preserved due to their efficacy; it is necessary that they do not drop below some minimal level.

Ethical values may affect the choice of goals not only in such explicit, conscious ways, but also in covert ways. This may occur when social policy commences with an unquestioned definition of a problem. The definition of the target of change is often based on this type of implicit, unexamined conception of where the problem is. For example, public policy designed to improve health care for an economically disadvantaged subculturally diverse group may be designed to change institutional arrangements that have led to the systematic exclusion of this group from the economic mainstream of the society. Conversely, it may be designed to reduce the educational, environmental, or psychological "deficiencies" of the disadvantaged group itself. The choice between these two primary goals may well depend on one's worldview, life experiences, ideology, and ethical values: A focus on removing systematic barriers is more reflective of the values of the disadvantaged group itself, while a focus on removing deficiencies suggests the values of the more dominant segments of society.

Ethical values play a key role in an evaluation of the means chosen to implement a particular social policy. Questions about the methods of inducing change in individuals typically involve a conflict between the values of individual autonomy and social welfare. To what extent and under what conditions is a government justified in imposing limits or rationing medical procedures that are designed to eliminate or reduce life-threatening conditions?

Conflicting ethical values enter into a judgment of the consequences of social policy. One of the latent consequences of scientific medical treatment for disease in subculturally diverse patients may be a weakening of traditional subcultural ideology, authority structures, and family bonds. The extent to which we are willing to risk these consequences depends on whether we are more committed to traditional values or those values inherent in biomedical ethics. Clearly, there are important trade-offs to carefully consider. Our assessment of the consequences of a policy depends on what ethical values we are willing or unwilling to sacrifice in the interest of social change.

Health and health care delivery both are major problems for minority elderly of color. This is part of a larger ethical question. Disparity in health and effective access to health services cannot be considered separately from other dimensions of life, especially where public policy plays a massive role. There has been progress in some areas; in other areas, social inequity still predominates. The elimination of blatant discrimination (e.g., involuntary racial segregation) through the legal system has not been parlayed into active inclusion and full social participation for many minority of color. This points us to another important context: stratification and ethnicity.

Ethnic background provides a unique historical calendar of life events for minority elderly. Ethnic-minority elderly face ageism, racial discrimination and prejudice, and prolonged poverty. Although white elderly may face ageism and health problems, they will not have problems because of the color of their skin.

This has been documented extensively by the numerous comparative data presented in this chapter. There is a need to examine the ethnic background and minority status of the elderly in terms of social class, income level, access to quality health services, education, gender, age, living arrangements, use of diverse health care systems (e.g., modern science and folk medicine), and social support systems in the family and community.

The delivery of health care in the United States is neither operated to provide nor designed to address equal access for the minority elderly and the poor. "There is no constitutional, statutory or regulatory 'right' to health care" (U.S. Department of Health and Human Services, 1990a, p. 19). National health care coverage still appears to be a long way off. President Clinton has steadily backtracked on his health care proposal in the face of vigorous opposition. We are again back to square one.

Overt barriers to health care for minorities of color (e.g., racially segregated health clinics and hospitals) have largely disappeared. However, institutional discrimination remains. This ranges from the sharp underrepresentation of ethnic-minority physicians to informal norms and practices and official policies. This effectively restricts access for minorities, the poor, and the uninsured. Racial-discrimination barriers to health care are illegal. Nevertheless, barriers to equal access for the minority elderly persist. There is rationing of health care, for example, for such procedures as renal dialysis and heart transplant and a limit on the number of days for mental health services per year. There is also a preference for private-pay-insurance patients; physicians claim that they do not profit off government-supported health care programs. Finally, there are restrictions on health care for the homeless and patients with a diagnosis of Alzheimer's disease or mental illness.

Folk illnesses and cures are frequently an element in an individual's particular ethnic identity (Chrisman & Kleinman, 1980). Ideas about health, illness, and healing are so closely tied to the values and behaviors of people's lives that knowledge about ethnicity may provide significant insight into the nature of the health ways of a minority elderly group in the United States.

Ethnic cultures can provide the elderly with the positive continuity of familiar and traditional roles (Holzberg, 1982). In the case of Mexican Americans, how does one argue against 500 years of sustained influence in the United States? When we lose the right to be different, it costs us our liberty. Further research on how ethnic background affects the process of aging would be valuable for making better-informed and morally responsible decisions on public policy.

3

Ethical Issues in a Religiously Diverse Society

Cromwell Crawford

Prema Mathai-Davis, commissioner of the New York City Department for the Aging, is one of the nation's most outstanding practitioners in her field and is the recipient of numerous awards for distinguished service. She holds a doctorate in human development from Harvard University, and among her many accomplishments, she is the founder of the Community Agency for Senior Citizens of Staten Island. In a recent interview, she was asked, "Do you think that your cultural background has played a role in your career as an advocate for the elderly?" Her reply: "I lived with my grandfather in a three-generational household. My value system has played a role in terms of enhancing my awareness of the issues" (Kripalani, 1993, p. 14).

This interview highlights the fact that issues of aging are more than biological and medical matters; they are social and cultural realities. As a researcher, Prema Mathai-Davis certainly understands the scientific facts of aging; but as a native of India, she interprets these facts from the perspective of the cultural world into which she was born and bred. "Facts" never stand as facts; they are always subject to interpretation. Among the interpretative elements of culture, religion stands out as the most universal and potent.

By "religion" is meant something more than institutional affiliation to some church, mosque, or synagogue. Religion and aging encounter one another on the experiential level. Following Tillich (1957), religion may be defined as the state of being grasped by an ultimate concern. That is, whenever a person speaks of the ultimate meaning of his existence, whenever he contemplates absolute duties and obligations, whenever he devotes himself to a cause he deems to be ultimately real, that individual is acting religiously, whether he is aware of it or not.

Ultimate concern is experientially expressed on two levels. First, ultimate concern is directed toward some truth about the world that is ultimately real. This vision of something that transcends the changing order of things provides the believer with the ground for confidence in the future.

Second, ultimate concern is directed toward that which is conceived as possessing final value. This "pearl of great price" supplies the norm by which to judge all other values. Belief in this *summum bonum* imparts to the individual not only a set of priorities, but also the hope for the endless flow of values into his or her life.

It was not so long ago that "ultimate concern" would have been understood in terms of Protestant Christianity by the average white, Anglo-Saxon American. The same would have been true for aging. Today the cultural milieu of American society has radically changed. A headline announces this demographic shift: "Asian Wave Is Changing U.S. Scene." The 1990 census shows that Asians are the nation's fastest-growing minority group, with higher-than-average incomes and education. According to economist Louis Winnick, author of *New People in Old Neighborhoods*, "Their impact will be far greater than their numbers" ("Asian Wave," 1990).

One impact that is already visible is the evolution of multiculturalism. Multiculturalism is "a new concept of American culture as a commingling of many distinctive strands, each equitably accepted within the fabric of our national life and all part of the rich interweaving of cultures that will be part of our emerging twenty-first-century civilization" ("Asian Wave," 1990, p. A3).

This chapter views the issues of aging from culturally diverse perspectives. Our multicultural stance is dictated not only by the fact that American society is fast becoming culturally pluralistic, but that technology is shrinking our world, so that the lives and destinies of all people are progressively being bound together.

The different viewpoints go beyond our customary Judeo-Christian traditions to include Islam, Confucianism, Hinduism, and Buddhism. They address our humanity, telling us how people care, how they cure, and how they cope with the vicissitudes of aging. They set before us windows through which to peer at the lives of others, and mirrors in which we may see our own lives in a new light. This provides occasions for self-reflection and self-reform. Long-held views of Western superiority must yield to alien insights from the East. A Bantu proverb says, "He who never visits thinks mother is the only cook" (Marty, 1987, p. ix). Visits to new worlds should enable us to acquire new tastes and thus expand our moral menus, but acquisitions of the new are not tantamount to rejections of the old. Home cooking may still be the best—for you—but there is a heightened awareness of the human spirit's ability to invent life differently; and amid all of life's passages, this genius for creation is demonstrated best is diverse approaches to aging.

To explain this diversity and creativity at work, we must examine the formal structure of ethics. Each religion begins with a philosophical a priori, a judgment about what is ultimately real, ultimately true, and ultimately good. This metaphysical assumption elicits basic commitments on the part of the devotee. The ethical task is then to show the bearing and relevance of this presupposition for human behavior. Ethics as a systematic discipline is the path whereby an individual reflects rationally and self-consciously on the fact of being a moral agent. Through the use of reason, he searches for ways to make his conduct consistent with his character. In this way he engages in coherent ways of deciding moral questions. Thus, on the one hand, ethics precedes morals, which have to do with actions; on the other hand, it logically follows metaphysics, which expresses the realm of finality. People are so constituted that they constantly ask moral questions: What must I do? What good shall I serve? Ethics informs these questions by making the individual aware of who he is, in order to regulate his conduct rationally, with reference to his total moral environment.

Since religious ethics operates on theoretical and scientific levels and attempts to explain the moral life in a thematic, systematic, coherent, and consistent form, it is generally not found as such in the scriptures of world religions. Instead, what we do find are moral teachings, dispositions, attitudes, virtues, and ways of life that are normative for followers of the way. The constructive task of delineating a system of ethics will therefore fall on us.

We now turn to the main task of this chapter, which is to explore the issues of aging from the perspectives of the following world religions: Judaism, Christianity, Islam, Confucianism, Buddhism, and Hinduism. Interspersed with the presentation, we shall suggest implications of these ideas and insights for contemporary problems of aging. Given the historical, philosophical, and literary expanse of the material to be covered, this chapter will be limited to essential considerations of the subject matter.

OVERVIEW OF THE ETHICS OF AGING IN WORLD RELIGIONS

Judaism

Jewish ethics must be understood in developmental terms, relative to its theological insights. It is therefore a theocentric ethics. The high-water mark of this progression is reached with the rise of the prophets, especially the later prophets such as Isaiah, Jeremiah, Ezekiel, Hosea, Amos, and Micah. In addition to the prophet, the Hebrew Bible is given shape by the priest and the sage. The priest centered religious life around the Torah and ministered to the numinous sense of the people. His chief virtue was love of God expressed through self-surrender and love of man expressed through self-giving. The sage functioned as counselor, giving moral lessons based on his reflections upon human experience. His central virtue was temperance in one's personal life and justice in social relationships. The prophet stands out as a religious personality who brings a fresh and passionate insight into the meaning of God's will for the present situation and grounds his appeal for right conduct in God's demand for righteousness.

Before we delineate the nature of prophetic ethics, we must identify its chief sources. Pivotal to Israel's theological understanding is the Exodus event. Through his servant Moses, God had mightily delivered the Jews from Egyptian slavery. This supreme event, through which God revealed himself in history, impelled the prophets to declare that Israel was thereby obligated to live in conformity with the divine act. For instance, against the unkindness, ignorance, injustice, and idolatry of his people, the Lord reminds them through Micah (6: 4), "For I brought you up from the land of Egypt, and redeemed you from the house of bondage" (Oxford Annotated Bible with the Apocrypha, Revised Standard Version, College Edition).

The Exodus event is followed by the Sinaitic Covenant, which serves as a second source of the prophet's ethical understanding. Through the encounter with Yahweh at Mount Sinai, the tribes of Israel acknowledged him as the sovereign over their life, and in return for his continued help, they owed Yahweh their supreme allegiance. Yahweh was a holy God, and by virtue of the covenant bond with him, Israel became a "holy people." The covenant not only bound the tribes to Yahweh, but to one another, forging bonds of solidarity.

A third source of prophetic ethics was the Covenant Code (Exod. 20:23–23: 33). The entire community was brought under the banner of "justice" raised by Yahweh's redemptive acts. The code legislated the equality of all Israelites before God (Exod. 21:23–25); respect for human life, regardless of rank and status; and the right to protection of the poor and weak, especially widows, orphans, and resident aliens. In sum, "The human being, called by God to freedom, is the indispensable form of wealth—this is the kernel of the whole legal ideology of the Old Testament. The equality of all members of the nation before the God who is no respecter of persons, demands the same rights in working life; it calls for voluntary sacrifice of all citizens, in order to avert the inroads of the inequality and oppression" (Eichrodt, 1949, p. 3).

A fourth influence upon the prophetic ethics was the awareness that Israel had been divinely elected. The notion that "God chose Israel for his people" is the key to the interpretation of the nature and history of the Jewish nation. This election does not refer to a single divine act but to a continuous providential control, conditioned in part on an inner capacity of the Jewish spirit for the task involved in this supernatural calling. The aim, as apprehended by the prophets, was that Israel was to proclaim the truth and righteousness of God throughout the world. "This centering of obligation in one God was of vast importance for ethical development. Moral development was possible because its source lay in the sovereignty and will of one God. It meant that the divine requirements had ultimate force for the holy people, and that no competing or rival allegiance could qualify or weaken them" (Muilenburg, 1952, p. 532).

Finally, the will for ethical action proceeded from the nature of the covenant relationship. For his part, God had initiated and faithfully perpetuated his promise to protect Israel. For their part, the people were to respond in gratitude and loyalty and meet the demands of the covenant by walking in "righteousness."

The nature of "righteousness" (*sedek*) was defined by the prophets with reference to the nature of Yahweh. Two terms stand out expressing the reciprocity of ethical relationship between Israel and Yahweh: justice (*mishpat*) and covenantal faithfulness (*hesed*). God is Lord of Israel, and yet, as party to the covenant, he participates fully in the life of the community as one of its members. Isaiah (30:18) proclaims, "the Lord is a God of justice." His holiness is expressed through justice (Isa. 5:16). It follows that all of the dealings of his people—in land, wealth, commerce, and civic and political affairs—must meet the standards of divine justice.

For Yahweh, your God, he is God of gods, and lord of Lords, the great God, the mighty and terrible, who regards not persons (i.e., shows no partiality), nor takes reward. He executes justice for the fatherless and widow, and loves the sojourner, in giving him food and raiment. Love therefore the sojourner [i.e., the resident foreigner], for you were sojourners in the land of Egypt. (Muilenburg, 1952, p. 537)

Yahweh sets the pattern of justice, and members of the Hebrew community are obligated to act as God acts. The divine cry for justice is heard par excellence in the prophecies of Amos (5:15). No room is left for compromise:

Hate evil, and love good,
And establish justice in the gate;
It may be that God, the Lord of hosts,
Will be gracious to the remnant of Joseph.

The reciprocity of ethical relationships between Yahweh and Israel is captured in a second term, representing covenant faithfulness. The Hebrew word *hesed* can also mean mercy, love, fidelity, and devotion. As Muilenburg explains, "*Hesed* is the community term par excellence." It can express relationships between kin, host and guest, friends, and the ruler and his subjects. The prophets also extend the word to include intimate relationships. "Here the mutuality of obligation between various persons of the same group is accentuated. It goes beyond justice and moves in the direction of grace and devotion. It becomes the interior disposition of the heart" (Muilenburg, 1952, p. 538).

If Amos is the supreme prophet of justice, Hosea is the compassionate voice of *hesed*. For him, personally, *hesed* springs forth from the experience of a loving husband and his unfaithful wife. Such also is the love Yahweh has for Israel, and when the relationship is finally restored, Hosea (2:19–20) hears God promise: "I will betroth you to me forever; I will betroth you to me in righteousness [*sedek*], and in justice [*mishpat*], in covenant faithfulness [*hesed*], and in love [*rahmin*]; I will betroth you to me in faithfulness [or steadfastness, *emunah*], and you shall know the Lord."

The covenantal relationship and the demands for righteousness that the prophets proclaim imply a distinctive Hebrew anthropology, which requires some explication. From the central tenet of Jewish theology that affirms the unity of God, there follows the central tenet of Jewish ethics of the unity of man. The ethical task of the human being is to achieve harmony with oneself, with others, and with God.

The task of becoming a fully harmonious being is met with many challenges. On the psychological level, humans confront an internal split between good desire, *yezer tov*, and evil desire, *yezer hora* (Agus, 1967). On the metaphysical level, humans experience the tension between their own autonomy and dependence upon the supernatural realm. On the sociopolitical level, there is the conflict between one's sense of belonging to the group and yet being independent by virtue of individual conscience.

Jewish ethics asserts that it is possible for humans to resolve all of these conflicts by making God the center of their lives. The home is the source of Jewish morals, and its values are the sum and substance of Jewish ethics. For the ancient Israelite, his foremost goal was maintenance of the integrity of his family. A child was reared to honor father and mother. This duty was revered as one of the Ten Commandments given to Moses: "Honor your father and your mother, that your days may be long in the land which the Lord your God gives you" (Exod. 20:12). In early life, to honor meant obedience to parents, and in later life it entailed their support in old age. The verse also points out that old age itself is considered a blessing. Long life is the reward for observing the Torah.

Veneration for old age is inculcated throughout the Hebrew scriptures. It is an essential part of the ethical code of Leviticus (19:32): "You shall rise up before the hoary head, and honor the face of an old man." Its antiquity gives it proverbial form: "The glory of young men is their strength, but the beauty of old men is their grey hair" (Prov. 20:29). Wisdom also comes from age. The Sanhedrin was constituted of elders. The composition of this body called for the exclusion of the very old, but this was based on ability, not chronology. All of the paradigmatic figures in Jewish history—Abraham, Isaac, Jacob, Joseph, Moses, Joshua—were men of age. The "book of the generations of Adam" (Gen. 5) celebrates age with potency—all of the generations of Adam were veterans with voracious virility. "When Methuselah had lived a hundred and eighty-seven years, he became the father of Lamech" (Gen. 5:25). This might have been wishful thinking, but it was thinking, nonetheless; and as the adage has it, "If you don't use it, you lose it." The ordinary length of human life is reckoned at 70 years, or, by reason of strength, 80 years. David died an old man at 70 (II Sam. 5:4; I Kings 2:11).

The teaching that age must be respected is derived from diverse considerations. Mention has already been made of the primacy of righteousness, justice, and covenantal love in the life of the people. These are the qualities of Yahweh, which must be embodied in his people. Persons cannot be excluded on the basis of age, because through allegiance to one God Israel is one people. A central motif of Jewish ethics is the sanctification of life. Life is holy, or more properly, life must become holy, and age is a time in which this transcendent dimension of existence is best developed. Learning is a virtue that comes with age, and the ancients in heaven are pictured as poring over the Torah. Spirituality aside, social justice demands that those with special needs have rights to special care that goes beyond charity. There is also the reward motif: veneration of the aged leads to the prolongation of one's own life.

In medical context, respect for age is mandated on the basis of the talmudic maxim that if a person is healthy, his mind can advance, regardless of age.

Respect is also due to the aged because of their added infirmities. David M. Feldman states: "Proper treatment and care for the aged is fundamental to the ethical code, and the individual mitzvah has, historically, been fulfilled both at home within the family circle and in institutions, known as *Moshav Zekenim*. The latter attend to routine needs, but the human ones come from personal attention by family in or out of institutions" (1986, p. 98).

Feldman also cites the case in a hospital ward where an elderly patient pushed the panic button because she was experiencing choking feelings. The interns on duty were overheard complaining in the corridors, "Imagine disturbing our sleep at night for a ninety-year-old woman!" The chief of interns heard it and gave them his reprimand: "A woman that age has as much right to her life, and to our vigorous efforts to preserve that life, as someone nine or nineteen" (Feldman, 1986, p. 98). In the light of covenantal ethics, the 90-year-old lady has even more rights than one who is 9 or 19. All life is sanctified, but the life of one who has acquired the wealth of old age is even more precious. In the end, it is not a question of what a person has or does not have, socially or economically, but who he is and to whom he belongs. Thus the Psalmist prays: "Now also when I am old and greyheaded, O God, forsake me not; until I have shewed thy strength unto this generation, and thy power to every one that is to come" (Ps. 71:18).

The Psalmist was assured that in old age or in death God would not forsake him. Expectation of a resurrection of the dead in the Days of the Messiah emerged as a major part of Pharisaic doctrine following the destruction of the Temple in 70 C.E., though the Sadducees rejected such notions. In general, rabbinic literature believes that after death our souls pass through a 12-month period of purifying punishments. Souls are then returned to a heavenly "treasury" to await the earthly return of the Messiah, when the purified bodies of the dead arise from their graves and are united with their souls. The righteous pass from God's final judgment into the beatific world, but the wicked can only enter following punitive purifications.

Modern Jews are skeptical of classic views of the afterlife, though their vision of the future is not without hope. A liberal Jewish outlook is expressed thus by Eugene Borowitz, reflecting the traditional this-worldly orientation of Judaism: "We can emphasize the good that people need to do while they are alive and can thus intensify our sense of human responsibility. We can find long-range satisfaction in the good we have done that will survive our death and in the knowledge that the Jewish people will carry on our ideals long after we are gone'' (1995, pp. 232–233).

Christianity

Christian ethics begins with the ethics of Jesus, specifically the Jesus whom we encounter in the synoptic Gospels (Matthew, Mark, and Luke). Recent studies of the Gospels demonstrate how problematic is the task of discovering the ethical teachings of Jesus because of the contributions of the early church. Evangelists not only gathered gospel material, but also presented it from precise theological perspectives of their own, and prophets, believing that they were possessed by the Spirit, brought forth the word of the living Lord for his church. Thus both of these sources made creative additions to the store of the tradition of Jesus' teachings, making it difficult to discern between the original and later additions. We are left with one stratum of material in which the theological improvisation of the church is clearly evident, another stratum that is ambiguous, and a third that, though not the *ipsissima verba* of Jesus, bears the marks of genuine Jesus material.

Jesus was a Jew, and as a son of Israel he incorporated basic Jewish ideas into the formation of his own moral axioms. Theological assumptions such as monotheism and the activity of the divine will in human history, the unity of morality and religion, and the values and virtues that proceed from that union— righteousness, justice, loving kindness, sacrifice, guilt, forgiveness, and individual responsibility—are all ideas within Jesus' Jewish heritage.

In addition to a positive attitude toward his heritage, there is reliable evidence that Jesus' attitude included some negative elements. The nub of this difference lay in his substitution of his message of the Kingdom of God for the Mosaic law that historically regulated the life of Israel. In the act of proclaiming the Kingdom of God, Jesus virtually nullified Pentateuchal law in repect to such matters as divorce (Mark 10:1–12; Matt. 19:1–9), oaths (Matt. 5:33–37), clean and unclean foods (Mark 7:1–23), retaliation (Matt. 5:38–48), and aspects of sabbath observance (Mark 2:23–3:6).

The structure of Jesus' ethical teaching was marked by vertical and horizontal dimensions. The vertical dimension represented a demand for radical obedience to God and complete trust in him. Allegiance to God was to have priority over all other concerns or commitments in life. In concrete terms, this injunction applied to a person's wealth. ''Lay not up for yourselves treasures upon earth, where moth and rust doth corrupt, and where thieves break through and steal: But lay up for yourselves treasures in heaven, where neither moth and rust doth corrupt, and where thieves do not break through nor steal: For where your treasure is, there will your heart be also'' (Matt. 6:19–21). The demand also extended to the family. When informed that his brethren and his mother were looking for him, Jesus replied, ''Who is my mother, or my brethren?'' And looking around at his audience, he said, ''Behold my mother and my brethren!

For whosoever shall do the will of God, the same is my brother, and my sister, and mother" (Matt. 12:48–50).

Radical obedience to God went beyond external acts to inner states. Going further than the command of the Decalogue, "Thou shalt not kill," Jesus said that even the harboring of anger toward another person incurs divine judgment (Matt. 5:21–22). Again, if one's hand causes one to sin, one must eliminate the offending part, because it is better to enter life maimed than with two hands to go to hell (Mark 9:43). Similarly, one must not make a display of pious acts. "Thus, when you give alms, sound no trumpet before you, as the hypocrites do in the synagogues and in the streets, that they may be praised by men. . . . But when you give alms, do not let your left hand know what your right hand is doing, so that your alms may be in secret; and your Father who sees in secret will reward you" (Matt. 6:2–4). A second facet of the ethical teachings of Jesus is the horizontal dimension. Experientially, the two are connected. When Jesus was asked which commandment is first of all, highlighting Leviticus 19:18, he answered, " 'You shall love the Lord your God with all your heart, and with all your soul, and with all your mind, and with all your strength.' The second is this, 'You shall love your neighbor as yourself.' There is no greater commandment than these" (Mark 12:30–31). Through this summary of the entire duty of man in the twofold command of love for God and neighbor, Jesus rejected the legalism of the Pharisees.

It is worthy of note that reference to the neighbor is in the singular. The focus is on the specific, individual case, not some abstract reference to humanity. Luke's version of the command is illustrated by the story of the good Samaritan (10:29–37), which makes the point that while all men are brothers, the person in a situation of need becomes one's neighbor and thereby has radical claims upon us. This concern for neighbor needs is expressed in the Golden Rule: "Whatever you wish that men would do to you, do so to them; for this is the law and the prophets" (Matt. 7:12). Jesus expresses God's concern for each individual, especially for the lost, the last, and the least. The parable of the lost sheep is a case in point (Luke 15:3–7). Human needs must be given priority over institutions. "The sabbath was made for man, not man for the sabbath" (Mark 2:27).

Finally, God's Kingdom brings about the reversal of values. The first shall be last and the last first. In the Kingdom of God, divine blessings are bestowed upon the poor, those who mourn and those who are persecuted (Luke 6:21–23). Life in the Kingdom is marked by freedom from anxiety about what we shall eat, what we shall drink, and wherewithal we shall be clothed. True greatness is to turn and become like children: to give up self-chosen goals and relate oneself to God as to a father, having a childlike attitude of humility and openness.

This brings us to the application of Jesus' ethical teachings. The reference to children shows that for Jesus, age was more a matter of attitude than of years. What gives our years their vital quality is a childlike mind, born of the Spirit.

Jesus said to Nicodemus, "You must be born again" (John 3:7). Nicodemus was old, but age could not deny the possibility of a new beginning.

A second application of Jesus' ethical teaching is his notion of the extended family. Jewish tradition had taught him to revere his parents, but his vision of life in the Kingdom of God dissolved tribal and familial boundaries to include other persons as his mother and father, brothers and sisters.

Third, Jesus believed that his mission was not only to teach but to heal, the two being theologically of one piece, as in the episode of whether it was easier for him to say to the paralytic, "Rise up and walk" or "Your sins are forgiven" (Mark 2:9). In his healing mission, Jesus demonstrated that everyone who suffered in body and mind the pain of disease and decrepitude was worthy of help.

Other implications of the ethical teachings of Jesus pertaining to the aged are derived from his description of the "neighbor" as anyone who is in need, and from the expectation of the reversal of physical fortunes, delineated in the Sermon on the Mount—"Blessed are the poor in spirit, for theirs is the kingdom of heaven," and so on (Matt. 5:3). The Beatitudes illustrate the fact that much of Jesus' message was eschatological, but his eschatological thinking was the temporal and traditional formulation of an overpowering sense of divine immediacy. In that sense, the coming Kingdom had come, the first fruit of the harvest was here, and people were invited to experience the power and presence of God for themselves. Hope therefore did not point to a speculative future, but to a present reality.

Finally, it must be squarely acknowledged that elders find the need to depend on family, friends, and professionals the most irksome and humiliating fact of aging. Throughout their lives they fend for themselves, stand on their own two feet, and learn to cherish their autonomy and independence as their most prized possessions. Then, like a thief in the night, age takes it all away, leaving only taunting memories behind. This bad dream is ended for the Christian when he or she comes to view human dependence as a sign of ultimate dependence on the providence of God. As part of the created order, no one stands alone. However, in order for the elder to trust life and the Creator of life, he or she must be able to trust the instrumental goodness of fellow humans whose friendship energizes and mediates that faith. This places a tremendous responsibility on those who minister to the needs of the weak and infirm, because it is their deed that transforms service into a sacrament that sustains both body and soul.

Paradoxically, this deepened dependence on God can make for independence. Only as humans acknowledge their creaturely dependence on God do they become fully human. Therefore, in the life of dependence, the elder Christian may find independence in dependence. Drew Christiansen, S. J., has developed this line of thought into a "theology of dependence" (McCormick, 1987, p. 159). It is eloquently summarized in the following prayer of Teilhard de Chardin:

> When the signs of age begin to mark my body (and still more when they touch my mind); when the ill that is to diminish me or carry me off strikes from without or is

born within me; when the painful moment comes in which I suddenly awaken to the fact that I am ill or growing old; and above all that last moment when I feel I am losing hold of myself and am absolutely passive within the hands of the great unknown forces that have formed me; in all those dark moments, O God, grant that I may understand that it is you (provided only my faith is strong enough) who are painfully parting the fibers of my being in order to penetrate the very marrow of my substance and bear me away within yourself. (McCormick, 1987, p. 160)

Islam

The message of Islam has a twofold basis: faith (*iman*) and right-doing (*ihsan*). The heart of religion is for a person to surrender his purpose to the divine while doing good to one's fellow humans. The Koran declares: "Lo! those who believe [in that which is revealed unto thee, Muhammad], and those who are Jews, and Christians, and Sabaeans—whoever believeth in Allah and the Last Day and doeth right—surely their reward is with their Lord, and there [in the other world] shall no fear come upon them, neither shall they grieve" (Koran 2:62).

In common with Judaism and Christianity, Islam affirms the unity of Ultimate Reality. Its first tenet is the Oneness or *tawhid* of Allah. The attributes of Allah are power, reason, and love. Allah is infinite, volitional, and rational. He is the creator, sustainer, and cherisher of all that is. He is transcendent, like the overpowering light of the heavens, and immanent, like the lamp enclosed within the niche. Allah has 99 most beautiful names, which become the basis for ethical reflection. He is the Beneficent, the Merciful, the Compassionate, the Provider, the Peacemaker, and the Just, among other attributes.

In accordance with the *tawhid* of Allah, true Muslims are *al-muwahhidun*, "those who maintain the Oneness."

The second basis of the message of Islam is right-doing (*ihsan*). The relation of *ihsan* to *iman* (faith) is one of cause and effect. Belief in the Unity of God gives meaning and direction to all of life. Since humanity's ideal nature is a manifestation of divine reality, loyalty to God is loyalty to one's own ideal nature. Human creation is unique because it shares the divine attributes, but this dignity calls for a corresponding responsibility. The Koran says: "God is He Who appointed you [mankind] His Vicegerents upon earth. Know, then, that he who fails to recognize this dignity and to act in accordance therewith shall be answerable for his neglect" (Koran 35:29).

Ihsan consists of righteous acts. The whole of Islamic law (*Shariah*) deals with righteous action, which forms the foundation for two chief principles: mercy (*rahmah*) and brotherhood (*ikha*).

Mercy is the most sublime characteristic of Allah. He is *al-Rahman* (the Merciful). It is also the chief feature of the Prophet Muhammad and his mission. In political affairs, mercy is the cornerstone of the organized state. It is not the preserve of humans only, but is extended to include the humane treatment of animals. The Prophet is reported as saying (*hadith*), "If you behold three mounting an animal, stone them until one descends."

Righteous action is also expressed through the principle of brotherhood. The Koran declares, "And remember Allah's favour unto you: how ye were enemies and He made friendship between your hearts so that ye became as brothers" (Koran 3:103). The Koran elevates brotherhood to include all of humanity. With mercy as their banner, Muslims are required to strive for universal brotherhood at all times and in all places.

Within domestic relationships, righteous action is sensitive to the needs of older members of the family. A general principle of the Koran apropos of social and domestic relations is "Act benevolently toward your parents and near of kin, the orphans and the needy and the next door neighbour and the distant neighbour and your partners in business and co-workers and wayfarers and travellers and those over whom you exercise authority" (Koran 4:36). More specifically, Islam holds to a gradation in our affections and attachments, and following the highest place, which must be accorded to God and His Apostle, aged parents are to be given greater affection than spouse or children. In comparison with the love of parent for a child, the love of child for parent is deemed superior, for whereas parental love is predominantly instinctive, filial love is born of gratitude and highlights the principle of reciprocity.

Sura 17, which resembles the Decalogue of the Hebrew Bible, moves immediately from the injunction against idolatry to care and honor of parents: "Thy Lord has decreed you shall not serve any but Him, and to be good to parents, whether one or both of them attains old age with thee; say not to them 'Fie' neither chide them, but speak unto them words respectful, and lower to them the wing of humbleness out of mercy and say, 'My Lord, have mercy upon them as they raised me up when I was little' " (Koran 17:22).

It could be the case that a Muslim son had Jewish or Christian parents, but age was to be given its rightful priority, regardless. Often, Muslim sons could be seen carrying their aged Christian mothers on their backs to churches. Respect for the aged goes beyond familial ties and derives its motivation from fundamental Koranic principles. Among these, the following stand out:

- The essence of the human self is divine, for God infused into Adam his own spirit.
- A corollary of the Unity of God is the unity of humanity. "A person has no faith unless he loves for his brother what he loves for himself."
- True piety is the giving of alms to kinsmen, the needy, the traveler, and the poor. *Zakat* is obligatory tithing; *sadaqa* goes beyond legal requirements to charitable giving for people in need.
- The Islamic demand for surrender signifies that the physical aspect of human life can be spiritualized and sublimated by subordinating itself to a higher ideal.
- The universe is an ordered whole in which no event is a product of mere chance and all of life's passages are goal-seeking activities.
- Life being a dynamic movement of the unfolding of immense potentialities, humans are destined to move to higher things by constantly dying in order to be constantly reborn.

- As "nothing is created in vain," so in human personality no aspect is created in order to be utterly repudiated or despised.
- The Islamic state is envisaged as a welfare state. Law and order and defense are not the sole functions of the state. Relief of poverty and suffering and care for the elderly are essential functions of the state.

Confucianism

The Confucian philosophy is preeminently a humanistic one. Its major preoccupation is with morality, which is squarely based on the notion of a common human nature. The paradigmatic individual for Confucian ethics is the *chun-tzu* or superior moral person. This ideal figure embodies the virtues of *jen, li, i,* and *shu* and serves as the exemplar of practical morality. Our purpose is to investigate the significance this Chinese understanding of the *chun-tzu* holds for questions pertaining to aging.

The basic virtue a person must cultivate the Confucians call *jen* (Analects IV, 5). The Chinese character *jen* combines the symbols for *man* and for *two*, thereby conveying the idea of a relationship between persons. The word carries the meaning of "human-heartedness." It implies a shared humanity that finds its expression best in human relationships. It is thus the moral hub around which society revolves. *Jen* defines the nature of morality. Its five ingredients are gravity, generosity of soul, sincerity, liberality, and kindness.

Jen belongs to the internal side of morality. It is more a matter of self-cultivation than of conduct, though the two belong together. The man of *jen* is one who, desiring to develop himself, develops others, and in desiring to sustain himself, sustains others. To be able from one's own self to draw a parallel for the treatment of others; that may be called the way to practice *jen*.

The second virtue that defines the *chun-tzu* is *li*. It means "educated behavior" and provides the form of the moral life. Confucius said, "The superior man, extensively studying all learning, and keeping himself under the restraint of the rules of propriety (*li*), may thus likewise not overstep [the boundary] of what is right" (Analects VI, 25). The Taoists attacked the Confucianists for the importance they attached to rituals, ceremonies, and rules of etiquette as productive of social conformity and decadent artificiality. But the intent behind the practice of *li* was to develop character along the lines of conventionally accepted styles that made for poise, dignity, and decorum. In the words of the *Hsun-tzu* (third century B.C.E.), "The rules of proper conduct begin with primitive practices, attain refinement, and finally achieve beauty and felicity. When *li* is at its best, man's emotion and sense of beauty are both fully expressed. When *li* is at the next level, either the emotion or the sense of beauty overlaps the other. When *li* is at the lowest level, the emotion reverts to the state of simplicity" (Smart & Hecht, 1982, p. 309). By way of illustration, Confucius held that upon the loss of a parent, one ought to express feelings of sorrow, and the rites of mourning were there to provide dignified forms of mourning. Of course, in the absence of sincere sorrow, the rites would amount to meaningless mumbo jumbo.

A third virtue of the *chun-tzu* is *i* or righteousness. "The superior man holds righteousness (*i*) to be of highest importance" (Analects XVIII, 23). The "just action" in some difficult circumstance is called *i*. Once the facts have been weighed in the balance of *jen*, the decision to act must be carried out because of the "oughtness" of the situation. It functions as a categorical imperative. It demonstrates that Confucian justice goes beyond law and principle to include compassionate wisdom.

Fourth, the *chun-tzu* is a person of "catholicity and neutrality." The superior man is "broadminded, with many interests and wide-ranging abilities" (Analects II, 14; VII, 30). This nonpartisan attitude arises out of his humane concerns for the predicaments of other moral agents. The same *jen* morality causes him to maintain a neutral attitude in the face of novel and abnormal situations. In order to do justice within specific cases, he must remain flexible. Moral actions cannot be directly deduced from moral rules. Confucius said of himself, "I have no course for which I am predetermined, and no course against which I am predetermined" (Analects VIII, 8).

Finally, the *chun-tzu* is a person who harmonizes his words and deeds. He is modest in his speech, but exceeds in his actions. Thus Confucius declared that a *chun-tzu* "acts before he speaks, and afterwards speaks according to his actions" (Analects II, 12; IV, 2; XIV, 29).

Confucius grounded his moral teachings in the obligations that arise out of the family structure. "Filial piety is the root of all virtue and the stem out of which grows all moral teaching. It commences with the service of parents; it proceeds to the service of the ruler; it is completed by the establishment of character." Confucius viewed the state as the extension of the family, wherein the same attitudes toward authority and obedience that were valued in the family were also valued in the state. Thus the family functioned as matrix and model of all relationships and contributed to the value assigned to age. The demands of righteousness (*i*) reach their high point in the principle of reciprocity, which is the Confucian version of the Golden Rule. "Tzu-kung asked, 'Is there one word which can express the essence of right conduct in life?' K'ung replied: 'It is the word *shu*—reciprocity: Do not do to others what you do not want them to do to you'" (Analects, 1982, p. 315). Thus, with reference to the senior members of society, the superior person exhibits the virtue of conscientious altruism (*chung-shu*) by putting himself in their place as he deliberates his own choices, and in making his choices he is guided by the principle of the Golden Mean.

Buddhism

In Buddhism the issues of aging are frontally addressed. This is because the Buddha shifts the locus of reality from the permanent to the impermanent, from substance to process, and from eternity to time. These ideas, along with the ethics to which they give rise, are found in his first sermon delivered to five recluses who had earlier been his spiritual partners.

While yet a youth, Siddhartha began his spiritual odyssey through contemplation. Fearing that these contemplative tendencies might someday lead the prince to espouse the life of renunciation, King Suddhodana arranged for his marriage at the age of sixteen. His father also tried to isolate him from the stark realities of mortal existence, typified by old age. However, these efforts only served to spark the surging curiosity in his young mind. The deep desire to know eventually precipitated his "four visions." Though a young man, through the expansive powers of his heightened sensitivities, he indeed became an old man, a sick man, and even a dead man. He would not allow anyone or any circumstance to isolate him from experiencing life in all of its tragic forms.

The legend of the four visions provides us with a psychologically graphic view of the evolutionary process of Siddhartha's thought. There is a movement from the objective to the personal, from the general to the particular, from the abstract to the concrete, from observation to involvement, from information to responsibility, and from what one has to what one is. The last point is highlighted by the vision of the *bhikku* (holy man), gracious, having no desires, no possessions, looking on young and old with equal eyes. Deeply touched by him, Siddhartha says: "He is a happy man. The learned praise such a man. I would like to be such a man" (*Dhammapada*, 1972, p. 6).

Siddhartha's decision to renounce the life of royalty was a supreme response to the equanimity that the *bhikku* embodied. His search finally led him to the bo tree (tree of wisdom), under which he received his enlightenment. The sum of that experience is found in the Four Noble Truths.

The First Noble Truth is that *dukkha*, translated as suffering or ill, is universal. "Birth is ill, decay is ill, sickness is ill: likewise sorrow and grief, woe, lamentation and despair. To be conjoined with things which we dislike: to be separated from things which we like—that also is ill. Not to get what one wants— that also is ill. In a word, this body, this fivefold mass which is based on grasping—that is ill" (Vinaya, 1982, p. 236).

The First Noble Truth treats the issue of old age as one facet of the larger issue of universal suffering. Two concepts are relevant for us: *anitya* and *anatma*, or impermanence and nonsubstantiality.

The Buddha says, "Whatsoever is an arising thing, all that is a ceasing thing." Suffering arises from the fact that everything is impermanent and in a process of becoming. The youth of the present generation become the elders of the next generation. All things are bound to the wheel of change and decay.

Since everything is impermanent, there can be no permanent soul (*atman*).

Humans are embodied collections of five *skandhas* or components. When these components disintegrate in death, it marks the end of that particular configuration of *skandhas*, and no permanent *atman* or soul carries on. What continues after death is a person's karma, which is the sum of all the good and bad results of his previous existence. This karma takes on embodied existence and lives on as another individual. The Buddha's mission was to free individuals from bondage to the wheel of continued existence.

The Second Noble Truth states that everything happens according to a causal principle. *Dukkha* in human existence is consequent upon some cause, and when that cause is removed, the effect ceases. Passion, desire, and emotional involvement with things all combine as the cause of suffering and of rebirth. People crave (*tanha*) for all manner of things, based on the hope of permanent existence, here or in the hereafter. What gives this "thirst" its karmic force is its function as a mental volition.

The Third Noble Truth is about the extinction of thirst. "It is the utter passionless cessation of, the giving up, the forsaking, the release from, the absence of longing for this craving" (The First Sermon, 1982, p. 236). This is to say that Buddhism is not ultimately a pessimistic philosophy in respect to aging or any other facet of suffering. Evil is man made; hence it is eradicable. The solution to the problem of life is in identifying and removing the cause, namely, "thirst."

When the veils of ignorance and attachment are removed, and the craving for permanent satisfaction, existence, and individuality is shed, the person becomes an Enlightened One. Enlightenment is not annihilation of the self, but annihilation of the illusion of the self. The person who sheds that illusion enters the state of "Thusness," which Buddhists call nirvana, a state that surpasses human description.

The Fourth Noble Truth is about the practice that leads to the ceasing of ill. It enshrines the Noble Eightfold Path. It incorporates ethical conduct (*sila*), mental discipline (*samadhi*), and wisdom (*panna*). For this study, ethical conduct is important. *Sila* embraces the conception of universal compassion for all creatures, human and nonhuman, and is based on our common creaturely condition. "All tremble at weapons; all fear death. Comparing others with oneself, one should not slay, nor cause to slay" (*Dhammapada*, 1972, p. 129). This calls for empathy in all our relationships, as did Siddhartha in his vision of the old man, which set him on his spiritual quest. That quest culminated in the creation of a religion that is essentially a mind culture. "We are what we think, having become what we thought." The primacy accorded to wisdom in Buddhism ultimately relativizes all issues of age. "Though one may live a hundred years with no true insight and self-control, yet better, indeed, is a life of one day for a man who meditates in wisdom" (*Dhammapada*, 1972, p. 106).

Hinduism

Hindu views on aging were formalized in classical times with the development of the institution of *ashramadharma*, the ethical organization for the individual. Shrinivas Tilak describes the Hindu view as a compromise on the part of the Dharma Shastra writers such as Manu (100 B.C.E.–100 C.E.) between the Vedic desire for a healthy, happy, and long life and the otherworldly ethics and aspirations of Upanishadic and Buddhist seers (Tilak, 1989).

The new ideal that emerged through the positive integration of the elements of *pravritti* (this worldly life) and *nivritti* (renunciation) was the Hindu view of the stages of life (*ashrama*). The humanistic significance of this scheme lies in its attention to the psychological and moral dynamics of human existence. It starts with the presupposition that the individual is a complex organism, having four basic needs that naturally arise within the course of the human life cycle. The *Kamasutra* (400 C.E.) urges their acquisition in a timely manner: "Man, the period of whose life is one hundred years, should practice Dharma, Artha, and Kama at different times and in such a manner that they may harmonize, and not clash in any way. He should acquire learning in his childhood; and in his youth and middle age he should attend to Artha and Kama; and in his old age he should perform Dharma, and thus seek to gain Moksha, that is release from further transmigration" (*Kamasutra*, 1963, p. 5). There is a clear correspondence here between age and the acquisition of capacities that arise with time.

In addition to the four *purusharthas* or values of life, the *ashrama* scheme presupposes the individual's sense of certain social obligations, formalized in the ethical concept of the "Three Debts" (*rinas*). Before a person qualifies for *moksha* (liberation), he must pay off vital obligations incurred as a member of the human family. There is the debt to the *rsis (rsi-rina)*, who have served as the revealers of truth contained in the Vedas. This is repaid by passing through the *brahmacharya-ashrama*, in which the Vedas are studied according to the prescribed rules (*vidhivat*). Then there is the debt to the ancestors (*pitri-rina*). This is repaid by passing through the *garhasthya ashrama*. The householder procreates many sons in accordance with *dharma* and thereby ensures the perpetuation of his own family and that of the human race (S. C. Crawford, 1982). The third debt is to the deities (*deva-rina*). It is reciprocated by performing the sacrificial duties of the *vanaprasthya ashrama* according to one's ability (*shaktitah*).

Ashramadharma has several elements of gerontological significance. First, the *ashrama* scheme supplies an age-specific structure through which all of the variegated forms of human needs (*purusharthas*) are actualized in a timely manner. For instance, the student must not indulge in sexual pleasures, but must submit to rigorous discipline, not because sex is bad, but because at the student stage the growing child must first learn the meanings of responsibility and self-control. Once he becomes a householder, the young man is encouraged to give full expression to his sexual desires through procreation. In addition, the householder is to pursue the delights of wealth within the bounds of moral law. Thus there is no denial of the claims of the flesh, so long as the body feels the need for senate satisfaction. With age, changes in the body diminish the intensity of the needs of the flesh and set the stage for hungers that transcend the body. All hungers are therefore valid and are deserving of equal respect, and the mark of a full life is the extent to which a person has allowed a capacity to flourish when its time has come. Each time is the best time, because it uniquely demarcates a different slice of life—life that is new, even as it grows old.

Second, this holistic view of the person, which recognizes a congeries of human needs that are brought to fruition on successive levels of maturation, has a moral correlate that states that a person is *right* for a particular stage when he is *ripe* for that stage. Here ethics is seen as being connected not only with philosophy and theology, but also with biology and psychology. This cautions against the sort of moralistic reasoning that passes judgments on the wants and wishes of the elderly and that is long on philosophy and theology, but short on psychology and biology. The principle of ripeness should also help us understand some of the sudden decisions that old folks make, especially the decision that it is time "to go." It is not that they are overcome by some suicidal urge; they are tuned in to an internal clock. To thwart the individual's decision at this point could mean that conventional ideas of "rightness" have blinded us to nature's rules of "ripeness."

Third, virtue, wealth, and pleasure function as principles of conduct and are regulated by age, in addition to caste and gender. These principles function both on the horizontal and vertical levels. In the first instance, they uphold communitarian concerns and are expressed in terms of a network of mutuality. A strong sense of mutual obligation is reinforced by the doctrine of the three *rinas* and is solemnly practiced through each succeeding age. The vertical level is reached when life in this world loses its charm and the individual seeks freedom from the cycles of birth and rebirth. Negatively, *moksha* is deliverance from the sufferings of old age and the limitations of finite being; positively, it is becoming a perfect spirit like the Supreme Being.

Thus the aged person is seen as active to the end, with *moksha* functioning as the culminating principle of human action. Often the last two stages of life are described as states of "disengagement," presumably because communitarian ties are cut off (Tilak, 1989). But this image of the recluse in retirement is false. It overlooks the fact that disengagement on the horizontal level is only the means to reengagement on the vertical level. Life's most difficult tasks, requiring all of one's reserves of body, mind, and spirit, are reserved for the end. This conjures up a strenuous and optimistic image of old age.

This image proceeds from the fundamental Hindu principle of the progressive realization of the spirit, a principle that vivifies all of *ashramadharma*. The model of the stages of life is therefore to be commended for its faith in human dignity and capacity, even of the aged.

Contrary to the moral systems that claim to be realistic, believing in the depravity of man, *ashramadharma* assumes that given the proper nurture, every person has the inner ability to meet all debts and duties to nature, God, and humanity and to advance through progressive nonattachment to states of spiritual freedom. Theology aside, the elimination of notions of retirement from *ashramadharma* should, on the secular level, make us reconsider the values we uncritically place upon retirement. Retirement could be one way we shorten life. The Hindu tradition says that the only true retirement is that of the ego. Outside that, rest is for the dead.

CONCLUSION

Our review highlights the fact that the issues of aging are fundamentally religious realities that must not be medicalized or reduced to objects of biology. Each religion speaks to our humanity in its own distinctive voice, shedding light on how we must care, cure, and cope with our mortality. On the one hand, there is profound trust in the goodness of God; on the other hand, there is acceptance of nature's laws. Therefore, what counts is not longevity but quality of life. To have this sense of spiritual creativity is the great happiness and the premier proof of being alive.

4

Ethical Issues in Spiritual Care

Patricia Suggs

It is by facing the terrors of one's own old age, by launching out on the final night-sea journey, that a person finds the courage and insight to be profoundly wise for others in elderhood.
—Bianchi, 1982, p. 188

As we enter into old age, we are facing a future of opportunities, but also one of challenges. The advantage for older adults in dealing with these opportunities and challenges is that they have a wealth of experience behind them. With maturity and a healthy perspective, the adverse as well as the prosperous conditions can be confronted.

An aspect of an individual's life that is often neglected or ignored completely is that of the spiritual realm. In all realms of life, but especially the ethical, spirituality is at the core of a person's being and therefore very much a part of decision making and lifestyle. In this chapter, we will give a definition of spirituality and examine its place in the older adult's life and the part it does, or should, play in making major ethical life decisions.

THE SPIRITUAL DIMENSION

The spiritual core can be considered the deepest center of the person. Here the person is open to the transcendent dimension; and it is here where he or she experiences ultimate reality. *Spirituality* is composed of those attitudes, beliefs, and practices that enable us to reach out toward that part of reality that is transcendent. According to L. A. Burton (1992), there are basic assumptions with regard to spirituality: (1) Tillich calls it "the existential awareness of non-being." Spirituality is grounded in history where life events are being experienced and interpreted. (2) Human beings seek interpersonal connection and at the same time seek safety in and from that connection. Everyone is a self-in-relation. This relation may appear different to different people and finds its expression in different ways, including solitude. Whatever or whoever is construed as the Ultimate will be a part of this relation. The role of family history of belief, community, and cultural patterns of belief must be acknowledged as having a part in this relational development. (3) Spirituality is experienced and expressed in the context of physical structure, social class, ethnicity, gender, age, and sexual orientation. Each offers possibility and limitation. Each is a potential source of creativity as well as a reminder of personal finitude. Embodiment (and its potential limitations) is a primary context for the development and expression of spirituality. Spirituality represents our essence. All aspects of our lives make up our spiritual being. Thus, as we age, our spirituality takes on different dimensions.

According to Blazer (1991), there are distinct dimensions of spirituality and aging. These include the following:

1. Self-determined wisdom: knowledge of the larger system in which one lives.
2. Self-transcendence: crossing a boundary beyond the self.
3. Meaning: the meaning of aging, of living to an age when we gradually lose physical and mental capacities. Answers for this meaning are individual. Spirituality often provides the framework within which the elders evaluate.
4. Acceptance: accepting the totality of life, of one's only life cycle and of the people who have become significant to it. Upon reflection, there is no room for ifs. This is very often a spiritual task.
5. Revival of spirituality: one of the pleasures of aging is relaxation of defenses, freeing individuals for new tasks. The wisest of the aged are advocates for the aged. Hope tends to accompany advocacy; it is the hope that is experienced not only in providing a better life for oneself but providing better treatment for older persons in general.
6. Exit from existence: one of the developmental tasks is exit from existence. Death is a part of life and must be accepted as such in order for a person to be at peace with himself or herself and his or her world.

Spirituality is not limited to any one tradition. All religions have their spiritual aspects. These "spiritualities" directly influence the way aging is looked at and defined. In the Islamic view of aging and death, for example, the followers are very realistic about the human condition. There is no sentimentality or evasion. Old age is like a window through which we glimpse the reality of our situation. The Islamic vision has hope and faith, not just loss and disintegration. Faith is a fulfillment of intelligence, with death seen as a return to the origin. Old age and death bring to light what is the basic human situation at all times: complete dependency upon God and his mercy. Aging and death are but "signs" of the divine order of the cosmos. Old age, or the last stage of life, is seen as a period of religious maturity and personal transcendence (Lapidus, 1978; Moody, 1990). In a similar vein, Christian spirituality concerns and embraces the whole life. The inward person is not the only aspect of the person considered; the body is also important. Christian spirituality includes in its scope both humanity and nature.

As we look at our own society, there is real evidence that spiritual issues are becoming more and more important. Born between 1946 and 1964, baby boomers have already shaped American culture in many ways that have been documented in the popular media. One effect is the transforming of America's religious landscape (Roof, 1994). This generation is genuinely seeking a transforming, unifying vision of life as a spiritual journey. Of the group studied by Roof (1994), 80% believe in God or a higher power, but want to make direct contact without commitment to religious orthodoxies and institutions. The majority seem to prefer turning inward in solitary meditation instead of engaging in public worship. Roof calls what they have an open, exploring approach to religion; they seek knowledge and experience of the spiritual realm of existence through many different religious and spiritual traditions. Younger generations can profoundly affect older generations. Many older adults (in informal surveys) are showing interest in explorations of personal simplicity. According to Roof (1994), the "children of the sixties" know that religion, even with all of its institutional limitations, holds a vision of life's unity and meaningfulness. Therefore, it will continue to have a place in their life story.

Books can be and have been written about spirituality in the various cultures. This chapter will be grounded in the Western tradition and will utilize the following definition:

> Spirituality is the acceptance of life in relationship with one's God, self, community, and the environment. It can be demonstrated through the desire to be at peace with one's self or a higher being; or by simply listening to music, reading, praying, and searching for the meaning and purpose of life. (Fahey, 1994, p. 1)

MIND/BODY DUALITY

"There is a fundamental human conflict that intensifies as one grows older: the tension between infinite dreams, wishes, ideas, and hopes on the one hand, and limited, vulnerable, fleeting physical existence on the other." Some celebrate the spirituality of the human body; others emphasize the embodiment of the human spirit; and still others articulate visions of transcendence (Cole & Winkler, 1994, p. 325).

With regard to the mind/body duality, W. F. May (1983) has identified two distinct camps: (1) There are those who see life as sacred. Death is synonymous with evil. The resulting belief is that one should save a life as long as possible. Conflict can arise within those with this belief. For example, how does one ever accept death, which is a very natural part of our existence? (2) There are those who see suffering as synonymous with evil. Quality is valued over quantity. The resulting belief here is that one does not prolong suffering any longer than is necessary. How many years a person lives is not the critical factor.

Ethical decisions will be critically different, depending upon the belief system to which the individual gives her or his loyalty. Certain questions naturally arise: Will these differences be allowed in the future, for example, with managed care and scarce resources? Should they be? What part will or should spirituality play?

IMPACT OF THE SPIRITUAL REALM ON THE WELL-BEING OF OLDER ADULTS

> Nobody grows old by living a number of years.
> People grow old from lack of purpose.
> Years wrinkle the skin.
> Lack of purpose wrinkles the soul.
>
> —Author unknown

How we evaluate our lives with their successes and/or failures depends upon the meanings we attach to them. This is much more a spiritual process than a physical one. In a broader sense, spiritual becoming in elderhood consists of a "lifelong growth in creativity and wisdom" (Bianchi, 1982, p. 190).

"They know that in God's creative and sustaining love for each of them, they *are* much more than they do, for what they do is necessarily limited by time and space, while who they are is rooted in the infinity of God's unique love for each of them" (Magee, 1988, p. 78). From a spiritual perspective, losses experienced in the aging years have no bearing on the older adult's self-worth. One's basic view of aging (the meaning of growing older and the proper approach to it) is not a medical, scientific matter, as is often portrayed in this country. Rather, it is a philosophical/theological question—a question of value and therefore of ethics (Sapp, 1995). Our human worth does not derive from what we do but from who we are. Harry Moody (1994, p. 2) captures the situation of many older adults well when he states, "Are we not struggling with a persistent illusion that crops up again and again on every spiritual path: the illusion that I must go somewhere else, that I must go beyond my present condition, must become, somehow, other than myself?"

During the "sabbath" stage of life, spirituality provides refreshment, inspiration, renewal, and growth, moving the aging and elderly into an ever-deeper experience of wholeness, peace, and spiritual well-being or "shalom." "Far beyond the psychological subjectivism of mere 'feelings of well-being,' it involves peace with God, others, and oneself" (Moberg, 1990, p. 19).

Spiritual well-being is a significant source of psychological well-being, both a meliorating and therapeutic force in physical and mental health. "Spiritual wellness is the search to create a personal sense of life's meaning, value, and purpose in relation to the process of spiritual connectedness with family, community, society, and the world'' (Seicol, 1997, p. 4). While we come to depend upon these connections to the community for support as we grow older, it is also important to remember that our aging in and of itself does not allow us to relinquish our responsibilities to other individuals and/or to the community. Older adults have an ethical obligation to plan for their aging, hopefully minimizing the burden on those who will assume responsibility (Sapp, 1995).

Spiritual maturity cannot be attained in isolation. It is an ongoing process of relational interdependence between God, self, and others, not merely independence or dependence. No one can be fulfilled or whole except as a person-in-community. The community can help persons "harvest" their past experiences and put them into perspective. Even the negative aspects of one's life, for example, burdens and losses, can become the means for quality aging and spiritual gain. Spirituality demands community. A sense of belonging is one of the most powerful forces in human experience. This need touches and strengthens our basic humanity. According to J. P. Gilbert (1986), there is power in belonging in the sense we have of who we are because we belong. It is belonging where we find the strength to be creative and resourceful. Persons belong to organizations and groups, formal and informal, because they want to belong (J. P. Gilbert, 1986).

But for a person to become stronger in his or her spirituality, he or she must have times of solitude. God always addresses us in our individuality. Faith is found in the values we affirm in our politics, in the activities we participate in, in our spending patterns, and in everything we consider important (J. P. Gilbert, 1986). As we age, we take more time to look inward and discover our true identity and our purpose in life.

I finally came to the place where my tendency to "look in" was replaced by the desire to "look out." Growing older with physical hurt has not been easy.... There have been times when I resented this affliction ... but with the help of family, friends, and doctors, and the unexpected kindness of children and strangers, I have come to accept it; and I have learned much from the experience.... I deeply cherish the lives that have nurtured me: my parents and husband, our children and their spouses, our grandchildren, relatives, and teachers; co-workers, students, and strangers.... All of these have helped me to affirm my faith, strengthen my hope, and motivate my love. (McCulloh, 1990, p. 2)

SPIRITUAL NEEDS OF OLDER ADULTS VERSUS YOUNGER ADULTS

Each developmental stage presents us with unique opportunities and challenges. As children, we are, for the most part, taken care of by adults. Our basic survival needs are met in addition to our need for love and nurture. As we enter into adolescence, we begin to formulate our own belief systems and attempt to separate ourselves from our parents or guardians. Young adulthood has us pursuing our dreams, entering our career paths, and marrying and having children. When middle age approaches, we are confronted with some physical problems, maybe for the first time in our lives. Our careers are in full swing, or we decide to change career paths. We are caring for our children, and some of us are even caring for our elderly parents. Life may become complicated. We begin to anticipate our own mortality. As we enter into our elder years, we may need to address the negative stereotypes of aging and physical disabilities, and we are more certain than ever of the reality of our mortality. As we age physically and mentally, we also need to develop spiritually. In the words of an older woman (93 years of age): "When I was five years old, I had and needed a simplistic faith. I could not handle anything else; however, now at age 93 that simplistic faith will not do. My needs are very different." This raises an important point: our spiritual needs must grow and develop as we grow and develop.

In our older years, we have the experience and time to focus on our inner beings. We can evaluate the direction our lives have taken and change our paths if necessary. Evelyn Butler McCulloh states this well when she says: "As my physical orbit has become smaller, my spiritual life has expanded in depth, quality, and meaning" (McCulloh, 1990, p. 5).

In the second half of life, persons experience role transformations, the loss of friends and loved ones, physical change and decline, and other inevitable outcomes of the aging process. These experiences often oblige older adults to reorder their priorities. This reordering is more likely to occur in the older years because by this time persons have grown cognitively and emotionally. This growth helps them think abstractly, tolerate ambiguity and paradox, experience emotional flexibility, and commit themselves to a value system that is bigger than the conventional one (Labouvie-Vief, DeVoe, & Bulka, 1989). All changes, particularly the losses, produce opportunities for the deepening and widening of spiritual integration in the second half of life.

A perspective that has proven to be effective as we define the developmental stage of aging is contextualism (McFadden & Gerl, 1990). This perspective emphasizes plasticity or the potential for change. Suffering can bring one face-to-face with meaninglessness, but out of suffering, one can also emerge reintegrated with a renewed sense of spirituality. Aging individuals can actively choose to enhance their own spiritual development. Aging alone does not automatically confer integration within the self or with others. This potential for plasticity means that interventions can occur and enhance spiritual development even in very late life.

As we grow older, we seem to become more interested in issues related to the meaning of life and all of its mysteries. This happens regardless of our belief or faith system. As we participate in this process, we review our own lives. We engage in reminiscence. Victor Frankl (1992, p. 7) put it this way: "Only under the threat and pressure of death does it make sense to do what we can and should, right now. That is, to make proper use of the moment's offer of a meaning to fulfill—be it a deed to do, or work to create, anything to enjoy, or a period of inescapable suffering to go through with courage and dignity.'' Betty Friedan, in her book *The Fountain of Age* (1993), claimed that it took her years to put the missing pieces together, to confront her own age. But she moves now into the future with comfort, instead of being stuck in the past. She has taken account of her gains and losses, her failures and successes, and made them a part of her now: She claims she is herself at this age.

THE DISABLED OLDER ADULT

Aging does bring with it decline, to a greater or lesser degree depending upon the person. But even in this state the Scriptures tell us that we are not alone. "Even to your old age and gray hairs I am he, I am he who will sustain you. I have made you and I will carry you. I will sustain you and I will rescue you" (Isa. 46:4). This Scripture gives the gift of hope. The Scriptures also give a basis for value that is independent of productivity. Feeling valued by God can give a person enough self-esteem to be able to reach out to others, despite his or her own limitations.

In his article on religion and health, H. G. Koenig (1995) relates how the Scriptures address the topics of suffering, disability, and sickness (for example in James, Job, and the Psalms). There are those passages that state that suffering is an important means by which to refine one's character. Although these are often debated, it is common knowledge that suffering can have a positive effect on one's life. If life were always smooth and easy, we would have little motivation to search for God. It is when life puts up barriers that we have to reassess our view of the world and our own priorities. A strong spirituality can enable even the most disabled adult to perform great ministries by supplying him or her with a purpose and a meaning to his or her existence. No medicine could accomplish this.

According to Fahey (1994), older adults can cope with and change their view of their own circumstances through spirituality. An example he gives is of an older adult who suffers from a disability. This person may experience a perceived or real loss of love, esteem, and value by others because he or she cannot fully contribute to situations or relationships. Spirituality, or establishing a loving relationship with one's God, knowing that one is valued by a supreme being, can help one develop a sense of self-worth. This helps the older adult focus more on being supportive to others and less on his or her own situation.

SPIRITUALITY AND END-OF-LIFE DECISIONS

As we explore the ethical issues in the spiritual care of the older adult, we must take a look at more than the elderly and their needs. We must look at the system in which they will find themselves. For example, the biggest system in which the older adult will find herself or himself is that of health care. Older adults find themselves immersed in a system that is all too often confusing and misleading. The values of the older adult and the values of the practitioner do not always coincide. As we age, our attitudes about death and dying begin to take on new form.

In Bianchi's book *Aging as a Spiritual Journey*, he quotes Albert Outler: "None of us like the shadow or the pain that surround death but death is part of the natural, God-established cycle of things. To overcome death through science, as some 'immoralist' writers project, smacks to him of 'hubris,' that Greek sense of pride by which humans inflate their egos in destructive ways" (Bianchi, 1982, p. 250). Outler concludes with a statement of confidence in God's providence, but rather gently accompanies our journeying, luring us toward good from beginning to end:

To overcome death? No. This seems to me to be hubris, for death is a natural and inevitable thing. It seems to be in some important sense a constructive part of the whole experience of existence. I'm scared in the sense that I don't like pain, and it upsets me mightily to have things and my family upset. If there were any assurance that I would die with my boots on, or go out quietly with peace at last, then it seems to me that death is neither friend or foe, but simply God's way of bringing to be and passing on into whatever is provided by his providence. (Bianchi, 1982, p. 250)

Changes in values, expectations, and capabilities of aging patients raise ethical issues in geriatric care (H. Koenig et al., 1992). The values and practices of medical practitioners provide an additional impetus for ethical issues. The conflicts between paternalism and the autonomy of the patient represent complex issues of control. When more importance is given to cost containment than to individual patient benefit without the patient's awareness, the physician's advocacy role for the patient's well-being is undermined. Patient trust in the profession is threatened.

"Care for the elderly can impose upon the physician unusual demands and high moral obligations" (Pearlman et al., 1993, p. 398). High technology has blurred the distinction between life and death. Quality of care is another ethical concern in geriatric medicine. Good care often requires a comprehensive, interdisciplinary approach. However, acute care continues to receive a higher priority than long-term care (Pearlman, 1994). Cost-containment strategies, competitive interests, and consumerist behaviors are thrust upon providers and patients before policies guaranteeing a just rationing of resources can be generated. A careful process of reasoning is often the most effective means of resolving cases and ascertaining the best thing to do. Barriers that can interfere with this method are time constraints and a lack of cultural understanding of risks to the patient.

The major barrier, however, to effective and efficient care of the older adult is communication. Studies have shown that physicians are both less aggressive and less comprehensive with older patients (Wetle, 1987). Physicians often overemphasize the contribution of health to overall quality of life and underestimate the importance of not only material concerns, such as finances, but also social concerns, such as relationships, and spiritual concerns. Physicians need to shape their interactions with their patients to the patients' values and goals.

"As matters of both legal and medical professional responsibility, the primary obligation for ensuring morally justified processes of decision making lies with the physician. He/She must provide complete and realistic information regarding prognosis and the potential benefits and risks with various therapeutic options, especially those involving withholding or withdrawing therapy" (Pearlman, 1994, p. 402). Withholding or withdrawing life-sustaining therapies is one of the most troublesome ethical issues in geriatric care. Physicians may inadvertently override the wishes of their patients. It is essential that a competent and informed patient be allowed to determine whether or not life-sustaining therapy will be undertaken. If there is a lack of evidence as to the person's wishes, then surrogates must try to protect the patient's best interests.

The medical profession unfortunately defines itself by the effort to prolong life at any cost. Instead, it should respond to the patient's requests to cease and desist in the medical struggle when the patient has no more strength to fight and cannot serve his or her health (May, 1983). At the same time, neither physicians nor society ought to prize quality of life so highly that they solve the problem of suffering by eliminating the sufferer.

The role of the health care provider is sometimes cure, occasionally relief, and always comfort (May, 1983). The spiritual beliefs of the patient should always be respected and considered as care plans are written and decisions are made. Any procedure should be evaluated in terms of whether it offers optimal care or merely maximal treatment. Full efforts to keep a patient alive may actually neglect the patient, overlooking the patient's real needs or wants. This type of negligence treats the dying as if they are going to get well or might get well.

With more and more control by third-party payers regarding health care decisions, the nature of real choices made can be distorted. For example, bias may be shown toward elaborate technology or life-prolonging attitudes and not necessarily toward support for patient decision making. Free communication and deliberations about choices become difficult, if not impossible. "The natural weaknesses of age are compounded by the structural dependency of old age" (Moody, 1992, p. 39).

A demand for self-determination and autonomy in geriatric health care fights all forms of domination. However, according to Moody (1992), autonomy is not the whole answer. Open and free communication about the various ethical dilemmas in which persons find themselves can help us state and deal more honestly with the real problems we face. For this process (which Moody, drawing from the perspective of Jürgen Habermas, calls "communicative ethics") to be effective, it must be based on discussion among persons who respect the position(s) of others in the communication process itself.

Many proponents of euthanasia doubt the patient's ability to cope once terminal pain and suffering have appeared. Their view is that life has peaked somewhere in the past, and all ahead slopes downward toward oblivion. However, this does not take into account the fact that even if a person is terminal, quality of life can and should still occur. A person's deepest relationship with God and/or family may actually occur during his or her final stages of life. Preempting a life too soon may take away a person's opportunity to come to terms with his or her life as he or she has lived it, thus enabling him or her to leave this life in a peaceful, tranquil state.

RESPONSIBILITY OF THE INDIVIDUAL

When we talk about ethics and the rights of individuals, we must not fail to discuss the individual's responsibility. It is the patient's responsibility to inform others of his or her decisions. A living will provides an excellent way of doing this. It allows individuals to state a preference for no heroic measures. However, because it is uncertain whether or not health professionals must carry out the terms of the living will, some states have enacted natural-death acts. The only patients truly covered are those on the edge of death. To help those who may have to endure a prolonged death, some states have established a durable power of attorney for health care.

Advance directives can serve as an educational device to stimulate discussion about lifesaving treatments. Patients must be competent, and documents must assure that professionals following their directives are not later subject to criminal liability. Certain questions of administration must be addressed: What are the time restraints on these documents? How may they be initiated? How are decisions arrived at when some third party contests the document?

The most effective way to assure that patient choice is supported is advocacy. When decisions are being made, caregivers should act as advocates and honor the wishes of the patient. The advocate pleads the cause of the patient. He or she supports the patient's decision and calls for its hearing in the health care system. Various groups have identified themselves as patient advocates (self-help groups, friends, and several health groups, e.g., social workers, nurses, and hospital ethics committees). If the patient's choice is to be carried out, advocates must recognize the person within the patient. They must keep uppermost the inherent dignity of the individual, seeing the person within the context of caring.

Because of the diversity of belief systems in our society, regulations and laws must be made to protect us from ourselves. In any society there are those who push laws to the extreme. The ethics of death and dying presents special problems: there will be those who are dying and want to die naturally, but family and/or friends along with the health providers will not allow this to happen; and there will be those who are not necessarily terminal but are very ill, and someone may make the decision to engage in euthanasia. It is imperative that persons make their decisions without being manipulated or unduly influenced in any way. These distinctions are often difficult, if not impossible, for the physician to make. That is why it is essential that older adults really know their physicians and let the physicians know their desires and needs. It is common knowledge that when this relationship is intact, all parties can have their needs met.

POWER OF DECISION MAKING

The individual makes the decision when he or she is cognitively intact. The family, guardian, or agent designated by a durable power of attorney for health care makes the decision when the individual is not cognitively intact. If the family is not in agreement, medical staff will do what is least likely to result in a malpractice suit. If no family and/or friends exist to aid in the decision, the medical profession's views will have precedence.

Decisions when the patient has cognitive problems (such as dementia) are often extremely difficult to make. The possible scenarios are too numerous to mention here, but the following is an excellent example of one such scenario that could begin to occur more and more as the number of persons with Alzheimer's disease continues to increase:

Margo, when fully competent, had executed a formal document directing that if she developed Alzheimer's disease, she did not want treatment for any other serious life-threatening diseases she might contract. She even stated that if she contracted such a disease, she should be killed as soon and as painlessly as possible. A resident who was taking a gerontology elective began visiting Margo every day and learned about her life with dementia. She appeared happy, active in her painting, reading, and listening to music. According to the resident, "Margo is undeniably one of the happiest people I have known."

Ronald Dworkin offers a new way to interpret disagreements over abortion and euthanasia. According to Dworkin, Margo executed her formal document when she was fully competent. He believes that she should be granted her prior wishes, despite the value she appears to obtain from her present life with dementia. Dworkin believes that our lives are guided by two kinds of interests: (1) experiential interests, those we share with all creatures; and (2) critical interests, hopes and aims that lend genuine meaning and coherence to our lives (Dresser, 1995). Those with dementia cannot express their interests; they cannot articulate their hopes and aims. Thus Dworkin's view effectively leaves out cognitively impaired persons.

D. Callahan (1995) agrees with a position that states that the "self" continues to exist even in a demented state. It is possible that we may find acceptance of a life we earlier thought unacceptable. He proposed three contextual and background considerations: (1) No one should live longer in the advanced stages of dementia than he or she would have in a pretechnological era; (2) the likely deterioration in a late-stage demented patient should lead to a shift in the usual standard of treatment, that of stopping rather than continuing treatment; and (3) there is as great an obligation to prevent a lingering, painful, or degrading death as there is to promote health and life. However, there are a few major problems with decisions to terminate treatment. These are how and when to use available technology that could sustain the life of a patient; how and when to turn upside down the traditional standard that when in doubt, treatment should be provided; and how to determine when to invoke the duty of the physician to help the patient avoid a poor death. Many of these decisions can only be made with a clear understanding of the patient's whole self, his or her external and inner self, his or her spiritual dimension. Ethics is much more than politics and economics. Ethics represents our values and goes to the very core of our spiritual being.

The physician must have a quality relationship with the patient and thus be able to discern the wishes of the patient and to act in his or her best interests. If this is not the case, the physician should talk with someone who can give an assessment of that person. In addition to family and friends, this very often is the patient's pastor and/or spiritual mentor. This person is often privy to the most intimate thoughts of his or her parishioners, some that not even family members know. His or her perspective can be extremely helpful in these times. When no other family member or close friend is available, the physician should speak with the clergy person or spiritual mentor, when one exists, in order to make the appropriate decision. The task for the professional is to demonstrate caring and vicarious decision making, not to deliver candid instruction (May, 1983).

The impact of this type of care, holistic care, is an individual issue. What is quality to one is not quality to another. However, it can be assumed that persons whose whole being is taken into account in their medical regimen will feel more satisfied with their care.

Durnbaugh (1988) offers the following paradigm for managing our choices in health care:

1. Know yourself. Healthful living and stress reduction decrease need for medical care. Know the medical problems of your parents. Become self-caring; take control of your health while you are healthy.

2. Know your health resources. The primary health resource is your physician. Select wisely based on your health history. For example, if you have a history of heart disease, find a physician with special skills in treating that problem. Ask your physician for information on drugs, treatment alternatives, second opinions, and use of consultants. Health professionals have personal and professional guidelines of conduct based on professional codes of ethics. Beyond the code is a sense of personal commitment to the patient. Relationship at this level leads to a sense of loyalty and mutual trust, or a covenant.

3. Know your legal rights in the health care system. Legal issues are malpractice, incompetence, and negligence. The law is concerned with conduct and good of com-

munity. Ethics deals with individual good, involves matters of conscience, and is concerned with motive and attitudes. Various health professionals are concerned with patients' rights. The Patient's Bill of Rights is one group's attempt to increase patients' awareness of their rights in the health care system. Knowing your legal rights will go a long way toward protecting your rights in decision making.

I would add a fourth principle: Know what is most important to you spiritually and communicate this to your family, friends, and health care providers.

With regard to the use of ethical principles in decision making, we must continue to ask ourselves several questions (May, 1983): Do older adults respond to these principles differently than other adults? What is their perspective? Do we make decisions differently as we age? Is this appropriate? Should policies reflect this? As we work with older adults and, indeed as we age ourselves, we must strive to find answers to these critical questions.

ISSUES OF EUTHANASIA

A very difficult area to understand and discuss is that of suicide. As May (1983, p. 86) well puts it, "The suicide reminds us of the deeper fault of a medical profession defined exclusively by the fight against death. Its sins are not simply those of excess in battle, a too-fanatical commitment to life at all costs, but also those of defect, a too-limited sense of the way beyond the battle to life and health."

There are a number of writers and philosophers in the Christian era who have defended man's freedom to commit suicide, for example, David Hume (1963) in his *Essay on Suicide*. The arguments that have been used in favor of voluntary positive euthanasia include the following: (1) The life of the suffering person has become useless to his family, society, and himself. A healthy person may not commit suicide because he has many duties he is morally obliged to fulfill toward his family, society, and his own development. The terminally ill have no more duties because they are incapable of carrying them out. (2) One has to choose the lesser evil. The prolongation of useless suffering is a greater evil than procuring immediate death, a death coming anyway within a short time. (3) It is inhuman and unreasonable to keep a terminally ill patient alive when he does not want to live. (4) One who does not believe in God can reasonably conclude that man is the master of his own life; therefore, he can freely choose. (5) Man's freedom to act should not be restricted unless there are convincing arguments that his freedom to act comes into conflict with the rights of others. (6) Voluntary positive euthanasia is an act of kindness toward one's family and society because the terminally ill person chooses not to burden them with his or her prolonged illness, expenses, and all the work of caring for a gravely ill patient. It is better to free scarce medical and financial resources to be employed in curing those who can lead a useful life. (7) Believers hold that God gave us our life, but it does not follow from this that we may not interfere in our lives, because God made us stewards of our lives. It is reasonable to assume that God does not want us to suffer unnecessarily when we can easily terminate our misery.

In the Western tradition, theistic philosophy has opposed direct killing of self either alone or with help from others. The main argument for this position is that God has direct dominion over human life; we are managers of our lives but do not own them; we may not destroy them. We cannot decide our beginning and we cannot decide our end. Although this is valid on the basis of theistic philosophy, it does not convince everybody, possibly not even the believer. The question that persons must answer for themselves is this: What are my spiritual values?

Voluntary passive euthanasia is the refusal of treatment. The right of a competent patient to refuse treatment is generally recognized in Western legal tradition. Is it morally justifiable? We have a moral duty to restore our health to fulfill our duty in life; however, many believe that it is not wrong to refuse treatment that is useless. Is there a natural right to die when our time comes? Rights are derived from natural needs and duties.

One of the practical difficulties of exercising the right to die is the fact that many patients are taken to the hospital in a critical condition that prevents them from revealing their will not to be placed on life-supporting machines. The living will is intended to remedy this situation. Questions that routinely arise around this issue include the following: Is it moral to let an incompetent terminally ill patient die by not starting or by stopping useless treatment? If a terminally ill and mentally competent patient may refuse useless therapy, shouldn't the guardians of a mentally incompetent patient have the same right? Is it morally right in the case of a terminally ill, mentally incompetent patient not to start useless treatment or to stop such therapy by turning off the machine or "pulling the plug"? Who is entitled to make such a decision?

The controversy over euthanasia is about the moral difference between action and inaction, commission and omission. According to sound ethical principles, we are never allowed to perform an act that directly violates the rights of others, but we are not always obliged to perform an act that would save others from injury.

Patients cannot make a well-informed decision about whether or not to refuse treatment unless doctors tell them the truth about their illness. A solid ethical principle is that everyone has a right to the truth unless he or she has forfeited his or her right to it or indicates that he or she does not want to hear the truth, does not want to be informed.

Embedded in all of these positions and arguments is one overarching fact: the terminally ill have spiritual needs that will play an important role in their impending death and when it will or should take place. These needs include a search for meaning in life and death, a sense of forgiveness for oneself and others, a need for love, and a need for hope (Conrad, 1985). For many, their spiritual needs include a trust in a higher power, a sense of connectedness with the world, and a need to live to the fullest (Mudd, 1981).

RECOMMENDATIONS TO IMPROVE POLICY, PRACTICE, AND RESEARCH

No discussion of ethics in our society should occur without taking into account the spiritual needs of the individuals. There needs to be more involvement by religious/faith institutions in wrestling with these issues and in helping with ethical decision-making processes. These institutions must help individuals to develop their spirituality. Above all, it is critical to remember that a person's spirit is his or her essence. Take that away or disregard it, and you have ceased looking at the individual as a person.

Our society is changing at such a fast pace that it is often difficult to stay ahead in areas of policy. However, the whole arena of ethics and health care demands that we do just that. Because of the increasing aging population, major decisions will be made regarding health care and death and dying issues. These decisions will affect all generations. Some direction must be taken.

In D. Callahan's (1987, p. 223) controversial book *Setting Limits*, he made three proposals that in our day and time seem to make sense:

1. Resist the urge of pursuing, with no limits, medical goals that combine the following: beneficiaries are primarily the elderly; indefinite life extension is sought, costs are high, and the population-wide benefits are slight. Instead, we should seek to advance research and health care that focus on quality, not quantity, of life.
2. Those working for the elderly should shift their priorities from "more" toward the development of an integrated perspective on a natural life span, one that knows where the boundaries are.
3. Try to enter a cultural agreement to alter our perception of death as an enemy to fight at all costs and instead accept it as a condition of life to be accepted.

While Callahan's points make sense, caution is needed. There is the implication in Callahan's book that policies can be made for all of the elderly, seeing them as homogeneous and not the heterogeneous population they really are. For example, bypass surgery in a 90-year-old is justified if that 90-year-old is otherwise healthy, active, and could benefit from the surgery. Another 90-year-old may not benefit because of multiple problems that would prohibit an acceptable recovery from the surgery. There should be no policy that states that bypass surgery will be done on no 90-year-olds.

In terms of the individual's responsibility, Callahan claims that a person who cares about his or her society should value more than just medical progress. Each element of progress can bring expenditure of resources. Thus medical progress and increased life expectancy have both good and bad elements.

Stephen Post (1992) takes a somewhat different stance. While he agrees with Callahan's sense of justice, he believes that it has to come from the hearts of those who grow old, and not through public policy. We should not legislate this aspect of morality.

Moody (1992) has a proposal that appears to lend support to Post's view. In his book on ethics and aging, he describes an "ethics of responsibility." This ethic takes seriously a fact of moral life: actions coming out of good intentions can lead to bad results. With a system based on self-determination and social justice, the key is to devise a communicative ethics that takes into account human capacities and deficiencies. When we intervene in the areas of advocacy, empowerment, persuasion, and deciding for others, we are involving practitioners. This requires not only following rules and/or principles, but also prudent judgment. A dependence on the discretion of virtuous practitioners is not enough. We must have principles and ideals in order to prevent opportunism, improvisation, or worse. Human rights are important; however, there are many (e.g., nursing-home residents) who cannot exercise basic human rights. Moody argues for a "communicative ethics" (described earlier in this chapter) that is adequate to meet the challenge of an aging society.

A required virtue for any ethical decision is practical wisdom. Its principles include deliberation, consultation, self-questioning, openness, and respect for others. Bioethics must also look more closely at the material circumstances, for example, power relationships, reimbursement incentives, and the bias of medical technology available. Instead of focusing on abstract rights and isolated individuals, we must look at the social setting in which communication takes place (Moody, 1992). American society is truly a melting pot of cultures. These cultures must be understood in order to communicate effectively with persons concerning their spiritual life and how this impacts on their beliefs and demands for health care. At times there seem to be more questions than answers. Where will we be with regard to managed care? What will advance directives look like? Will we go in the direction ethicists such as Callahan or Moody think we should?

No matter what direction we may find ourselves going in our society, it is vital that we understand the spiritual elements of older adults' lives. Their "being" is far more spiritual than physical. Only a truly holistic approach to the care of the elderly can be ethically sound.

5

Ethical Issues in Medical Care

Anthony Back and Robert Pearlman

Medical care of older persons raises ethical issues because the nature of medical care is being transformed by biomedical technology, spiraling costs, and increasing oversight by third-party payers. An aging population requires more medical care, but over the past 50 years this care has changed from a casual house call to a highly regulated, technological, and expensive system of care delivered mostly in medical clinics. The complexity and invasiveness of sophisticated medical interventions have led many patients to question how much they want life extended if the quality of that life will be compromised. While patients struggle with these decisions, managed-care organizations are strictly controlling costs by limiting the interventions they will cover.

Since its inception, bioethics has championed individual autonomy, using a method of case analysis based on the principles of autonomy, beneficence, and nonmaleficence. More recently, though, ethicists and corporate executives have pointed out that unrestricted medical expenses can work against the public good. The resulting tension between the primacy of personal autonomy and social good is forcing bioethicists to look beyond established principles to professional and social responsibility or to new concepts, such as an ethic of caring. The principles of autonomy, beneficence, and nonmaleficence remain important, but in analyzing individual cases, reduction to principles can sometimes isolate an ethical problem from the cultural and psychological context that clinicians and patients face. Thus in this chapter, we present five cases that raise paradigmatic problems in the care of older persons, and we indicate areas in which principlism is giving way to new types of ethical analysis.

CASE 1

Alan is an 80-year-old man who presented with hemoptysis and was subsequently diagnosed with unresectable non-small-cell lung cancer. He and his physician decide to proceed with palliative radiotherapy with the intent of controlling the hemoptysis. During the second week of radiotherapy, Alan becomes confused. A head computerized tomography shows multiple brain metastases. The physician notes that whole-brain radiotherapy is possible but recommends against it, calling it futile. Alan, who has long been interested in alternative health care remedies, asks his physician to supervise his use of oral shark cartilage.

Clinical Issues
Medical futility
Alternative medical therapies

Ethical Principles
Nonmaleficence, beneficence
Nonmaleficence

Medical Futility

When can a medical treatment be considered medically futile, and what are the implications of determining that a treatment is futile? In certain instances, medical therapies that are efficacious are not beneficial. Although this occasional discrepancy between efficacy and benefit has long been recognized, it has been rediscovered by physicians and patients using medical technology of increasing complexity. New medical technology has made curable diseases that were once hopeless. However, the indiscriminate use of new technology has alienated patients, who fear being kept alive in the condition of vegetables, and physicians, who resent being viewed as technicians pushing buttons on ventilators. The problem is in defining which medical therapies fail to provide benefit in specific clinical contexts. Such therapies are often described as medically futile.

A widely accepted, practical definition of medical futility does not yet exist (Youngner, 1988). In the bioethics literature, futility has been used to describe situations in which a medical therapy has an extremely low chance of providing (1) some physiologic effect (Lantos et al., 1989; Youngner, 1988), (2) prolongation of life, (3) a minimal quality of life (Schneiderman, Jecker, & Jonsen, 1990), or (4) a goal pursued by the patient (Lantos, Miles, Silverstein, & Stocking, 1988). Some definitions of medical futility require agreement by physician and patient; some definitions do not require that the physician even discuss the therapy with the patient. Perhaps the most influential definition of medical futility has been proposed by Schneiderman et al. (1990), because it lays out clinically useful guidelines for determining when a medical therapy fails to provide benefit.

The Schneiderman definition of futility specifies independent quantitative and qualitative criteria. If an intervention is expected to have less than a 1% chance of patient benefit, which must be distinguished from a strictly physiologic effect, the intervention should be considered medically futile. In Alan's case, palliative radiotherapy for brain metastases would not be futile by the quantitative Schneiderman criterion. Alternatively, if an intervention is expected to result in an unacceptable quality of life, the intervention should also be considered medically futile. Because many patients would consider life during and after brain radiotherapy to be acceptable, the qualitative Schneiderman criterion for medically futile intervention also does not cover Alan's radiotherapy.

The significance of judging an intervention to be medically futile is that physicians are no longer obliged to offer that intervention. Schneiderman notes that medical futility determinations are specific to particular therapies and would not apply broadly to medical care. Once an intervention has been determined futile for a particular patient, the physician would not be obliged to consider it further, although the physician has a responsibility to explain to the patient and family why the intervention is futile. Thus futility determinations raise issues of accuracy, accountability, physician respect for patients, and information disclosure, which perhaps explains why some ethicists and physicians remain skeptical that medical futility will help limit medical care appropriately.

The Schneiderman definition of medical futility has been widely debated, and several objections have been raised (D. Callahan, 1991b; Honegger, 1991; Lantos et al., 1989; Truog, Brett, & Frader, 1992; Youngner, 1990). The 1% quantitative standard has been criticized as lacking consensus from the medical community and as clinically inappropriate. Outcome data are not available for many situations in which physicians raise questions of futility, although the quantitative standard lays out a framework for future outcome studies. The qualitative standard is problematic because patients and physicians disagree about how an "unacceptable" quality of life can be defined. Most seriously, critics of the Schneiderman definition object to the withholding of futile treatments as paternalistic and inimical to shared decision making. These critics foresee a potential problem in physicians making unilateral, value-laden decisions, such as the decision made by Alan's physician. One study describing how futility is used in establishing do-not-attempt-resuscitation orders showed that medical residents sometimes make futility determinations inappropriately (Curtis, Park, Krone, & Pearlman, 1995). For instance, qualitative futility was determined without discussing quality of life with communicative patients in one-third of the cases where this type of futility was the basis for an order to withhold cardiopulmonary resuscitation.

In the case here, Alan's physician uses futility in a casual sense that fails to engage the ethical implications of futility determinations. Rather than entering into a discussion about medical futility, Alan and his physician ought to discuss the risks and benefits of radiotherapy for brain metastases. Although Alan's lung cancer is incurable, radiotherapy confers some palliative benefits in both survival and control of symptoms such as confusion. Although some patients in Alan's situation might decide to forgo radiotherapy, that decision ought to rest on medical information about the outcomes of radiotherapy and Alan's personal values and goals.

Futility determinations are often viewed as a conflict between medical authority and patient autonomy. However, discussions about interventions that may be medically futile can often be reframed within an ethic of care. As described by Schneiderman, Faber-Langendoen, and Jecker (1994), an ethic of care would stress end-of-life care designed to emphasize comfort, dignity, and nonabandonment rather than the application of lifesaving treatments. This ethic of care differs from beneficence in stressing a process of care, rather than a treatment outcome, that is based on an ongoing relationship with a medical care provider. Reframing goals of care in this way might allow Alan and his family to separate further intervention from further care and allow Alan to think more clearly about what he would want near the end of his life.

Complementary Medical Therapies

What is the physician's responsibility to a patient who uses alternative or complementary therapies? Only recently have physicians realized how frequently patients use alternative medical therapy (Eisenberg et al., 1993). In one study, almost 50% of cancer patients sought complementary therapy at some point during their illness (Cassileth & Berlyne, 1989; Cassileth, Lusk, Strouse, & Bodenheimer, 1984). The actual practices range from discussion groups to injections of serum to coffee enemas. The reasons that patients pursue these alternatives to allopathic medicine include a distrust of biomedical science, a need for caring that these patients often fail to find from traditionally trained physicians, and a need to believe that a nontoxic cure of a life-threatening illness is possible. Complementary therapies are most prominent when traditional medical treatments, often described as allopathic, are toxic or have limited efficacy.

Ironically, the major difficulty that physicians have in dealing with alternative treatments is the lack of efficacy data. The Office of Technology Assessment (1990) after an extensive review of alternative cancer treatments concluded that most have little scientific data to recommend them. For instance, most alternative practitioners base their claims on anecdotal cases that do not have a diagnosis of cancer established by a biopsy. The patients are not followed systematically. The causes of death, when noted, are not established. This absence of evaluable data is the major reason that complementary therapies have not earned the respect of the medical establishment (McGinnis, 1991).

The sole complementary therapy that is backed by scientific data is the use of discussion groups for metastatic breast cancer (Spiegel, Bloom, Kraemer, & Gottheil, 1989). Spiegel and colleagues demonstrated that survival appeared to be prolonged in patients randomly assigned to peer discussion groups facilitated by a psychiatrist; the paper generated much interest, but these findings have not yet been replicated. While this example is often cited as a foothold for complementary therapies amid the usual allopathic armamentarium, it scarcely begins to address the issues that physicians face in dealing with complementary therapies.

The challenge for physicians is twofold: first, proponents of alternative therapy charge allopathic physicians with holding cultural biases derived from their professional training. For instance, alternative practitioners charge that allopathic physicians overemphasize physical aspects of health and devalue mental and spiritual aspects of health. A second challenge for allopathic physicians is that well-informed patients may prefer alternative forms of care. These challenges can be examined using approaches developed in the bioethics literature. With regard to allopathic biases, we will first examine how a physician's obligation to a patient depends on how both parties conceive the physician-patient relationship. Next, we will examine preferences for complementary therapy as one type of multicultural medical encounter, drawing on an ethical framework that has been proposed for evaluating professional responsibilities for providing care.

A physician's obligation to a patient who seeks complementary therapy depends on how both parties consider the physician-patient relationship. The four models of physician-patient relationships proposed by E. J. Emanuel and L. L. Emanuel (1992) highlight different levels and types of physician obligations.

In the Emanuels' paternalistic model, the physician assumes that the patient shares the same values as the physician and acts to promote the patient's well-being independent of the patient's current preferences. The paternalistic physician is, for purposes of health care, the patient's guardian. Although this physician would probably not have inquired about use of complementary therapy, he or she would be obliged to prevent or discourage the patient from using it. The problem with this approach is that it fails to adequately respect patient autonomy and may, paradoxically, encourage some patients to try complementary therapy.

In the informative model, the physician acts as a source of information and allows the patient to decide what treatments should be given. If a physician were approached by a patient with a request for complementary therapy, the physician would be obliged only to state what he or she knew about the efficacy of the complementary therapy. The physician would not be obliged to make a recommendation, nor would one be expected by the patient. This model fails to acknowledge two aspects of most physician-patient relationships. It assumes that patients have fixed and known values that allow them to make decisions about their treatment, but often patients are uncertain about what they want. A crucial role for the physician is in helping patients figure that out. In criticizing this model, the Emanuels stress the human capacity for "second-order desires," or the capacity to reflect on one's wishes and even revise preferences. This is particularly important for patients with life-threatening illnesses, who often reorder their priorities in life. The other aspect of physician-patient relationships that this model fails to address is the importance of a process of care in discussing treatment alternatives.

In the interpretive model, the physician acknowledges that patient values can be inchoate and conflicting and that an important physician role is to help the patient sort things out. The physician's obligations are to inform the patient, as in the informative model, but further, to bring the patient to a level of self-understanding that will help him or her make good medical decisions. Thus, for a patient who inquires about complementary therapy, a physician would be obliged to help the patient determine why he or she is seeking it. For instance, is the patient seeking complementary therapy because he is depressed about his metastatic colon cancer? Perhaps acknowledgment and treatment of depression would be more useful for this patient than coffee enemas. The physician ought to probe more deeply to better understand the meaning of the patient's request. The major problem here is whether physicians are actually capable of doing this, and there seems a clear danger that physicians will use their own values in making such decisions, which undermines patient autonomy in a pernicious way.

The Emanuels' deliberative model includes the features of the interpretive model and adds a physician obligation to help the patient achieve a type of moral self-development by instructing the patient in good health-related values. In discussing complementary therapy, this model would oblige the physician to discuss the rational basis and scientific justification for medical therapy. This model embodies most of the features patients and physicians value in their relationships. The emphasis on physician values, in particular, makes explicit the basis for specific recommendations. There is no pretense that a scientific recommendation is value free. The problem with the deliberative model is its complexity. This model of physician-patient relationships goes far beyond rules of nonmaleficence, beneficence, and respect for patient autonomy (Beauchamp & Childress, 1994). The deliberative model appeals to a consideration of virtue. Virtue, as used in the context of the physician-patient relationship, would be based on an idealized physician who would act in a virtuous way. A focus on virtue-based ethics, as propounded by Alasdair MacIntyre (1981), would move beyond rules to considerations of an individual physician's integrity and character. However, virtue-based ethics tends to be short on explicit recommendations for paradigmatic cases.

A different approach for a physician asked to provide complementary therapy is to consider it a multicultural interaction. Not all Americans, for example, subscribe to allopathic beliefs about the role of technological interventions in healing. Bioethicists have documented distinct cultural differences in patient preferences for receiving bad news and for exercising personal autonomy. In one large study conducted in Los Angeles, Blackhall and colleagues demonstrated that Korean Americans reported a markedly lower desire to receive news of metastatic cancer, compared to Mexican Americans, black Americans, or European Americans (Blackhall, Murphy, Frank, Michel, & Azen, 1995). In an ethnographic study of Navajo Indians, Carrese and Rhodes (1995) demonstrated that advance care planning, for instance, would constitute a dangerous violation of traditional values. For a Chinese man to request acupuncture may represent simply a traditional ethnic belief rather than distrust of allopathic medicine or a particular physician provider.

A framework for using multicultural experiences as a perspective for an ethical analysis of physician interactions with complementary therapy has been described by Jecker, Carrese, and Pearlman (1995). They describe an approach to multicultural ethical problems that consists of three steps: identifying goals; identifying mutually agreeable strategies; and meeting ethical constraints. The process of identifying goals and strategies could serve as a safeguard for caregivers, requiring them to step back and ask what they are trying to achieve for patients with nonallopathic beliefs about medicine and healing. In caring for a patient like Alan, caregivers will rapidly progress to an examination of their own ethical constraints. At this level of analysis, a physician may refuse to supervise shark cartilage and justify refusal because the practice would violate professional integrity, which requires that the physician act in accordance with his or her own ethical convictions and beliefs. Ultimately, these authors recommend that differences be adjudicated through a procedure that begins with a nonjudgmental stance and that recognizes inequalities of power in the physician-patient relationship. The authors do not specify details of the adjudication procedure, but presumably all parties would be represented, including third-party payers. Further empirical work could define the nature of multicultural problems that patients and physicians encounter, as well as the effect of a process such as the one Jecker, Carrese, and Pearlman describe.

CASE 2

Earl is a 71-year-old man who completed an advance care directive and has developed severe dementia. He no longer recognizes his family, but is comfortable and seems to be content with life in a skilled nursing facility. However, Earl begins to refuse food, and his advance directive states that he would never want to have a feeding tube or any type of artificial nutrition. His physician, citing the advance directive, feels that a feeding tube should be withheld. Earl's wife thinks that he should have a feeding tube. Earl's adult son is torn between the physician's opinion and the wife's.

Clinical Issues	Ethical Principles
Advance care planning	Autonomy, beneficence
Interpreting advance directives	Autonomy

Advance Care Planning

There are different approaches to advance directives. The principal goal of advance care planning is to promote good medical decisions for patients who become mentally incapacitated. Advance care planning is a two-step process. In the first step, persons formulate preferences for future medical care in the event of mental incapacity. These preferences are based on personal values, outcomes of treatments, and quality of life. In the second step, these patient preferences are communicated so that they may serve as an action guide for future caregivers. This communication is the patient's advance directive (Pearlman, Cole, Patrick, Starks, & Cain, 1995).

Advance directives can take many forms: verbal or written, formal or informal, and legally approved or unofficial. The validity of a patient's advance directive is based on thoughtful reflection, authentic preferences, and unambiguous communication. Two general types of advance directive currently exist: instructional directives, which are documents specifying patient preferences in various future situations; and proxy directives, which designate a spokesperson for decision making. Instructional directives, popularly known as living wills, appeared after California's Natural Death Act specified that terminally ill patients could issue directives to their physicians to withhold or withdraw life-sustaining treatment that merely postponed the moment of death. One well-known instructional directive is the medical directive (L. L. Emanuel & E. J. Emanuel, 1989), which includes brief clinical scenarios such as coma, terminal illness, and dementia and asks patients to express their preferences for numerous life-sustaining treatments under each condition. Proxy directives, usually called durable power of attorney for health care, empower a specified decision maker, who may be a family member or nonfamily person. The power of attorney ought to be instructed to use substituted judgment, which is to use the patient's values to make decisions as the patient would have decided for himself or herself. Many current directives contain both instructional portions and appointment of a proxy decision maker.

The theoretical limitations of advance directives are largely consequences of the difficulty in eliciting and understanding patient preferences. Patients may have concerns about expressing their preferences for future medical care. Some patients think that advance directives represent techniques to limit health care expenditures, especially if they have been economically disenfranchised; others decline to complete directives because of fear that the directive will later be misinterpreted (Lynn, 1991). In addition, the preferences that a patient expressed in a directive may not be relevant to the future situation, as in the case of Earl. It is legitimate to question whether Earl's previous preferences should outweigh the positive aspects of his current quality of life, despite his cognitive impairment. Using the standard of best interests, one could argue that Earl ought to have a feeding tube because he did not predict accurately his future condition (Dresser, 1994).

Although patients may also change the content of their advance directives, this does not invalidate the process of advance care planning. The process of thinking through advance care may help patients and caregivers understand important values and goals. In addition, the preferences that patients indicate in advance care planning are stable over time. However, the possibility that a patient may change his or her preferences can lead to legitimate questions about the accuracy of an existing directive. If a patient has changed his or her preferences without also changing his or her directive, that patient may be overtreated or undertreated. Thus advance directives ought to be reviewed and updated with every significant change in health status or social situation, prior to discharge from a health care facility, and during outpatient follow-up.

Logistical questions about when an advance directive should be implemented may occur when a patient is at risk for transient mental incapacity. For instance, if a patient has lost mental capacity in the setting of a nonemergent acute illness, such as a urinary-tract infection, it may be medically prudent to evaluate the etiology and treat the confusion rather than simply declare the patient incapacitated and invoke the advance directive. This issue may benefit from the development of practice guidelines for evaluating mental incapacity that could maximize respect for patient self-determination when timely medical decision making may be important for patient well-being.

Finally, advance directives may be ignored by caregivers. In a prospective study performed in one nursing home, care was inconsistent with an existing directive in about 25% of the outcomes, which included hospitalization or death in the nursing home (Danis et al., 1991). These findings suggest that decisions occur during end-of-life care that place priority on considerations other than patient autonomy.

Earl's case, though, represents an instance in which an advance directive warrants reevaluation. Based on the principle of beneficence, it is ethically acceptable for his family and physician to agree that his current quality of life may take precedence over autonomous statements that Earl made in the past because they are not directly relevant to his current condition.

Interpreting Advance Directives

Patients and health care providers often formulate advance directives using colloquial terms that can be interpreted variably. For instance, a patient may state that she "would not want to live like a vegetable." While the physician may assume that living like a vegetable refers to coma, the patient can be simply describing a condition in which she is unable to work. The variability in patient interpretation of common remarks, such as living like a vegetable, requires further delineation.

Often caregivers are faced with statements in a living will that may not pertain to the situation at hand. For example, many living wills only specify treatment withholding or withdrawal if a terminal diagnosis is present, so that this type of advance directive would be irrelevant in a nonterminal situation. Another problem arises when patients express their preferences using simplified value statements, such as "I want all treatment as long as there is hope." Hope is a subjective, affective state that may have little to do with clinical outcomes for possible medical interventions, and the relationship between hope and prognosis is nonlinear. Patients may assume that the living will can take care of any situation; however, a narrow interpretation of the advance directive could result in a treatment plan that fails to take clinical realities into account. Conversely, physicians may assume that they should extrapolate from a patient's wishes as stated in the living will, which would undermine the patient's decision-making authority. In a study of dialysis patients, there was wide variation in the amount of leeway that patients wished caregivers to use in interpreting their advance directives (Sehgal et al., 1992).

Empirical research suggests that physicians more often take too much leeway in interpreting advance directives. Even those physicians who engage in advance care planning discussions do not always understand what their patients would want under circumstances of mental incapacity. Thus physicians may project their values for medical care onto patients (Schneiderman, Kaplan, Pearlman, & Teetzel, 1993). Similarly, limited understanding may exist between patients and proxies, as demonstrated by poor concordance of preferences (Uhlmann, Pearlman, & Cain, 1988). These problems do not invalidate the idea of advance care planning, but simply underscore barriers to implementation that currently exist. This type of planning is more complex than it initially appears.

Because of the problems in eliciting patient preferences and interpreting written advance directives, research has focused on facilitating the deliberative process of advance care planning and improving communication about directives. For instance, many people seem to want an advance directive to avoid receiving life-sustaining treatment in circumstances they consider to be "worse than death" (Pearlman et al., 1993). States worse than death may include severe dementia, permanent coma, or long-term mechanical ventilation, and discussions about these states could be a core element in advance care planning. Further barriers to be addressed in advance care planning include patient and caregiver reluctance to talk about death and dying, limited clinician training in discussing advance care planning, differing cultural meanings around advance care planning, and limited time available for discussion.

Earl's case illustrates the importance of clear communication and shared understanding in advance care planning. It may be helpful for Earl's physician to ask the son to think about how Earl would have decided for himself, using Earl's values. More specifically, it may be helpful to ask Earl what aspect of living with dementia he found unacceptable. Fear of being a burden might not provide as compelling a justification for a family with ready economic means to provide care, whereas a fear of loss of personhood might need to be evaluated with respect to changes in cognitive ability that have occurred. In Earl's case, it is worth questioning whether his previous statements, made without knowing his future life, should take priority over his current quality of life. If Earl's family does not know what he would have wanted, the principle of autonomy may not be relevant, and some ethicists would then argue that a comfortable but demented patient might reasonably have parts of his or her advance care plans reinterpreted by caregivers (Dresser, 1994). Although Earl's wife, as the designated proxy, is legally authorized to make a decision, family dynamics and social roles can make this authority difficult to exercise, and an ethics committee may be helpful in facilitating timely decision making.

CASE 3

Denise, a 70-year-old woman with non-small-cell lung cancer widely metastatic to bone, asks her physician for a medication she could use to hasten her death. She has a long history of depression, although she is not currently taking an antidepressant. Although her pain is well controlled with oral morphine, she recently refused radiotherapy to a painful lesion in a weight-bearing area of the pelvis. Her husband is shocked at this request.

Clinical Issues	Ethical Principles
Evaluating decisional capacity	Autonomy
Physician-assisted death	Beneficence, nonmaleficence

Determination of Decision-making Capacity

How should a physician determine whether a patient is decisionally incapacitated? Decision-making capacity is a central determinant of a person's ability to exercise his or her autonomy and direct his or her care. Respect for the right of competent adults to choose what is done to their persons is a well-established principle of American medicine. Moreover, autonomy requires that "individuals critically assess their own values . . . and then be free to initiate action to realize their values" (Emanuel & Emanuel, 1992). When decision-making capacity is compromised, a patient loses the opportunity to fully engage in informed consent for medical treatments or advance care planning.

Decisional incapacity is of particular interest in geriatric medicine for several reasons. Older persons have an increased prevalence of delirium associated with intercurrent medical problems. Age is associated with increasing rates of dementia. Many patients lose decisional capacity in the final stages of dying. Finally, many older patients are inappropriately judged as being mentally incapacitated.

Decision-making capacity differs from competence. Decisional incapacity is a clinical determination, whereas mental incompetence is a judicial one. Clinically, decision-making capacity refers to the ability of an individual to demonstrate to a health care provider that he or she understands the nature and consequences of a specific health care decision. Legal incompetence refers to tests of decision-making capacity specified by law, which are sometimes administered by mental health professionals. Thus no simple boundary exists between clinical decisional capacity and legal incompetence.

The questions facing a health care provider are the following: (1) What circumstances or clinical data should suggest an evaluation of decisional capacity? (2) What criteria should be employed to judge a patient's decisional capacity? The clues that should trigger an evaluation of decisional capacity include problems with cognition or functional status, psychological states that affect reasoning such as depression, appearance of unreasonable choices often involving high burden or low benefit, or a shift in long-standing values or preferences.

The appropriate criteria for the determination of decisional incapacity continue to be debated. Three types of criteria have been used: when a patient is unable to understand the reasons for treatment, including the nature of the treatment and its risks and benefits; when a patient is unable to understand the existence and implications of a choice between treatments; and when a patient fails to exhibit reasoning consistent with his or her values. The latter criteria reflect a linear, rational orientation to decision making that may not always work in clinical practice. For instance, patients who are disinclined to explain their reasoning or values might be judged by this standard to be mentally incapacitated.

A commonsense approach to assessing mental incapacity considers the relative burdens and benefits of the medical treatment under consideration. With medical interventions that provide large benefits with few side effects, it seems reasonable to accept a low standard of decisional capacity. For example, provision of antibiotics for a bacterial pneumonia is a straightforward choice for many patients with decisional capacity. Refusal of antibiotics ought to prompt an exploration of patient understanding and reasoning. With medical therapies that have less clear benefits and high burdens, it seems reasonable to require a high standard of decisional capacity. In addition, a patient decision to forgo one medical therapy does not imply that the patient would forgo all therapies. Denise's physician should not interpret her decision to forgo palliative radiotherapy as meaning that she would refuse other therapies aimed at pain control; her decision may have been based not on therapeutic nihilism but on other factors such as personal experience with a friend or logistical problems in getting to the radiotherapy facility.

Evaluation of Denise's request for physician-assisted suicide entails an evaluation of decisional capacity, which might include psychological assessment for depression, a social assessment of secondary factors that could underlie this request, and a medical assessment of alternations in cognition caused by illness. In Denise's case, it would be crucial for a physician to address this assessment before making a decision to provide a prescription for physician-assisted suicide.

Physician-assisted Dying

Should patients be allowed to have a physician-assisted death? The debate over physician-assisted death could be described more accurately as a debate over assisted suicide. The term *assisted suicide* is used to refer to situations in which a physician provides a patient with a means of committing suicide, such as a prescription for barbiturates (Humphry, 1991), which the patient uses independently. Assisted suicide differs from voluntary euthanasia in that the patient must be physically capable of suicide; the physician does not administer the means of death (Battin, 1992). The term *euthanasia* generally refers to situations in which a physician provides medication intended to cause death, often intravenously, at the request of the patient.

Four types of philosophical arguments are used in debates over physician-assisted dying; the first three were categorized by Fins and Bacchetta (1995). Deontological arguments are often religious, especially Judeo-Christian, and promote sanctity of life and an individual's relation to God in rejecting physician-assisted death.

Another deontological argument, presented as secular even though it has roots in Judeo-Christian belief, is that humans are stewards and not absolute masters of life, and even suffering may have meaning as an experience that reflects man's place in the cosmos. Brock (1992), however, uses a different type of deontological argument, based on a principled respect for autonomy, to argue that a competent individual can waive his or her right to life.

Consequential arguments are the second type of philosophical position invoked in ethical analyses of physician-assisted dying. These consequential positions generally predict the impact of legislation or policy on patients, physicians, and family members. For instance, F. G. Miller et al. (1994) contend that legalization would divert resources away from optimal palliative care for patients near the end of life. Others raise the concern that a layer of regulation spread over end-of-life care would promote expediency while undermining compassion and intimacy. Numerous ethicists have noted risks for frail, disabled, and poor members of society. Some consequential arguments split assisted suicide and euthanasia because of the balance of risks and benefits to society; because assisted suicide requires a patient to self-administer a medication, for instance, the potential for unwanted or involuntary euthanasia is reduced, and error, coercion, and abuse seem less likely.

Clinical pragmatism represents an empirically based approach to physician-assisted dying. This type of approach analyzes clinical details of actual cases to negotiate between ethical theory and clinical practice. Foley (1991), for instance, cites research suggesting that a relationship exists between inadequate pain relief and requests for physician-assisted suicide. Miles (1994) explores the psychological dimension of the doctor-patient relationship in these situations. Most of the empirical data have come from the Netherlands (van der Maas, van Delden, Pijnenborg, & Looman, 1991) and are difficult to extrapolate to the United States because of differences in access to health care and patient relationships with primary-care providers. However, our empirical study of physician behaviors in Washington State indicated that patient requests for physician-assisted death are not rare, and that physicians often perceive nonphysical concerns underlying these requests (Back, Wallace, Starks, & Pearlman, 1996). Thus clinical pragmatism brings a dimension of clinical experience to bear on the debate and highlights the need to assure adequate evaluation and palliative care for these patients.

Finally, there are virtue-based approaches, as in the F. G. Miller et al. (1994) analysis of professional integrity and physician-assisted death. They view as inadequate arguments about the ethical appropriateness of physician-assisted death that are based solely on respect for the principles of respect for autonomy and beneficence, and argue that the internal values of medicine must also be met. They contend that physician-assisted death could only be justified if professional integrity is not violated. Recognizing that professional integrity does not encompass the whole of bioethics, they nonetheless view integrity as a crucial goal for physicians.

Denise's case raises issues for each type of argument. At the level of clinical care for an individual, caregivers would be prudent to use a clinical approach such as that described by Block and Billings (1994) to explore her reasons for requesting physician-assisted death, to assure adequate palliative care, and to address psychological issues. Caregivers and patients may then need to explicitly discuss deontological issues that place personal beliefs squarely in the provider-patient relationship. The difficulty may be in having explicit discussions about a practice that is currently illegal in most places. Physicians will probably continue to deliberate in silence and occasionally act on the basis of professional conscience. If Denise persists in her desire for physician-assisted death, she may turn to a patient advocacy group. Like other issues in which public and professional opinions are polarized, such as abortion, the ethics of physician-assisted death may be overtaken by its politics.

CASE 4

Frances, a 67-year-old woman, is evaluated by her primary-care physician for a breast mass. Her physician decides not to refer her for a biopsy, but to reexamine her in two months. The physician works for a preferred-provider organization that uses monthly productivity reports specifically detailing the number of subspecialty referrals. If a physician makes too many subspecialty referrals, his income will be affected and eventually he could be dropped from the list of preferred providers. As a contractual obligation, the physician has agreed not to inform his patients, including Frances, of this arrangement.

Clinical Issues	**Ethical Principles**
Managed-care practices	Justice, beneficence
Analyzing institutional structures and policies	Justice

Managed-Care Practices

How does managed care affect the physician-patient relationship? Managed health care plans have quickly become major players in medical care because they appear to control the cost of medical care. In order to contain costs, managed-care organizations use a variety of techniques that affect both subscribers and physicians, and these techniques alter the physician-patient relationship in ways that ethicists are just beginning to understand. The physician-patient relationship that ethicists have traditionally analyzed has usually been idealized in that patients and physicians both were assumed to have unlimited choices and few restrictions based on cost. In a managed-care relationship, however, both physicians and patients have restricted choices, and the purpose of these restrictions is cost control.

Perhaps the most problematic ethical issues arise from the techniques that managed-care organizations use to direct physician behavior (American Medical Association Council on Ethical and Judicial Affairs, 1995; Miles & Koepp, 1996). By using financial incentives to encourage physicians to make cost-conscious decisions, managed care creates loyalty conflicts for physicians. In one type of loyalty conflict, managed-care organizations may encourage physicians to view expensive tests or interventions as a limited resource within the plan. Consequently, physicians managing a panel of patients may be expected to balance the interest of one of their patients against the interests of their other patients in order to preserve the economic interests of the plan. In another type of loyalty conflict, physicians must balance their own financial interests against the interests of their patients. For instance, a physician who orders tests not approved by the plan may have his salary bonus withheld. Consequently, an unlucky physician with a panel of patients who are sicker than average may feel pressure to inappropriately limit care, a practice sometimes called bedside rationing. In addition, managed-care organizations sometimes explicitly prohibit physicians from disclosing the type of incentives the organization is using or medical therapies that may be available outside the managed-care plan. These so-called gag rules encourage physicians to shift their primary responsibility from the patient to the organization. Thus a physician no longer acts solely as patient advocate: he or she is also accountable to the health organization, which may include shareholders, or to peers within the organization. Specific examples in which medical care has been limited inappropriately have been widely reported in the media, but systematic effects on patient care have been difficult to document.

For Frances's physician to explain that her breast mass simply requires observation is inappropriate and misleading. If Frances delayed her follow-up, not realizing the gravity of her situation, diagnosis of an early-stage breast cancer could be delayed, and her chance for curative therapy could be lost. This sort of phenomenon would be impossible to detect within most current medical information systems; increased mortality from breast cancer might never be detected among health-plan enrollees.

Managed care is not inherently evil, but in examining its effects on the physician-patient relationship, the effects of cost control need to be weighed against patient advocacy using a broad set of outcome measures that should include cost and quality (Loewy, 1996; Sorum, 1996). These analyses will start with individual cases but will likely conclude at the level of institutional policy.

Addressing Institutional Structures and Policies

Analyses of managed care have led some ethicists to conclude that bioethics ought to be oriented toward institutional structures rather than individual cases. The first generation of guidelines for managed-care organizations tends to address role responsibilities within the organization. For example, in order to preserve the physician's role as patient advocate and discourage physicians from bedside rationing, allocation decisions should be made at a policy level within organizations. These allocation decisions ought to be visible to potential patients who are considering a contract with that organization. Patients and physicians should be actively involved in the development of policy, and either physician or patient ought to be empowered to initiate a challenge when a particular test or intervention is denied. Financial incentives meant to encourage physicians to limit care should be designed to minimize their effect on individual treatment decisions.

Some ethicists feel that early identification of potential conflicts may enable institutions to minimize conflicts of interest faced by caregivers. Emanuel (1995) has commented on six structures that could potentially counter conflicts of interest: (1) professionalism, (2) disclosure, (3) competition, (4) prospective review of financial incentives, (5) prospective review of guidelines, and (6) mediation and appeals procedures. Whether this preventive approach could be effective may depend on the authority accorded to ethicists within health care institutions. Justice considerations may not be a high priority within institutions struggling to maintain market share and economic viability. An alternative approach is for ethicists to bring issues to the forefront of public debate, in what Zoloth-Dorfman and Rubin (1996) call a "medical commons." In their view, the medical common good may be protected by a vigorous public press, individual moral agency, legislative regulation, and collective civil discourse. This approach depends less on authority but more on the media, which may not be inclined to provide much analysis of complicated issues such as health care.

In other words, a complete ethical analysis of Frances's case ought to go beyond what her physician said in the exam room to the institutional structure of her managed-care organization. This type of problem does not represent a classic type of ethical dilemma that results from the conflict of two different ethical principles. At the individual case level, there is the issue of the physician's failure to disclose the seriousness of Frances's breast mass. Frances's physician faced a situation in which his interests competed with his patient's interests. In resolving this situation, a professional ethic that outlines standards of professional behavior may be more likely to encourage creative solutions than an approach that insists on balancing principles. At the institutional level, the issues concern the structure of physician incentives and the quality of care for specific clinical syndromes such as workup of a breast mass. Here ethicists can influence public discourse by articulating standards for comparison, as in the proposal by Showstack, Lurie, Leatherman, Fisher, and Inui (1996) for a socially responsible managed-care system.

CASE 5

Zelda is a 68-year-old woman in good health. However, she is worried about developing dementia because her mother died of Alzheimer's. Her physician refers her to a university research unit that evaluates the family pedigree and suggests initial genetic linkage studies. The researchers explain that their work may or may not result in a predictive result for Zelda and her family, and that a predictive DNA test may or may not be available. However, Zelda's daughter is extremely alarmed because of the costs of long-term care and because of her own potential risk, and she contacts a commercial lab advertising a DNA test for early Alzheimer's disease.

Clinical Issues
Presymptomatic genetic screening
Intergenerational responsibility

Ethical Principles
Beneficence, nonmaleficence
Justice

Presymptomatic Genetic Screening

Zelda has not been diagnosed with dementia, but her concern that she may carry a genetic susceptibility for dementia is a new type of health issue. The availability of predictive genetic testing has created a new class of patients, those who have a disease susceptibility but not yet the disease. Thus Zelda might be found to have a familial form of Alzheimer's dementia, and as genetic testing improves, presymptomatic screening tests will soon be available. As physicians acquire the ability to give genetic bad news to a patient, ethicists will need to address questions of appropriateness and timing in the disclosure of this type of information (Post, 1994).

Counseling patients about genetic risk will present formidable challenges for caregivers. Patient susceptibility for Alzheimer's dementia can probably be caused by several different genes (Plassman & Breitner, 1996). Not all of the susceptibility genes for Alzheimer's have been identified at this time, and in the near future it is likely that any genetic test result will represent incomplete information about disease susceptibility for an individual patient (ter Meulen, 1996; Weisgraber & Mahley, 1996). Consequently, a patient who has a negative test for apolipoprotein E first needs to be counseled about the technical issues of false negative test results. Then the patient needs to be counseled that a negative genetic test result for dementia does not mean that he or she will never develop dementia. Alzheimer's dementia most often occurs in individuals without a known genetic susceptibility. Thus the negative test result means that the patient carries a standard, or average, risk of dementia. Finally, the patient will need to understand that he or she could still have a familial susceptibility for Alzheimer's based on some other gene. Eventually, a detailed profile of risk may be obtainable from a panel of genetic tests, but for the near future the genetic information available is likely to be fragmentary. The patient education required for a level of understanding adequate for decision making about test results will obviously require substantial health care resources.

Like Huntington's disease, an inherited neurodegenerative disorder, the inexorable course of Alzheimer's dementia cannot be halted by a medical intervention at this time. Thus the initial endpoints for genetic screening programs for this disease will be psychological rather than medical. Research following disclosure of linkage for Huntington's has demonstrated that this type of information can often be disclosed without causing psychological damage or permanent loss in quality of life (Wiggins et al., 1992), but these studies have also shown that individual reactions to risk information are extremely diverse. For instance, about 15% of individuals at risk for Huntington's who receive test results indicating that they are not at genetic risk experience intense psychological discomfort and require extensive follow-up care. The same diversity of patient reactions is likely to hold true for Alzheimer's. However, identifying the disease-specific concerns requires further study.

Some ethicists question the value of providing disease susceptibility information when no effective therapy exists. Certainly the most powerful reason to provide a patient with information about genetic disease susceptibility is if an intervention exists to modify that patient's risk. But even in the absence of a disease-modifying intervention, genetic information still enables patients to plan for the future, allay anxiety, and reduce uncertainty. Research with tests for familial breast and ovarian cancer has shown a high level of patient interest, although these initial studies may represent patients with high levels of motivation and understanding.

The handling of genetic information thus creates many potential patient harms. Inadequate education about the meaning of test results may cause inappropriate fear of disease or inattention to health status. Insensitive counseling could result in psychological harm after disclosure of test results. Inadequate quality controls could result in inaccurate tests. Lack of confidentiality about test results could compromise medical insurance coverage. Despite these problems, commercial firms are rushing to offer genetic screening tests because of the huge potential market, although the complexity of the clinical issues suggests that some type of regulation will be necessary to protect patients. The first mass genetic screening program has just begun for a type of familial breast cancer associated with a specific gene mutation in the breast cancer gene BRCA1 in women of Ashkenazi Jewish descent. These programs should provide useful information for screening programs that will need to address a much larger group of patients than have been addressed in the Huntington's experience.

Finally, medical insurance coverage for patients with genetic susceptibility for serious illness has not yet been guaranteed by insurance companies or mandated by the federal government. In the research studies published to date, the genetic information has been recorded only in research charts. How insurance companies and other third-party payers use this information ought to depend on studies of patient outcomes, but the intense public interest in knowing genetic susceptibility—even when no further interventions are available—suggests that the test cases will occur in the near future (Pokorski, 1997). Because resolution of these issues will require institutional policy or legislation, ethicists will need to address the institutions as well as the individuals involved.

At the level of policy, public priorities for genetic services are emerging as a patchwork of disease-specific and state-specific documents. Genetic services have not previously been accorded high priority compared to other health services. However, commercial enterprises are planning to create public demand through consumer marketing, and these will no doubt highlight the new technology in the public mind. Consequently, genetic screening will come up against other priorities in spending for health care. Future public priorities are likely to rest on well-defined, attainable goals, including the accuracy and reliability of the test, the seriousness of the condition, and the availability of an effective intervention.

Intergenerational Issues

The reaction of Zelda's daughter in this case underlines one aspect of the intergenerational issues raised by genetic testing. Clearly, test results for one family member may have clear implications, albeit unintended, for other family members. If Zelda is truly at risk for dementia, Zelda's daughter will face personal and economic burdens that are not directly accounted for by most health economists. If Zelda develops dementia, her daughter will need to devote time, energy, and money toward Zelda's future care in ways that could adversely affect the daughter's own interests. Zelda's daughter's expenditures might be considered part of the true cost of Zelda's future illness, but it is not clear how these expenditures ought to be considered in relation to Zelda's current decision to pursue genetic testing. While many children want to care for their parents, it seems unjust to require Zelda's daughter to suppress her own needs and desires in carrying out Zelda's care. In addition, in our society these burdens fall disproportionately on women, many of whom are elders caring for their very elderly parents. Arras and Dubler (1994) propose that accommodation and mediation of the legitimate interests are the appropriate models for addressing the interpersonal and intergenerational relationships in these settings (see also Collopy, Dubler, & Zuckerman, 1990). They suggest a trial of mediation with the goal of finding a mutually agreeable accommodation and recognize that there are limits to what can be expected of a caregiver.

CONCLUSION

Although this chapter has covered a broad range of ethical issues evolving in the medical care of the aging, these cases illustrate ways in which bioethicists and medical caregivers are critically evaluating ethical problems. The principles of autonomy, beneficence, and nonmaleficence provide initial guidance for ethical analysis; however, empirical data from outcome studies, psychological studies, ethnographic research, and basic science also contribute to ethical decision making. The multifaceted nature of the resulting ethical analyses will not always fit comfortably into a model of ethical decision making based solely on weighing principles. Thus we have tried to indicate ways in which ethicists have looked beyond principles to concepts such as caring, virtue, and even institutional structures. As the costs of medical decisions increase, bioethicists, caregivers, and patients will experience increasing pressure to justify their decisions about medical care. An ethically informed view will be essential to health care providers and policymakers in evaluating these decisions.

6

Ethical Issues in the Quality of Care

Kathy A. Marquis and Bette A. Ide

With the passage of Medicaid and Medicare legislation in the 1960s, quality-assurance systems received a focus of attention in the health care delivery system that had never before existed. Initially, quality-assurance activities were concentrated in hospitals, but they have now expanded into ambulatory care, primary care, long-term-care settings, and community and public health care programs. Even in the present period of debate regarding health care reform, every health care initiative, no matter how diverse, contains explicit commitments to quality care in some form.

In the 1970s, major right-to-die cases such as Quinlan and Saikewicz (*Superintendent of Belchertown State Sch. v. Saikewicz*, 370 N.E. 2nd 417 [Mass. 1977] and *In re Quinlan*, 355 A. 2nd 647 [N.J. 1976]) were decided. Since then, ethical debate and analysis have become commonplace in the health care delivery system, though ethical decision-making systems are not fully integrated into it. While ethics has always been an acknowledged and essential component of professional practice, the impact of medical technology and the sociopolitical evolution since World War II have resulted in an increasing awareness that ethical questions and issues arising in the health care environs extend far beyond a "professional" code of ethics and touch each individual within society and society as a whole. Organ transplantation, the use of fetal tissue for research and treatment, abortion, assisted suicide, genetic manipulation, and health care rationing are just a few of the issues confronting the health care delivery system. What is not always evident is that quality assurance and ethics are irrevocably interrelated and interdependent, conceptually and practically, when they are applied to the health care delivery system. The major purpose of this discussion is to demonstrate (1) the fundamental and indivisible relationship between quality assurance and ethics at both the national and clinical levels and (2) the significance and impact of this relationship upon the health and welfare of the elderly.

Historically, quality-assurance issues and decisions focused primarily upon clinical practice questions and dilemmas arising from individual patient and family interactions and/or upon the quality-assurance systems utilized within various health care institutions and agencies. The prototypic quality-assurance model developed by early leaders such as Donnabedian (1989) addressed three parameters: structure, process, and outcome. The model viewed the health care system as three subsystems consisting of (*a*) the client/patient; (*b*) the provider, which included not only the physician but health care organizations with their respective facilities, procedures, and skills; and (*c*) the environment, which included the social, genetic, physical, and psychological factors impacting health care interactions. In the model, the provider system was identified as the structure; process referred to the interaction of the patient/client with the provider; and outcome focused on what happened to the client as a result of the interaction of the three subsystems.

Initial quality-assurance efforts concentrated upon structure and process. Methods employed to measure structure included (and still include) licensing, credentialing, continuing education, accreditation, and like approaches to assure the continuing qualification of providers. Tools used to measure process include medical-record audits, peer review, and utilization review. Medical malpractice is also viewed by the legal profession as a quality-assurance tool for structure and process because it arguably acts as a deterrent to substandard practice. Today the dominant focus of quality-assurance efforts is outcome, even though systems approaches such as continuous quality improvement and total quality improvement intend to address all three parameters.

The focus upon outcome has, in great part, been stimulated by the continuous exponential increases in health care costs. Health care costs have increased at double-digit rates since the mid-1960s. In 1960, only 5.3% of the gross domestic product (GDP) was spent on health care. By the 1980s, that figure had increased to more than 12%. Projections indicate that by the year 2000, at least 19% of the GDP, more than $1.6 trillion per year, will go to health care. To put that cost into perspective, consider that the average family of four could be spending $30,000 per year for medical care, more than for food, clothing, transportation, and housing combined (Kassler, 1994). Some statistics indicate that we have already reached a level of $1 trillion per year, twice as much as in almost all other comparable nations (Kalb, 1996; Reinhardt, 1994; Sage, Hastings, & Berenson, 1994). Why? As is always true, there is no single answer.

For at least 20 years, much of the public, as well as physicians, hospitals, and insurance companies, has indicted the legal tort system and costly medical malpractice actions. The so-called medical malpractice crisis was precipitated, in this view, by ever-increasing medical liability insurance premiums. The rising premiums were, in turn, caused by outrageous and egregious compensation for injuries resulting from specious claims of negligent medical care. As is so often the case, the truth lies somewhere in between.

As recently as 1991, medical liability costs accounted for only 1% of health care expenditures (Billings et al., 1990; Sage et al., 1994). According to the Harvard Medical Practice Study, a full 1% of all hospital admissions actually do result in injuries caused by negligent medical care. In actuality, only 1 in 8 such incidences give rise to a medical malpractice claim, and of those only 1 in 16 receive any compensation. Unfortunately, of the suits that are filed, only 1 in 6 are based on persuasive evidence of actual negligence (Sage et al., 1994). In other words, there really are cases of injury that are not being compensated, but of the cases that are being compensated, many are not valid. Nonetheless, because of the practice of "defensive medicine," the calls for legal tort reform continue.

Defensive medicine is the performance of tests and procedures that would not otherwise be performed but for the fear of litigation. While it is not possible to accurately measure the cost of defensive medicine, estimates of savings from malpractice reform range between $25 billion and $75 billion in a five-year period (Reinhardt, 1994). Even assuming that these figures are accurate, medical malpractice costs would amount to less than 3% of the overall health care costs per year. Further, the reasons for the use of unnecessary tests and procedures are far more complex than "defensive medicine" alone.

Industry waste and fraud have also received significant attention as major causes of escalating health care costs. The General Accounting Office estimates an annual cost of $80 billion per year, or 10% of health care spending (Sage et al., 1994). But it is medical technology that is the overwhelming trigger of ever-increasing health care costs.

Medical technology accounts for as much as 50% of all health care–sector inflation. At least half of the increased hospital costs is due to an increase in the intensity of medical services that are required by the technological changes (Kalb, 1996). In fact, medical services account for nearly one-third of the rise in all health care costs. In 1992 alone, health care employment figures topped 10 million, an increase of 43% in just four years. That total does not include those working in the insurance, pharmaceutical, or medical equipment and supply industries. In other words, one-seventh of the nation's economy was linked to health care (Kassler, 1994).

But what is most alarming is that the Office of Technology Assessment estimates that less than 20% of all present medical services and procedures have ever been shown to have any positive impact on patient outcomes (Billings et al., 1990; Jost, 1989; Kalb, 1996; Mariner, 1995). The growing recognition and acceptance of this fact, both within and outside the health care delivery system, coupled with the cost issues, have resulted in growing support for the development and use of clinical practice guidelines and outcomes research.

Clinical practice guidelines are defined by the Institute of Medicine as "systematically developed statements to assist practitioner and patient decisions about appropriate health care for specific clinical circumstances'' (National Health Lawyers Association [NHLA], 1995, p. 4). The primary focus of clinical practice guidelines is to enhance the quality, appropriateness, and effectiveness of health care and to facilitate the adoption of treatment approaches that are not only medically effective but also cost efficient (NHLA, 1995). Although clinical practice guidelines have been available to some extent for years, it has only been in the past decade that prestigious medical groups such as the American College of Obstetricians and Gynecologists, the College of Surgeons, and others have both supported them and become intimately involved in their development.

In 1989, the Agency for Health Care Policy and Research (AHCPR) was officially established with the mandate to develop broad-based studies directed toward improving the organization, financing, and delivery of health care. Established within the AHCPR was the Office of the Forum for Quality and Effectiveness in Health Care. Through the forum the AHCPR is responsible for facilitating the development, review, and updating of (1) clinically relevant guidelines to assist the health care provider in the prevention, diagnosis, treatment, and management of clinical conditions and (2) standards of quality, performance measures, and medical review criteria through which health care providers and other appropriate entities are assessed in order to assure the provision of quality health care (NHLA, 1995).

Because the goal of clinical practice guidelines is to promote treatment approaches that have the most effective outcomes, the guidelines are becoming core considerations for many quality-assurance programs in spite of concerns about "cookbook medicine" and the potential for rigid legalization of guidelines as standards of care. Physicians and other health care providers vary significantly in (1) the use of tests to make diagnoses; (2) the choice of treatment or management approaches such as watchful waiting versus medical or surgical intervention; (3) the decision to admit to the hospital; (4) resources available in each setting; and (5) timing of hospital discharge. The reasons for these variances range from simple disagreement to uncertainty as to the best way to proceed (Billings et al., 1990). This marked degree of variance is one reason why clinical practice guidelines and outcomes research will remain essential components of future quality-assurance efforts.

Though the present commitment to clinical practice guidelines and outcomes research is definitely a constructive step in the quest for improved quality of care, it is still but a piece of the quality puzzle. While outcomes research should eventually help in more appropriate use and adoption of medical technology, costly new technology continues to be introduced and adopted with little or no demonstrable evidence of its actual effectiveness. Further, the question of whether a given technology should be developed initially is not even being raised. Even the developing science of technology assessment, which addresses questions of technology efficacy and value, does so only after the technology is on the market, not prior to its development (ten Have, 1995).

Further, while clinical practice guidelines may assist in greater consistency of care, most efforts are directed toward the cure and/or treatment of medical illnesses or diseases, while minimal study is directed toward preventive efforts. The major diseases that confront the health care system today arise from social circumstances and lifestyle choices upon which present medical intervention strategies have little overall impact, at least regarding occurrence. Major chronic illnesses such as coronary artery disease, hypertension, and even some cancers are strongly correlated to lack of exercise, inadequate nutrition, smoking, and alcohol. No less challenging and resistive to medical intervention strategies are the morbidity and mortality associated with illicit drug usage, AIDS, motor-vehicle accidents, domestic violence, homelessness, homicide, suicide, and environmental toxins, known and unknown.

Quality-of-care questions also relate to issues of availability and accessibility. What care shall be provided to whom? Who decides? What can our society afford not only regarding money per se, but also the use and direction of resources? Unfortunately, while there is little disagreement regarding the need for quality in health care, "the debate on how it is to be measured has increased inversely with the decline in resources to support health care in the United States. As those resources have become scarce, conflicts have arisen in the health care system between responsible provision of service to all and the highest quality of care for selected populations" (A. G. Taylor & Haussmann, 1988, p. 84). Integral to this debate, whether it is addressing strictly clinical concerns or resource allocation on a national level, are the implicit and explicit value systems held by individual participants in the health care system and society as a whole. In fact, the very definition of quality is dependent upon, and is and will be derived from, these value systems.

As noted previously, the imperative for health care reform is being driven by a national concern for the exorbitant cost of just maintaining our health care system as it is. Besides the costs already discussed, major expenditures arise from publicly funded health care programs. Medicare and Medicaid cost approximately 15 cents for every tax dollar. Of the money spent on health care, it is estimated that eight times more is spent on those over the age of 65 than on the average citizen (Lamm, 1989). In fact, approximately one-third of the federal budget goes to programs to aid the elderly (Moody, 1992, p. 3). Some estimate that by the year 2050, 20% to 25% of the population will be over the age of 65, and as early as the year 2020, 1.7 million elderly over the age of 65 will eventually enter a skilled nursing facility (SNF) (Murtaugh, Kemper, & Spillman, 1990). Thus the impact of the care of the elderly population upon future health care costs cannot be overestimated. However, this distribution of resources to the elderly should not be viewed simply as a function of an aging society with its associated array of medical problems. It should also be recognized as a symptom of our unfettered advocacy for medical technology.

Consider the following data: Of insured persons, 75% of households accounted for 30% of total health spending, and another 5% for 38%, but 72%

accounted for only 9%. Roughly 6% of households absorb almost 70% of all health care spending. The increase in the degree of concentration of health care spending in fewer and fewer households is due, at least in part, to medicine's increasing willingness and ability to address catastrophic illnesses with bold but very expensive medical interventions whether in the young or old (Reinhardt, 1994, pp. 107–108). In view of these data, there is little doubt that allocation decisions are going to have to be made regarding the continued utilization of resources or technology, which benefits, in reality, fewer and fewer people.

One of the first issues, and perhaps the most fundamental one, to be addressed is whether or how resources will be distributed to the benefit of the individual versus society as a whole or vice versa. A certain tension has always existed between these two perspectives, primarily because of the strongly held ethic in American society respecting individual autonomy. In fact, the very predominance of medical technology is logically consistent with this ethic and the consequent value placed upon the life of each individual. Yet the values of individual autonomy and the sanctity of each life have themselves become antagonists because of the technological ability to maintain physical life even when this is contrary to the autonomous desires of given individuals.

A survey in 1995 reported that 47.8% of physicians were unwilling to withdraw life support from comatose or critically ill patients or remained neutral about it even when such action reflected the wishes of the patient and family (Asch & Christakis, 1995). Other statistics indicate that 40% to 70% of patients do not die until after do-not-resuscitate orders are written. This results not only in prolonged suffering for patient and family, but in expenditures greater than $2.5 billion per year (Mondragon, 1987, p. 441). Even with the U.S. Supreme Court decision in *Cruzan v. Director* (1990), which upheld the validity of refusing life-sustaining treatment, the varying ethical beliefs of providers and patients and continuing concerns regarding liability dominate end-of-life decisions.

Concern on the part of providers regarding the law is somewhat warranted by confusing messages generated recently in a few court decisions involving medical futility cases. For example, in 1991, 85-year-old Helga Wanglie was in a persistent vegetative state, unable to breathe or eat on her own. The family was informed that continued aggressive therapy would be of no medical benefit and should be discontinued. The husband disagreed, and eventually the hospital filed for the appointment of a conservator. The reason for the filing was to have a neutral person appointed so treatment could be stopped. The court appointed the husband and bypassed addressing the real issue in the case (*In re Wanglie*, 1991).

To date, in every known case where a provider has sought court approval for discontinuing treatment that offered no benefit, the courts have found for not discontinuing the treatment (Daar, 1995, p. 223). Though these decisions seem contrary to the intent of cases such as those of Cruzan and Quinlan, the consistency is that the courts are most likely to view all end-of-life decisions first from the apparent perspective of the patient and then the family, but not the provider. Arguably, such questionable ethical and legal decision making by the courts is also generating to some degree increased costs and human suffering. The reality, however, is that these legal cases are few, and providers do make such decisions daily, generally unhampered by legal intervention, with and without patient and family input, under the aegis of medical decision-making prerogatives. It is equally important to note that these decisions are, in effect, resource-allocation or rationing decisions; they are not confined to end-of-life scenarios.

Each day, again with or without full patient and family input, physicians decide who will receive an organ transplant, coronary angiography, end-stage renal dialysis (ESRD), or cardiopulmonary resuscitation. Though it is true that third-party administrators (TPAs) and other designated reimbursement administrators are having increased input into such decisions, the physician remains the primary allocator. Estimates indicate that almost 75% of such decisions are in the hands of the individual physician (Ficarra, 1989, p. 208).

To many, such decision making by physicians is a logical consequence and responsibility because they are the persons with the needed knowledge base to make these very decisions. But studies clearly demonstrate that a significant percentage of so-called medical decisions are based not on medical data, but on idiosyncratic behavior such as geographic location; personal or professional value systems regarding individual autonomy, professional autonomy, or cultural, racial, or gender biases; and/or beliefs or convictions about age or ability to pay. Note the following findings:

1. Since the 1970s the number of cesarean sections (C-sections) performed has increased 5.5% to 22% of all births. While the medical reasons for this are not evident, it has been noted that significantly more C-sections were performed in hospitals with higher malpractice insurance premiums and with larger numbers of malpractice claims filed against the hospital or physicians on staff (Localio, Lawthers, & Bengtson, 1993). Another study found that repeat C-sections were more likely to occur in for-profit hospitals (Stafford, 1991).

2. Some surgeons use management strategies for coronary artery bypass graft (CABG) procedures that impact costs far more than outcomes with no apparent medical rationale (L. R. Smith, et al., 1994).

3. A mother's race, early use of prenatal care, and insurance status may influence the likelihood that her very low birthweight (VLBW) infant will have access to neonatal care (Goldenberg, Bronstein, & Haywood, 1995).

4. Minority preschoolers, blacks and Hispanics, receive lower-quality overall asthma care than white children. While emergency-room treatment and hospital length of stay are essentially equivalent, nonwhites are less likely to be prescribed nebulizers for home use and are less likely to have taken inhaled steroids or cromolyn sodium (Finkelstein, 1995).

5. Coronary angiography and aggressive intervention strategies are employed far more often for men than for women (Gatsonis, Epstein, & McNeil, 1995).

6. When end-stage renal dialysis was originally implemented, few individuals over the age of 65 were considered candidates because of the decreased potential for positive outcomes. Presently over 42% of new ESRD users are the elderly, but without any substantive data that outcome has improved (Moss, 1994). It is also probable that once reimbursement was approved, there was an increased willingness to provide the technology to the elderly.

Another observation frequently made is that widely heralded new technologies that will supposedly save money by decreasing long, costly hospital stays actually increase overall costs. When coronary angioplasty was developed in the 1970s, the incidence of open-heart surgery was to have decreased. Instead, angioplasties increased from 26,000 in 1983 to 227,000 in 1988, and the number of bypasses increased from 191,000 in 1983 to 500,000 in 1993 (Kassler, 1994, p. 9). While the increasing number of aged and repeat surgeries can account for some of this escalation, the fact that internists do angioplasties and surgeons do bypasses is as probable a cause. Simply, each group chooses the approach with which it is most familiar. In any instance, the significant fact is that decisions are being made to a substantive degree based on other factors than objective medical rationales.

Another important consideration in analyzing these situations is that many decisions simply are not medical. If five people of varying ages are all "medically" qualified to receive a heart transplant, the decision concerning who receives it is no longer a medical question. Rather, it becomes a societal issue of how such decisions should be made, and who shall have what kind and amount of input. This question necessarily reflects back to the previously raised issue of the public good versus individual rights.

Richard Lamm noted in his speech "The Brave New World of Health Care" (1989) that "the sum total of all ethical medicine as currently defined is . . . unethical public policy. . . . Doctors consider a patient's health, but a society must consider the total health of its citizens." In other words, society has a responsibility to at least attempt to define or reach consensus on a set of principles or ethical guidelines by which resources can be equitably allocated. One of the major results of such guidelines is that quality-of-care parameters will be more easily defined and very likely significantly redefined from what they are today.

Because of the role that behavior plays in the occurrence of many of today's health problems, it has been suggested that many of these so-called health problems be demedicalized (B. Jennings, 1986). For example, illicit drug use, alcoholism, domestic violence, motor-vehicle accidents, and homicide are ills arising from and impacting upon the whole of society and not just the health care system. Demedicalization is intended to foster a multifaceted and integrated strategy for solving the given problem by utilizing and incorporating other relevant systems such as criminal justice, social rehabilitation, education, and/or employment. If such demedicalization occurred, outcome measurements for health would be established that specifically addressed only those activities and results for which the system could reasonably be responsible. For example, safe detoxification and/or supervised withdrawal for the chemically dependent could be one valid outcome measure.

If national ethical guidelines directed more resources toward the health of society generally, emphasis would be placed upon prevention, or at least mitigation, of commonly occurring sources of health care problems. However, a public health emphasis will frequently impinge, to some degree, upon individual rights. Historically, public health measures have included quarantine, mandated immunizations, and required reporting of certain communicable diseases. More recent examples include seat-belt laws, motorcycle-helmet laws, and prohibition of smoking in public places. Outcome measurements for these interventions should include epidemiologic data of prevalence and morbidity and mortality statistics as well as cost-benefit analysis from a societal perspective. Health care resources would be directed toward the educational programs and enforcement activities required to carry out the selected prevention programs. But two important ethical questions arise. How far do we want to go in regulating individual behavior? Again, whose or what ethical and moral values would dictate what these behaviors should be?

In addition to the redirection of resources toward prevention, decisions from a public perspective also mean answering questions about who gets the resources that are directed toward the well-being of the individual. If a service or procedure is "not clinically indicated," does this mean that the patient will not benefit from it or that limited resources should not be used for this person? Arguably there is no group for whom the answers have greater import than the elderly.

In a 1993 survey conducted by the Wirthlin Group for Mercy Healthcare Arizona, the general public slightly favored health care reform that emphasized the rights of the individual but really indicated a desire to have it all. The public wants quality, cost efficiency, availability, and protection for society as a whole. Physicians and insurers also preferred a system likely to emphasize individual rights, but administrators and ethicists were more likely to favor a system that promoted the good of society as a whole ("Public Professionals," 1993, p. 155).

The public and physicians agreed that it was ethically acceptable to put a cap on health care spending and to consider a patient's age, likelihood of survival, and the cost in deciding whether to withhold or give treatment options. All groups agreed that it was not appropriate to base decisions upon a person's expected contribution to society. Interestingly, none of the groups thought that rationing was appropriate even though both cost and age considerations are arguably rationing precepts. Perhaps it is the public's very perception of quality of health care that provokes this apparent contradiction.

For the past 50 years, quality medical care has been marketed as synonymous with sophisticated medical technology. The concept of rationing may provoke a sense of potential abandonment of these "lifegiving" technologies by passage of broad-stroked legislation. Specifically enumerated and limited allocation actions would thus be more palatable. In any instance, age, whether implicitly or explicitly acknowledged, is going to be, and already is, a primary consideration regarding health care reform nationally and the appropriate utilization of resources clinically.

The cost of care of the elderly is undisputed, as is the probability that these costs can only escalate if the health care system remains unchanged. More and more one reads or hears the growing fears that such costs are robbing our children of their future opportunities at life. Questions are also raised about the legitimacy of providing limited resources to an individual with short–life-span probabilities. But, as Daniel Callahan (1994) observes, there is no assurance that monies saved will be redirected for other health care and thus no reason to exempt any person from any treatment that may be of benefit. In other words, until there is a system that assures that the withholding of benefits for one person will result in an equitable distribution to others, there is no reason to limit anyone.

Related to these concerns are discussions about issues such as the ethics of advance directives, assisted suicide, euthanasia, "benign neglect," "slow codes," and appropriateness of specific treatment decisions in the context of caring for the aged. For example, how valid are advance directives obtained at the point of entry into an acute-care or skilled nursing facility when significant stress is present? If life is valued for itself, can age or functional capacity be valid considerations in end-of-life decisions? If quality of life is the guiding ethical principle, what guidelines and processes should be put in place to protect judgments of quality as defined by the person's culture, religion, or life choices?

Clearly, profound ethical questions and dilemmas exist within the health care delivery system in both national and clinical contexts that actually and potentially affect the health status of each member of society. Clearly, decisions about these dilemmas are being made daily, albeit often by no action or default rather than by thoughtfulness and discourse. Many of the individuals who are affected by these decisions are not aware that they are being made.

Over 20 years ago, Paul Ramsey insightfully predicted the ethical dilemmas underlying the political impasse that today has halted any real health care reform:

If there are moral dilemmas in modern medicine; if, as some would say, there is a moral crisis in the medical profession, this does not result from recent triumphs in medical research or the great promise and grave risks stemming from medical technology. The fundamental reason is the continuing moral crisis in modern culture.... It can no longer be assumed... that we are agreed on moral action guides, the practice of virtue, the premises and principles of the highest, most humane, most bracing ethics, or what a moral agent owes to anyone who bears a human countenance. (1973)

As O'Connell noted more recently, the present health care debate is symptomatic of our culturally diverse society and its increasing polarization of ideologies. "It should be no surprise then that politicians are incapable of crafting legislation on health care reform" (1994, p. 1).

Polarization of ideologies is not only the major obstacle to health care reform nationally, but, as has been noted, is also a significant reason for much of the diversity and inconsistency that exists at the clinical level. As long as the goals of health care remain ill defined both nationally and clinically, quality-of-care decisions will remain subject to health care delivery system nuances and lack of mutuality between providers and patients. The issue now is not whether there will be discussion, but the degree of depth, scope, reflection, and openness and the direction it will take.

7

Ethical Issues in Terminal Care

Dallas M. High

Dramatic advances in life expectancy and health care technology during the twentieth century have had a profound effect on death and dying, including when and where most people die and what constitutes care needs for those who are dying. In this chapter, the changing factors in death and dying are discussed, issues concerning prolonging life and forgoing life-sustaining treatments are confronted, and ethical issues in end-of-life decision making are explored. The chapter addresses the development of advance directives for care planning at the end of life and surrogate decision making for the terminally ill who can no longer make decisions for themselves. The special needs of dying persons are discussed, as well as whether euthanasia and assisted suicide should be legalized as choices for terminally ill patients. Ethical issues in palliative care and the hospice movement are discussed. Finally, seven ethical guidelines of terminal care are presented.

MORTAL ILLS

Within twentieth-century Western culture, comprehensive care of terminally ill persons has emerged as an almost entirely new phenomenon. The reasons for this are several and have given rise to many difficult ethical issues. First, we are living longer. Since the turn of the century, average life expectancy in the United States has increased from 47 years to over 75 years (Gardner & Hudson, 1996). In 1900, over half of all deaths involved persons 14 years of age or younger. Today only 2% of all deaths occur within this age group (Gardner & Hudson, 1996). As a corollary, an increase in the relative size of the older population (persons 65 years of age or over) is clearly evident. Elderly persons comprised 4% of the total population in 1900, 12.6% in 1990, and will be as much as 23% by the year 2050 (U.S. Bureau of the Census, 1989). The report of mortality statistics for 1993 indicates that 73% of all deaths were of persons aged 64 or older.

Second, since the turn of the century, there has been a dramatic shift in the causes of death. In the early part of the century, death was most often the result of short-term infectious, communicable diseases, such as influenza and pneumonia, tuberculosis, typhoid fever, diphtheria, and diseases of infancy. Today most people die from chronic, long-term degenerative diseases, such as diseases of the heart, malignant neoplasms, and cerebrovascular diseases. In 1993, for example, 62.8% of deaths were caused by these three classes of diseases (Gardner & Hudson, 1996).

Taken together, these two factors suggest that more often than not, the dying process will occur later in the life span, and that there is an increased probability for most of us that dying will occur progressively over a lengthy period of time due to long-term degenerative diseases. Indeed, a recent survey of patients receiving hospice care, mainly for malignant neoplasms and heart diseases, reports that the average length of hospice service from admission was over 80 days (National Center for Health Statistics [NCHS], 1996). For most of us, death most likely will not be rapid and sudden. The fact that many more Americans are dying of long-term diseases, experiencing a terminal illness over a long period of time, thrusts our society into the midst of serious ethical issues concerning care for terminally ill persons, care issues that are decidedly different from issues concerning acute care.

Third, it is clear that more and more people are dying in hospitals or other institutions. In 1900, 95% of U.S. citizens died in their homes attended by their families. Today about two-thirds of all deaths occur in hospitals, nursing-home facilities, or other institutions (NCHS, 1985). Often the dying are surrounded by an astonishing array of technological equipment designed to sustain life attended by professional caretakers.

Fourth, striking advances in modern medicine have generated a long line of biomedical technologies intended to prolong life. These life-sustaining technologies have also likely affected attitudes toward death and dying and, most important, have raised a number of difficult and confusing questions: In what situations should certain life-sustaining technologies be used? Do concerns for quality of life place limits on the use of such technologies? Who should decide on the use or refusal of life-sustaining technologies? Do patients have the right to refuse life-sustaining treatments? Who should decide for those who no longer can decide for themselves? The latter two questions also raise the general issue of control over the patient's final days of life. Special attention must be given to the ethics of final days since the dying process in a hospital or institution is removed from the familiar and friendly environs of the home. The final moments of life for many people may occur among strangers as an impersonal event.

PROLONG LIFE OR FORGO LIFE-SUSTAINING TREATMENTS?

The confluence of the factors of greater life expectancy, causes of death precipitating longer periods of disability and dying, and removal of death and dying from the home and the care of families to institutions have produced an unprecedented need to rebuke the unbridled use of life-sustaining technologies. As ethical debate has arisen over the last three decades, two opposing approaches have been used to treat dying patients: either to prolong life or allow patients to die by refusing life-sustaining treatments. A significant reason for the latter was a realization that treatment to prolong life was standard and virtually always utilized and that death was even considered to be the enemy of medicine. Of course, prior to this century, physicians had fewer therapies from which to choose in their efforts to prolong life. As more options became available and technologies, such as respirators and dialysis machines, became widespread, health care professionals, as well as patients and their families, came to face the question of whether some therapies should be used, refused, or limited. A landmark discussion on these issues by the President's Commission for the Study of Ethical Problems in Medicine and Biomedical and Behavioral Research bore the title *Deciding to Forego Life-sustaining Treatment* (1983).

Many essays and books defined the ethical debate in terms of active and passive euthanasia or distinguished killing from allowing to die (Bayles & High, 1978; Ladd, 1979; McCormick, 1974; President's Commission, 1983). Health care professionals and ethicists frequently employed and debated distinctions between acts and omissions that may lead to an early death; between withholding and withdrawing care; between an intended death and one that was merely foreseeable; or between ordinary and extraordinary means. Many health care professionals and ethicists thought that if such distinctions were carefully employed, then most ethical decisions on whether to prolong life or forgo life-sustaining treatment could be made.

It took more than a decade for health care professionals and ethicists to realize that such distinctions did not settle the moral quandaries of caring for terminally ill patients. While such distinctions may have a usefulness, albeit a limited one, what has emerged as more important is the reasoning and ethical deliberation behind the distinctions. For example, the ethics of what should be done in the care of a terminally ill person is not settled by labeling a treatment as extraordinary even if it is presumed that extraordinary treatment can be forgone. More important is the issue of why any treatment labeled extraordinary could be forgone. The highly publicized case of Karen Ann Quinlan, whose death came in 1985 nearly a decade after she was removed from a respirator, following a series of New Jersey court decisions, raised fundamental ethical issues concerning the reasons for actions (*In the Matter of Karen Quinlan*, 1975). Among them, the case caused serious rethinking of what should be done for patients with permanent loss of consciousness and medical responsibility toward those patients who are "hopelessly ill." In 1984 the *New England Journal of Medicine* published a remarkable article authored by ten experienced physicians from various disciplines and institutions on "The Physician's Responsibility toward Hopelessly Ill Patients" (Wanzer et al., 1984). The article not only affirmed the patient's right to refuse life-sustaining treatment, but acknowledged the physician's obligation to advise patients on end-of-life decisions and respect the wishes of patients, whether expressed at the time or by advance directive. The article took stands on providing appropriate care to both competent and incompetent patients. It argued that differences in patients' disabilities and illnesses should be a primary consideration in determining the form and intensity of care to be provided or withheld.

To focus our attention in this chapter on the elderly and their families is especially important since death occurs more at older ages and older people are at greater risk of terminal illnesses and dementing diseases than are younger people. As a result, elderly persons are more likely to become candidates for life-sustaining treatments as well as to face decisions to refuse such treatments. Consequently, decisions to withhold or withdraw life-sustaining treatments directly affect older people more frequently than younger people. Such decisions and other care decisions are likely to come at a time when cognitive impairment is present due either to a terminal illness, unconsciousness, or dementia. When one or more of these impairments occur, consent to or refusal of treatment must be made by someone other than the patient. Prior to the extensive use of life-sustaining technologies, families were typically called upon to make such decisions, or, alternatively, very few end-of-life decisions were made since short-term terminal illnesses left little time for long-term-care planning and decision making.

END-OF-LIFE DECISION MAKING

In recent decades, decision making at the end of life has moved far from the concerns of planning for the distribution of one's estate through a last will and testament, making funeral plans, or putting other financial and property matters in order. End-of-life decision making is more concerned with the attitudes and fears of patients toward the symptoms and conditions that may accompany the dying process, issues of the dignity of life of a dying person, and planning regarding acceptance or refusal of life-sustaining technological treatments. Not only are new technological treatments available that make end-of-life decisions necessary, but inappropriate use of these treatments can make death and dying additionally grievous. Ventilators, resuscitation, antibiotics, and artificial nutrition, for example, can be applied to save lives or can be used to support the remaining days of a life that in a manner that deprives that life of dignity and sufficient quality. Most, if not all, of us want to live out our remaining days as free of pain as possible and to have as high a quality of life as possible. Patients often do not fear death as much as they fear that dying itself will be a horrible, painful experience (Gallup & Newport, 1991; Saunders & Baines, 1989). Recent surveys report that only about 23% of Americans fear death per se. Such fear actually diminishes, rather than increases, with age. Eighty-three percent of persons 50 or older report that they have no fear of death, and over 75% of Americans believe that persons with a terminal disease have an absolute right to request that treatment be withheld so they can die (Gallup & Newport, 1991). When we realize that the time and manner of one's death and dying may be at the hands of medical science, we want to be protected against becoming a victim of the process and exert some control over it. We fear that life-sustaining treatments may merely prolong the dying process rather than life with some acceptable quality. The ethical issues of end-of-life decisions center on the use of various life-sustaining treatments, including medical provision of nutrition and hydration, and the underlying issues about the goals of care of terminally ill persons. The issues concern acceptance or rejection of life-sustaining treatments, including withholding and withdrawing treatments, and when, where, and how terminally ill patients should be cared for palliatively, that is, have care directed at symptom control rather than at treating the primary disease.

It is widely held that a competent patient has a right to make decisions about his or her own medical treatment, including a right to consent to treatment or a right to refuse treatment, generally so long as such refusal does not harm any third party or involve a communicable disease. That right is grounded both in common law, following from the ethical principle of autonomy, and in the constitutionally derived right of privacy. Ideally, that right is exercised when a diagnosis and treatment are evident and clear and the patient has been fully informed and is capable of making a decision. However, most situations, particularly for terminally ill elderly patients, are less than ideal. More often than not, unfortunately, many patients experience their final days like Mrs. D, who was treated aggressively for colon cancer, including a number of experimental therapies that caused her to endure intractable pain from the cancer as well as severe pain and nausea from the therapies. She was unable to make decisions for herself. Only after repeated pleadings from family members and after all medical therapies for life-sustaining efforts had been exhausted was medical attention given to treat Mrs. D's extensive and intense pain with opioid analgesics. She continued to have severe pain and died in pain, an everyday reality in many hospitals when pain is poorly managed or patients are undertreated for pain.

ADVANCE DIRECTIVES: LIVING WILLS AND DURABLE POWERS OF ATTORNEY

Many terminally ill patients will reach a point at which they will no longer be able to make decisions for themselves or their decision-making abilities will become significantly reduced. As a result, either someone else must make crucial end-of-life decisions for these people or at least substantially assist them. Substitute end-of-life decisions may reflect the judgments of physicians and families, who often make decisions to maintain aggressive treatment under the presumption that it is always best to act in favor of sustaining life. The issue then arises of whether a right of refusal of treatment may appropriately be extended to those persons now incapable of making decisions for themselves through a means of advance expression of wishes and direction.

The idea of planning for end-of-life decisions by advance directive first began in the late 1960s. Some patients, concerned that they might be forced to endure life-sustaining technologies that they might not want, wrote letters to their families, physicians, and others to express their wishes. Their wishes to refuse some treatments were often expressed vaguely and imprecisely in general terms about forgoing "heroic" or "extraordinary" means and through pleading to allow a "natural" death (see High, 1978). These informal documents were not intended to be legally binding but morally to exhort their readers to follow the expressed preferences of the writer in the hope of gaining dignity and appropriate care while dying.

In 1976 California passed the Natural Death Act, the first legally binding living-will act. In general, living wills are written documents that provide instructions to health care providers, family members, and others about the kinds of treatments an individual would want or not want to prolong life. A living will is executed while an individual is still capable of making decisions. Now most states have passed laws to sanction living wills, make them legally binding, and provide guidelines for their preparation. However, there are few, if any, assurances that the declarer's wishes will be carried out. Considerable differences currently exist among the state laws concerning the rights and responsibilities granted to patients and health-care practitioners for withholding or withdrawing life-sustaining procedures. Some of the laws limit the kinds of life-sustaining procedures a patient may refuse. For a living will to become effective, most statutes require that the patient must be terminally ill and unable to make health care decisions for himself or herself. Many states require that a patient must be certified by physicians as terminally ill. Some states require a designated form to be used to execute a living will, although frequently the type of form is merely suggested. The laws also require that certain technical procedures be followed in executing a valid living will, such as having the document witnessed and/or notarized. Some states have recently enacted provisions extending living will laws to make available a patient- or surrogate-executed directive to emergency medical services or paramedics regarding a do-not-resuscitate (DNR) order. The directive can inform an emergency medical responder of the patient's wishes not to be resuscitated via a signed and witnessed document or signed bracelet worn by the patient. Practitioners need to be aware of individual living-will legislation in their own states and keep abreast of changing and developing legislation.

As end-of-life decision-making instruments, living wills suffer the drawback of requiring the declarant to anticipate future health care circumstances and decisions. To anticipate such matters accurately is at best very difficult, if not impossible. Alternatively, if an instruction directive is written in a language general enough to cover a wide range of circumstances, it will likely be vague and ambiguous. If the document is drafted with sufficient specificity, that document will not be able to provide guidance for those circumstances not specifically anticipated. In any event, the instructions provided in a living will usually have to be interpreted by surrogate decision makers and health care practitioners in order to make use of them in withholding or withdrawing life-sustaining procedures.

The second mechanism for planning for end-of-life decisions under the generic category of advance directives is the appointment of a proxy or agent. When a proxy directive is created, an individual names and authorizes another person to make health care decisions for him or her in the event the individual becomes decisionally incapacitated. Again, most states have established statutory instruments for people to appoint proxies. Many have extended their statutes for the durable power of attorney to include health care proxies. A durable power of attorney can be designated to have authority to act as a proxy only when the principal becomes decisionally incapacitated. This is known as a springing durable power of attorney. Some states have preferred to establish separate laws for designating a proxy rather than extending the provisions of appointments of durable powers of attorney to include health care decisions. In whatever form, the majority of states empower a designated proxy to make a wide range of health care decisions, not just for those who are terminally ill.

One advantage the proxy-designation instrument has over the instruction directive is that the proxy can have knowledge of the contemporaneous medical circumstances when making the decision instead of having to anticipate these circumstances. However, if the proxy is expected to replicate the decision of the patient and decide as the patient would have decided, then anticipatory instructions from the patient will be needed. In instances when the proxy does not know the wishes of the patient, the proxy will have difficulty replicating the patient's own decision and will likely have to act on his or her own in the best interests of the patient.

In an effort to protect individual rights of decision making in health care, especially for end-of-life decisions, and to encourage the public to complete advance directives, in 1990 the U.S. Congress passed what has become known as the Patient Self-Determination Act (Public Law No. 101–508, 1990). Specifically, the federal legislation requires hospitals, nursing homes, home health care agencies, hospice programs, and institutions and agencies that serve Medicare and Medicaid patients to do the following: (1) provide each individual upon admission or enrollment written notice of his or her rights under state law to make decisions concerning medical care, including the right to accept or refuse treatment, and the right to formulate advance directives; (2) provide individual patients with written policy of the institution or agency regarding the implementation of their rights; (3) provide documentation in the patient's medical record on whether the individual has advance directives; (4) ensure that decisions are made freely by prohibiting conditioning medical care on whether the individual has executed an advance directive; (5) ensure compliance with requirements of state law (whether statutory or common law) by respecting advance directives; and (6) provide education for staff and the community regarding advance directives (Public Law No. 101–508, 1990).

By mandating these actions under Medicare Provider Agreements, the legislation does not grant new rights to patients. Rather, it affirms existing rights to accept or refuse treatment within limits provided by law and to execute advance directives as provided by statutory or common law. The impact of this legislation on the issues discussed in this chapter is currently under assessment, and the evidence so far suggests that the legislation is not achieving the ends hoped for by its advocates (Teno, Nelson & Lynn, 1994). Not only do people vary in their ways of dealing with health care decision making in general and end-of-life decisions in particular, but few people (less than 25%) are executing advance directives (American Medical Association, 1989; L. L. Emanuel, Barry, Stoeckle, Ettelson, & E. I. Emanuel, 1991; Gallup & Newport, 1991; Gamble, McDonald, & Lichstein, 1991; High, 1993). Moreover, the people who do write advance directives have little interest in the instruments per se. After all, advance directives are fallback measures and are needed only if rights are not respected and trusting relationships and communications fail. The ethical downside of advance directives, now reinforced by the Patient Self-Determination Act, is that an emphasis on legal and regulatory solutions tends to undermine any presumptive favoring of family decision making in caring for decisionally incapacitated elderly relatives (High, 1994a).

WHO SHOULD MAKE SURROGATE DECISIONS?

Whether or not a patient has completed an advance directive, if he or she becomes decisionally incapacitated, some other person will have to act for the patient when health care decisions, including end-of-life decisions, are demanded. Even if a patient has executed a living will, some other person will have to interpret and implement it. If a proxy or agent has been appointed, then that person will have the authority to consent to or refuse medical treatments for the principal in the event the principal becomes decisionally incapacitated. In some states those persons on a priority list of surrogates are authorized to act as decision makers in the event a patient has not completed an advance directive. Provisions for such lists are known as "surrogate/family decision-making laws." Conventional priority lists have the following order: guardian, if appointed, spouse, adult children, parents, and other relatives. Such lists follow a well-known and customary practice in medicine to turn to family members in the event a patient becomes decisionally incapacitated.

Although new forms of marriages, different lifestyles, and changes in the meaning of the nuclear family necessitate a contextual understanding of the concept of family to include partners and friends (Gubrium & Holstein, 1990), there are at least four good reasons for family members to act as surrogates for decisionally incapacitated persons, especially when they are terminally ill: (1) Family members usually know a relative's preferences, goals, and values. (2) Normally, family members are the most concerned for their relative's welfare. (3) In most instances, there are bonds between family members and the terminally ill relative generated by geographical proximity, frequency of contact, and affection. (4) Most important, the family, as the primary social unit, has within our society a latitude of self-determination. Accordingly, family members rightfully play an important role in decisions concerning care of a terminally ill relative, since the decisions made may have a major impact on their own lives. Beyond the theoretical reasons in favor of the presumption of family surrogate decision making, there is an accumulation of empirical evidence suggesting that family members are ordinarily preferred to serve as surrogate decision makers.

Though some national surveys indicate that a majority of people prefer family members to act as surrogates ("Poll," 1990; President's Commission, 1982), studies conducted at the University of Kentucky Sanders-Brown Center on Aging since 1986 on surrogate decision making for health care and end-of-life decisions provide additional evidence. In-depth interviews with elderly persons, statewide surveys of persons of all ages, and intervention studies among elderly persons have continually confirmed a strong preference for family surrogates (High, 1988, 1993; High & Turner, 1987). If this is so, and additional research continues to confirm such preferences, then this preference for surrogate should be honored, and the empowerment that families provide by good-faith surrogate decision making should be recognized despite arguments from some that families should be kept out of the decision-making process.

AUTONOMY OF THE DYING PERSON, BEST INTERESTS, AND SUBSTITUTED JUDGMENT

Driven by an understanding of autonomy indicating that an individual should have the freedom and right to accept or refuse treatment as an independent decision, the advance-directives movement has been seen as a positive step in caring for terminally ill patients. This strong sense of individual autonomy has held that surrogate decision makers should make decisions on the basis of what the patient would decide if the patient had been able to decide. On the other hand, for many years prior to the interest in advance directives, both the courts and the medical profession assumed *parens patriae* roles and acted according to what was considered best for decisionally incapacitated persons. Consequently, two standards for substituted decision making have emerged over the past two decades: *best interests* and *substituted judgment*.

Simply stated, the best-interests standard holds that surrogate decisions are acceptable on the grounds that they benefit the patient according to socially shared values of a hypothetical "reasonable" person. Factors such as relief of suffering, the usefulness or futility of an intervention, risks, benefits, and burdens are considered to provide an objective test. Such considerations may or may not reflect a patient's own preferences. By contrast, the substituted-judgment standard calls on surrogates to replicate the decision the patient would have made had the patient been capable. A substituted-judgment decision is based on the patient's own values, beliefs, and treatment wishes. For this reason, it is called a subjective test. The better a patient's own views and anticipated treatment decisions are known, the greater the likelihood that the surrogate decision can replicate the patient's decision. Patients may express their views through living-will documents, through conversations about the experiences of others, or through subscription to sets of beliefs, religious or not. Some persons may not have expressed such views or not have made them clear. In these cases, surrogates have no alternative but to use the best-interests standard.

Notwithstanding basic differences between the two standards, ethical and legal commentators, as well as the courts, have produced varying interpretations of each standard, particularly substituted judgment (Meisel, 1989). Some have held that substitute decisions require "clear and convincing evidence" of the prior wishes of the patient. For example, court opinions in Missouri (*Cruzan v. Harmon*, 1988) and New York (*In re O'Connor*, 1988) have imposed very high evidentiary standards concerning the principal's known wishes before allowing a surrogate to reject a life-sustaining treatment for a terminally ill patient. Other states have imposed less restrictive evidentiary rules. For example, the courts in Massachusetts have permitted surrogate, substituted-judgment decisions based on inferences of patient wishes and have sometimes extended the standard to surrogate decisions for patients who have never been capable of making decisions for themselves.

Because the substituted-judgment standard appears to promote individual autonomy more readily than the best-interests standard, it has been widely advocated as the ideal for surrogate decision making. For example, the aforementioned Patient Self-Determination Act was premised on that ideal. However, many ethicists and legal scholars continue to wrestle with the various interpretations of substituted judgment and sometimes attempt to bridge best interests and substituted judgment (Seckler, Meier, Mulvihill, & Paris, 1991). Arguments that the two standards cannot be easily separated in practice abound (Hamann, 1993; Harmon, 1990). Others have found fault with both standards (Rhoden, 1988) or have advocated for a modified version of the best-interests standard (Dresser & Robertson, 1989).

What have often been neglected in the debate are the preferences of patients themselves regarding the standards of surrogate decision making. Are elderly people mostly interested in having surrogate decisions made for them on the basis of substituted judgment, or are they more interested in who makes such decisions for them? Some empirical evidence is emerging suggesting that elderly people do not have a strong interest in having their own decisions replicated in surrogate decision making (High, 1989). Rather, it is frequently the case that elderly people prefer to rely informally on trusted surrogate decision makers without regard to whether the decision reflects one standard or the other. They are more interested in having the best decision made by whatever means. Frequently, elderly people believe that close family members, particularly spouses and/or trusted adult children, can make better decisions at the time of the medical crisis than they could by advance deliberation (High, 1988, 1990; High & Turner, 1987).

THE ROLE OF FAMILIES IN END-OF-LIFE DECISION MAKING

In general, a presumption in favor of families for surrogate decision making or even assisting with end-of-life decisions exists in law and in some ethical argument. It is also a widely known and commonly accepted practice in the medical profession to rely on family members to make treatment decisions for those relatives who never could or can no longer decide for themselves. Beyond that, families are faced with an enormous number of important decisions during the course of a terminal illness of a relative. In addition to crisis and end-of-life decisions, there are everyday decisions about care and treatment options, including financial decisions and family role responsibilities in relating to the dying relative. These decisions affect not only the patient but also the family members themselves. Moreover, end-of-life and care decisions are most frequently made by the family unit, rather than by the patient in isolation, even if he or she is capable. Ordinarily, family members and the patient, if capable, will discuss with one another decisions that must be made. Indeed, effective familial decision making enhances the ability of the patient as well as families to cope with a terminal illness by improving a sense of control.

The role of families in decision making for and with terminally ill relatives is not without some caveats. Family members may sometimes disagree about who should have the primary responsibility for surrogate decisions, or about particular decisions. In such cases, health care professionals and counselors working with the terminally ill patient have an ethical responsibility to ensure that such disagreements have not resulted from a lack of understanding of medical and care information or from other forms of miscommunication. Health care professionals always have an ethical responsibility to encourage effective communication to and among family members, even if there is an ongoing family conflict. Sensitive communication is key to assisting terminally ill patients and their families to deal effectively with end-of-life decisions and care.

A more serious problem may arise if family members, especially surrogate decision makers, have conflicts of interest or engage in other self-interested acts. Health care professionals and counselors should thoroughly investigate any biased surrogate decisions or actions of a surrogate of questionable competence. Health care professionals and counselors have an ethical duty to protect their patients from decisions and actions that are not in the best interest of the patient's well-being. Because some families abuse or otherwise fail to serve the best interests of their elderly members, a family surrogate's end-of-life decision making need not always be accepted.

ON DYING WELL

Whatever else may be said, dying is a highly personal process in the sense that dying affects one's personal being as a whole and immediately precedes the end of life. To recognize dying as personal entails that care of terminally ill persons should be based on respect for the inherent worth and dignity of persons. Unfortunately and all too frequently, persons with long-term terminal illnesses are referred to as hopeless cases that have to be managed under the conditions of life decline. The "life-decline" model often guides, even if tacitly, the outlook on care practices. More frequently it is taken as the major premise in developing an ethics of care of dying persons. That is why it is sometimes thought that terminal care can be based on efforts of making decisions to forgo treatment and allow persons to die or on medical management models of administering terminal care. Robert Morison, a physician, described the life-decline model in the following way: "The life of the dying patient becomes steadily less complicated and rich, and, as a result, less worth living or preserving. The pain and suffering involved in maintaining what is left are inexorably mounting, while the benefits enjoyed by the patient himself, or that he can in any way confer on those around him, are just as inexorably declining" (1971, p. 695).

While Morison is correct to claim that these are "the unhappy facts of the matter," in most situations, it is surely not an ethical claim that this is how matters ought to be (prescriptively), or that these are unalterable facts of the matter. The "unhappy facts" can be altered, at least to a significant degree, in many if not most cases, and the "decline" model does not have to preside over an ethic of care for the dying any more than aging should be confused with dying or an irreversible illness with insufficient well-being. An alternative approach can be taken without excessive commitment to programs aimed entirely at elimination of degenerative illnesses.

People should be enabled to "die well." Again, as noted earlier and contrary to some myths, people do not fear death so much as the loss of well-being and a painful decline (Gallup & Newport, 1991; Saunders & Baines, 1989). But decline is not simply equatable with physiological or biological deterioration. Decline in quality of life can occur quite without physiological or biological deterioration. Even the argument that a minimal condition of "health" is a necessary condition of "happiness" does not, and cannot, claim that "health" is a sufficient condition of happiness. Moreover, and perhaps more important, decline of "health" does not necessarily or for all persons entail diminishment of self and sense of self as an integral individual human being. Of course, there are a variety of contingent matters and conditions that can contribute to a loss of self-esteem and self-worthiness. These can, and often do, include environmental conditions, dependency, care conditions, relationships, and a cluster of inculcated values—right or wrong—that shape one's sense of self-image. The latter include such values as productivity, mobility, success, good looks, and so on. But the problems presented by these values and the measurement of a quality of life by these standards may be as much a problem of a culture as one relating to an individual dying patient. In fact, a reassessment of the prominence given to these values may be called for. Yet it still remains true that loss of physical activity, independence, productivity, and the like does not necessarily mean, even in a culture that values them highly, that life loses its meaning. Professionals (nurses and physicians) who work with the elderly and the dying regularly remind us of that experientially founded conclusion. The following case illustrates the reminder: Mrs. Z, an elderly, retired librarian, was being cared for by a hospice team for terminal cancer of the cervix. She was asked if there was anything she would like to do while confined to her bed. She replied that she had always wanted to study the German language and had never had the time or opportunity. A tutor was secured who met with her three times per week. Later Mrs. Z commented, "I am having a ball. These are some of the most meaningful days of my life."

In recent years, various attempts to defend and justify a medical ethic of "allowing a patient to die" have become moral, not medical, premises of caring (only caring) for the dying, whether tacitly or explicitly expressed as a subscription to "omissions" and withholdings or withdrawals of treatments. Sometimes such an ethic is defended as a corollary of "natural death," sometimes as an effort to draw a limit to aggressive and intrusive medicine, and sometimes as the morally and legally correct way to end pain, suffering, and meaningless life prolongation. These attempts, as an ethic of passive euthanasia, are sometimes offered as an alternative to active euthanasia. Indeed, the President's Commission (1983) argued for a moral distinction between actions and omissions that lead to death, concluding that many omissions in the medical context were acceptable (see also Beauchamp & Perlin, 1978; Ladd, 1979). While an "allowing to die" ethic was designed to resist aggressive and excessive use of life-sustaining treatments, it suffered a significant shortcoming if exercised alone. It could lead to the abandonment of the patient to his or her own autonomy, or to a position that "there is nothing more that can be done."

The prolongation of life should not be the exclusive aim of medical practice, nor should the withholding or withdrawing of life-sustaining treatment be the primary aim of ethics of care for the terminally ill. Appropriate care to the very end of life encompasses more and can result in an appreciation that the care of terminally ill persons is more than disease management. This neither argues for nor infers any subscription to the dictum "preserve life at all costs." An approach to care for the dying that takes its grounding in acceptance of death, imposing some moral categories of allowing to die and drawing general limits to the preservation of life by classification, suffers from imbalance. So long as it is possible to meet the needs of an individual patient, especially the dying and the terminally ill, it is neither morally responsible to kill the patient nor morally responsible to allow the patient to die. Moreover, so long as we also recognize that human beings are inherently mortal, it is neither the case that prolongation of life is the singular and chief need of a patient nor that properly relevant and pertinent treatment begins and ends on the principle of preservation of life. The question is not "to treat or not to treat" or "to treat or allow to die," but *how to treat*—even to the end of an individual person's life. Treatment of pain and symptoms and other palliative care must be recognized as forms of treatment.

Too often it is ignored or forgotten that personal well-being, which may well extend far beyond the dimensions of illness and health or even mortal ills, is a fundamental human value. That value was once expressed to me clearly and succinctly by a patient dying of cancer when she simply stated, "I want to live 'till I die." To value living well and individual well-being is not simply to value life as duration, that is, length of life, nor is it simply to value physiological function. Everyone will recognize that one does not need the body of a child or the physical abilities of an athlete to have a high quality of life, and, of course, it is evident that mere absence of disease by no means guarantees well-being. Even if we admit that total absence of health is death, is it possible that a person can be diseased to an extent, or even seriously so, and still have a high quality of life? Can a dying person who has a prognosis for a short length of remaining life still have a high quality of life for the remainder of his or her days? Both questions can be answered in the affirmative without accepting the "life-decline model" as a starting point or causing attribution of the "hopeless-case" role. Unless hope in fact does not have a dimension different from a quantifiable one, then one should be clear and unequivocal in claims, from the start, that all individual human beings are hopeless. All too often hope is mistakenly equated with cure or some wish to get out of life alive.

NEEDS OF DYING PERSONS

An ethic of care for terminally ill persons must be responsive to needs. Generally, the needs of dying persons will span the needs of life itself, from physical and medical care issues to psychological and social needs and often to spiritual concerns. To focus the point, consider persons dying from cancer. Sometimes these people will have to experience the deterioration of their bodies over a period of weeks or months. Anxiety, fear, loneliness, and depression are common. Most people can expect to experience symptoms from the primary disease. When a curative therapy is no longer possible, sometimes quite complicated medical care issues arise not only from the primary disease but from secondary sources, issuing in pain and discomfort. These may include appetite disturbance, fever, dysphagia (swallowing problems), persistent constipation, infections, dyspnea (difficulty in breathing), bladder dysfunction and incontinence, and metabolic disturbances. Quite simply and fully, dying persons have needs for relief of physical distress, including relief of pain caused by primary and secondary sources, relief from the fear of pain, and relief from other distressing symptoms.

In addition to the need for the relief of physical and mental distress, dying persons have a need for family, friends, and health care professionals to listen and make every effort possible to understand them and what it is like to be mortally ill. Dying persons need empathy (a sensitive understanding of another's situation), not sympathy (a feeling or expression of pity). Such a need may entail specific needs for opportunities to voice fears, to come to terms with oneself and illness, and to draw close to family and friends. Above all, dying persons will have needs to have their individuality and personal integrity maintained. For some, this will take on the character of spiritual or religious choices concerning the meaning of life and personal dignity. This may also entail a specific desire to live out one's remaining days at home or in an environment as homelike as possible. Indeed, most people would prefer to remain in their homes, an environment that is familiar and comfortable, not alien and additionally stressful, even though some people may choose an institution for care because of a lack of family care and the availability of high technology. Because home care most frequently meets the needs and wishes of dying patients, home care hospice programs have developed rapidly in the United States. Finally, dying persons have special needs for relief from the fear of being a burden, but not a relief from all responsibilities and decision making, if they are capable of these. The latter "relief" tends to exacerbate a dying person's sense of loneliness and isolation from everyday life and its decisions. Meeting all of these needs takes an integrated medical, nursing, and family team and does not simply constitute another medical specialty.

ARE EUTHANASIA AND PHYSICIAN-ASSISTED SUICIDE VIABLE ETHICAL OPTIONS TO STOP THE HURTING?

Perhaps the classical meaning of *euthanasia* needs to be reinstated. If one draws on the Greek etymology, euthanasia means "good or happy death," and that is only possible if the remainder of a patient's days constitute a life worthwhile with personal well-being until death. Unfortunately, the term *euthanasia* has taken on a very different meaning in contemporary culture: mercy killing. Refusals of life-sustaining treatments must be distinguished from the modern meanings of euthanasia as well as suicide and physician-assisted suicide. However, some ethicists and medical professionals have sought to classify withholding or withdrawing of treatment as passive euthanasia and mercy killing as active euthanasia. In any case, euthanasia would have to be understood as either an omission (passive) or an act (active) by another person and not by the patient. In that case, active euthanasia is an act by another person to end a patient's life. Refusal of treatment is a decision made by the patient simply to forgo treatment.

Suicide is an act by a patient to end his or her own life and should not be confused with euthanasia nor with refusal of treatment. In assisted suicide, a patient is provided a means to take his or her own life. These simple but important distinctions are often overlooked and have frequently been the source of confusion and obfuscation in public policy debates.

Most public debate has focused on mercy killing (active euthanasia) and physician-assisted suicide. Among the most prominent ethical arguments advanced by individuals and advocacy groups, such as the Hemlock Society, an organization dedicated to legalizing voluntary euthanasia and physician-assisted suicide, is that patients have a right to free choice (autonomy) over their lives, including a right to die. Further, euthanasia, if allowed legally, would reduce suffering and prevent cruelty among those enduring a terminal illness with intractable pain (Williams, 1978). Opponents of euthanasia regularly argue from an ethical principle that sanctity of life is primary and that no killing of another human being should take place. Opponents also plead that any effort to adopt standards for controlling or limiting the use of euthanasia would likely create a slippery slope in which standards will erode and deteriorate (Kamisar, 1978). As is ordinarily the case, ethical principles and arguments are advanced to favor or disfavor legalization of euthanasia. The ongoing debate is an ethical one since it is the case that just because some act is illegal, that does not make it unethical, or if some act is legal, that does not necessarily make it ethical. However, all good and sound laws should be supported with sound ethical principles and argumentation.

The Netherlands is the only country as a whole to embark on a grand social experiment explicitly to permit active euthanasia as well as physician-assisted suicide by custom and agreements with prosecutors, though the practices are not codified by statute or law. Euthanasia is carefully distinguished from homicide and is available only to persons who have a preexisting medical condition or problem. In practice, physicians will not be prosecuted for euthanizing patients if very specific guidelines are followed: (1) the patient's request must be voluntary; (2) the explicit wish of the patient to die must be repeatedly expressed; (3) the patient must have refused all the medical alternatives, and all care options must have been exhausted; and (4) the physician may not act alone; that is, an independent professional colleague must be consulted. Then, and only then, may a qualified, licensed physician carry out euthanasia. It is clear that other countries are watching the Dutch experiment closely. In 1996, the Northern Territory of Australia made it legal for physicians to assist terminally ill people with death by prescribing or preparing substances for self-administration or to administer a substance to a patient as a form of euthanasia. Some states within the United States have in recent years considered euthanasia legislation. Although the states of Washington and California narrowly defeated referendums that would have made euthanasia legal in certain circumstances, active voluntary euthanasia currently remains illegal in all states.

In recent years, an explosive debate has ensued over the morality and possible legalization of physician-assisted suicide. In assisted suicide, the doctor helps plan and provide the means for a patient to commit suicide. The state of Oregon passed an initiative in 1994, known as Measure 16, that would permit physicians to prescribe medications for use by terminally ill patients to commit suicide. It was subsequently challenged in the courts, but in 1996 a ruling by the 9th U.S. Circuit Court of Appeals, based in San Francisco, overturned Washington State's ban on physician-assisted suicide as unconstitutional and thereby decriminalized assisted suicide. That ruling affects 9 western states, including Oregon. On the other hand, by 1996, 33 states had enacted statutes against assisted suicide, and 10 states and the District of Columbia had banned the practice under common law.

Some of the statutes recently passed in various states banning assisted suicide were legislative responses to the much-publicized activities of Dr. Jack Kevorkian, a retired pathologist from Michigan who has assisted many patients to commit suicide. Medically the issue of physician-assisted suicide was pointedly raised in the *New England Journal of Medicine* with a disclosure by Dr. Timothy Quill (1991) that he had provided barbiturates to a woman suffering from terminal, acute leukemia. Many have taken this case as a medical turning point in the discussion, prompting others to join Quill in developing clinical criteria and regulatory proposals for legalizing physician-assisted suicide (Quill, Cassel, & Meier, 1992; F. G. Miller et al., 1994). Public opinion polls show that approximately 60% of Americans favor some legal reform allowing physician-assisted suicide (F. G. Miller et al., 1994). While the delegates to the American Medical Association annual meeting voted on June 25, 1996, to go on record opposing physician-assisted suicide (Sandrick, 1996), surveys among practicing physicians indicate that support for such legal reform is increasing, especially if appropriate safeguards are enacted (J. S. Cohen, Fihn, Boyko, Jonsen, & Wood, 1994; Lee et al., 1996). The 1994 Oregon initiative attempted to provide ethical regulations. As enacted, the measure would allow terminally ill patients who have less than six months to live to request from their long-term physician a prescription for lethal drugs to end their lives. The measure would require patients to make oral and written requests, to have their requests witnessed, and to have a consulting physician certify that the patient is terminally ill. In addition, the physician must ensure that the patient's decision is informed and voluntary. Further, a 15-day waiting period must occur between a patient request and the release of a prescription for medication.

Permitting death by physician-assisted suicide raises deep ethical concerns. Of course, it allows patients self-determination over their existence and provides a way to end intractable suffering and pain. Proponents believe that standards and regulations can be implemented to fully protect patients and society against abuse. Most advocates hold that physician-assisted suicide should be seen as a last resort when comfort or palliative care is no longer possible and all possible means of relieving pain, suffering, and symptoms have been exhausted. This means that voluntary physician-assisted suicide would be permitted only in those cases when all alternatives of care and comfort are inadequate (F. G. Miller et al., 1994). Proponents of physician-assisted suicide think that such cases would be relatively infrequent. This judgment does not differ from that of those who oppose legalizing euthanasia or assisted suicide on the grounds that the focus of attention ought to be directed more at improving palliative and symptom care measures in hospice-type ways. Such improvement, it is argued, would result in there being so few cases for which palliative care is not successful as not to warrant legalizing either euthanasia or physician-assisted suicide. The difficulty in such judgments is that little empirical research exists on the frequency of cases in which palliative care is unsuccessful as well as the lack of availability of such care to terminally ill patients who suffer from intractable pain or untreated pain. Indeed, much more research should be conducted on the needs for palliative care, practices of pain and symptom control and prevention, and their availability to terminally ill patients (Logue, 1994).

Aside from further discussion of opponents' arguments that standards and guidelines for physician-assisted suicide will deteriorate or that legalization of assisted suicide would jeopardize the physician-patient relationship, it seems that the debate is at an impasse and will not be further illuminated until more is known empirically about the current practices in the United States regarding care and pain relief for terminally ill patients. In the meantime, persons concerned with the ethics of care can continue to address the issues of comfort care, including palliative and supportive treatment and pain control and prevention, that should be made available and delivered to terminally ill patients. Hospice care is the best-known example of good palliative care, and many hospice advocates argue that appropriate palliative care precludes any need for euthanasia or assisted suicide.

THE HOSPICE MOVEMENT

Borrowed from a medieval term referring to wayside inns for pilgrims and other travelers needing help and assistance, *hospice* represents a variety of programs to assist and care for terminally ill patients. Much of the inspiration for the hospice movement in North America, which began in the 1970s, came from programs developed in Great Britain, especially at St. Christopher's Hospice under the direction of Dr. Cicely Saunders (Davidson, 1985; Zimmerman, 1986). Often working outside the established health care delivery system, many of the early hospice programs instituted palliative care services to meet the medical-symptomatic and psychosocial needs of dying patients and their families. These service practices have continued and have developed into a widespread network of hospice programs that utilize interdisciplinary teams of caregivers to enable dying persons to live as fully and comfortably as possible until death. Hospices have become an accepted part of the American health care field even though they serve a relatively small percentage of terminally ill patients (Rhymes, 1990).

Hospice programs are premised on several principles that may be understood to be ethical in nature. The programs stand in sharp contrast to the standard "medical model" of care and treatment since palliation or comfort care is a primary treatment goal. Uncontrolled and intractable pain is one of the most feared problems for terminally ill patients. Hospice programs aim to alleviate, control, and prevent pain based on symptom manifestation rather than relying on pathological characteristics usually addressed in acute-care situations (Saunders & Baines, 1989). To control and prevent pain, for example, medications are normally administered on a regular, four-hourly basis. The object of such an approach to pain and symptom control is to maintain functioning human beings who are as normally alert as possible. Second, in hospice care, patients, families, and their closest companions constitute the unit of care. Problems encountered by patients are seen as dynamically affecting others within a social context. Care is directed at seeing the patient as part of a social unit and community rather than as an isolated individual. Dealing with human relationships and issues of how relationships are affected by a terminal illness is intrinsic to hospice care. To treat a dying person as an isolated individual may only exacerbate the patient's sense of loneliness. In turn, relatives and friends who are not part of the primary care may feel cut off from any means of adapting to the impending loss of a loved one.

As a third principle, hospice care includes support for the survivors throughout their bereavement. Proponents of hospice principles recognize that many family members need ongoing support both during their care for terminally ill relatives, including respite care and experiences of anticipatory grief, and after the death of the patient. Finally, as a significant principle in hospice care, dying persons are treated as ends in themselves and not as means to something else. Dying persons, if cognitively alert, have purposes and goals of their own, and these should be recognized and facilitated. Further, dying persons should have their autonomy and abilities to be self-determining maintained and enhanced for as long as possible. Hospice care attempts to understand illness and dying from the perspectives of patients, including listening to and learning from patients and giving primacy to biographical stories of patients over clinical stages of dying. Stories refer to the narratives of individuals' lived experiences (Churchill, 1985). Allowing stories to be told and hearing them enable caregivers to come closer to the lives of patients and to meet the needs of dying persons in ways that may more fully meet their personal wishes.

TOWARD ETHICAL GUIDELINES OF TERMINAL CARE

The analysis of this chapter so far has emphasized that morally appropriate care of a terminally ill person should always involve care for a person as an integral human being until the end of life even though a primary illness may not be successfully treated. It can be further argued, on ethical grounds, that more can and should be done toward improving the care of the dying person than is presently the case in North America. Given this premise, in what follows, a general principle and some ethical guidelines are presented. As ethical reflections, arguments are made concerning how terminally ill persons should be cared for, not what is actually practiced in all cases.

While it may be true that a terminally ill person has reached a point at which no known cure is possible, it is never true that "nothing more can be done." As a normative principle, one can always care for a terminally ill person until the end of that person's life and provide palliative treatment relevant to the patient's condition. It is never true that the only ethical alternatives for a patient are either to give consent to an experimental therapy or to choose death. In many instances, the ethical priority is to assist a person in living out his or her remaining days, weeks, or months as meaningfully and peacefully as possible. Under proper care, a dying person's remaining days can be some of the most meaningful, including significant relationships with family and friends. Unfortunately, the principle here presented can be platitudinous or empty unless it is supported by specific guidelines for implementation. Consequently, the seven guidelines that follow are intended to promote the well-being (quality of life) of those persons who are terminally ill. Further, they are open ended and are also intended to promote discussion rather than foreclose it.

Guideline 1: Respect and Self-Integrity to the End of Life

The dying person should be accorded respect, dignity, and a sense of self-integrity with purpose and fulfillment to the end of life. Respect is both an attitude, which is commonly thought to be fundamental, and a principle of individual conduct and social organization. It is to value persons intrinsically. It is to have regard for a human being independent of particular characteristics. Some have argued that such respect is best described as love-agape (Downie & Telfer, 1969). In this sense, those who care for dying persons are being asked to be responsive to the highest level of relationship to another human being. Mere sentimentality and smothering care, on the other hand, are neither adequate nor appropriate. As much as a healthy person, the terminally ill patient has the need to be seen and treated as a self-integral individual. In practical terms, care of the dying cannot afford to be impersonal or insensitive to the lifestyle of the individual and his or her individual needs. Without such attention, respect and regard for the benefits of otherwise important medical techniques will be vitiated.

Guideline 2: Symptom Control

All symptoms should be treated and controlled as long as possible and as long as such treatment provides comfort to the patient. For the well-being of a dying person, it is important to realize that an appropriate therapy (and often the only proper therapy) is symptomatic treatment. The comfort and well-being of an individual patient may often hinge on effective relief from symptoms and having each symptom treated as it arises. Symptoms may range from minor irritations to serious distress, including dysphagia, anorexia, constipation, nausea, vomiting, incontinence, hiccup, cough, breathlessness, restlessness, and confusion (Enck, 1994; Saunders & Baines, 1989). Attending to the details of each symptom is important. Indeed, it has been shown that relief of minor symptoms often goes a long way to relieve the pain accompanying any serious illness. A patient who is terminally ill with cancer and is at the same time suffering from untreated constipation is a neglected patient, however much effort is or has otherwise been extended on that patient's behalf. Such treatment may not be heroic or dramatic, but is nevertheless important. Often those who compile lists of ways of relieving symptoms are apologetic for their simplicity, but it is all of the niggling things that can detract so much from the dying person's well-being. Consequently, it is important to exercise imagination and perseverance in relieving symptoms. Such care is, indeed, a positive approach to the treatment of a dying person.

Guideline 3: Pain Control and Prevention

A dying person should be assisted to live out his or her remaining days or weeks with minimal or no pain and remain, as fully as possible, normally alert. Among all the factors associated with dying, pain is probably the most dreaded and feared. Moreover, expectation and anticipation of pain is itself self-perpetuating pain. In most cases, the pain endured by a dying person serves no useful purpose. It does not serve as a warning or protective signal or as a diagnostic aid, as in the case of injury. Sometimes, pain associated with dying is categorized as long-term, chronic pain or as terminal pain. Professionals who care for terminally ill persons frequently describe the pain experienced by patients as "total" pain. The designation is intended to indicate not only that pain has multiple components, but that patients may feel that "everything is wrong," meaning that one's whole being is consumed by pain.

In recent years, significant advances have been made in pharmacological research and in care practices to control and prevent pain in terminally ill patients (Corless, 1994; Enck, 1994; Saunders & Baines, 1989). Considerable evidence exists that successful pain control is fully possible with proper employment of a variety of available therapies (drugs, surgical procedures, radiotherapy, and so on). Unfortunately, too many patients are denied relief or are improperly treated. Undertreatment with narcotic analgesics of patients with severe pain is common. Failure to follow basic and enlightened principles of pain control as well as prevention and lack of training in terminal care are major contributors (Enck, 1994). In addition, there are misconceptions about the use of strong analgesics, including misconceptions about addiction, tolerance, and fear of escalated dosages. These misconceptions and fears are the basis of the most prominent ethical issues on pain control and prevention in terminally ill persons.

Frequently patients, relatives, physicians, and nurses express fears of "addiction" to strong analgesics, especially morphine and morphinelike agonists. There is often an ethical wish for the patient or relative not to die experiencing the remaining days of life as a "drug addict." Although some have wanted to alleviate such fears by suggesting that it should not matter in the final days of a terminally ill patient if pain relief is obtained at the expense of addiction, the fears of addicting patients to opioid analgesics are scientifically unfounded (Enck, 1994; Saunders & Baines, 1989; Twycross, 1974). That is to say, empirical study evidence suggests that so long as appropriate doses of opioid analgesics are administered on a regular basis, such as every four hours, to control and prevent pain of cancer and other chronic diseases, the risk of either psychological or physical dependence is almost nil. The ethical issue of whether the use of opioid analgesics will cause addictive side effects is vastly overblown, and fears are misplaced if care in controlling and preventing terminal pain is provided with proper doses of drugs. Current terminal-care practices do not recommend the use of drugs to control pain on an "as-needed" (p.r.n.) basis since that causes a "peak and trough" effect and a lack of around-the-clock pain management and prevention (Enck, 1994). Administering a narcotic like morphine "on demand" places additional burdens on the patient, who will often try to endure the pain as long as possible or engage in clock watching for the next injection. Patients should be relieved of such burdens as well as enabled to forget about any possible pain and enjoy life that is left (Corless, 1994).

It is also a very common fear and argument that use of narcotic drugs with terminally ill patients will turn them into "zombies." If a patient is given sufficient drug therapy to relieve the pain, it is argued, this will likely be at the expense of a rational or normally alert existence. Again, if drugs are properly administered for maximum benefit and dosages are continually reassessed and adjusted accordingly, there is no evidence to suggest that pain cannot be controlled while maintaining patients' normal alertness. Likewise, the issue of tolerance may have precipitated an unfounded ethical claim about caring for terminally ill patients. Some patients and physicians fear that the use of strong analgesics "too soon" will limit the effect of such agents later when they are perceived as absolutely necessary. Again, studies suggest that such a fear is unfounded and that tolerance is at best a minor problem that can be managed by gradual increases in the dosages of narcotics (Enck, 1994; Saunders & Baines, 1989; Twycross, 1974).

Evidence suggests that technology is currently available to control and prevent pain in terminally ill patients if it is administered fully, properly, and with continual assessment. Nevertheless, more can be done for terminally ill patients in control and prevention of pain than is currently the case in the American care system. The predicament is due in part to inadequate training of clinicians in pain assessment and management. Significant ethical priority should be given to correcting these inadequacies as well as continuing the advances in research on effective pain control and prevention.

Guideline 4: Providing the Opportunity to Clarify Relationships

The dying person should have the opportunity to clarify relationships, to continue and develop normal friendships, and to know the truth. A terminally ill patient should be cared for both as an individual and as a social being. The importance of family, friends, and the atmosphere of community, whether a dying person remains at home or is admitted for inpatient care, cannot be overemphasized. Social interchange is just as much an ordinary function of life with the dying person as with the healthy. Physicians and nursing staff cannot afford to be impersonal. Loneliness and isolation due to or perpetuated by a particular care system are inexcusable. Together with adequate physical care, the dying person who has sufficient human companionship will be relieved of much anguish.

The dying person should know the truth about the diagnosis and prognosis unless, of course, that person explicitly requests not to be told. Personal autonomy should be honored, but helping patients to realize and accept the truth will many times require extensive skill at communication and patience. It is, therefore, important how one communicates to the dying person, and even more important, that one listens to the dying person. Attending persons (the care team, relatives, and friends) should not engage in evasions and deceptions. These can only add to a sense of loneliness, frustration, and abandonment.

Guideline 5: Rights to Care

The dying person should be accorded all rights due to any patient, including the right to make care requests, to refuse treatment, to be consulted about types of care, and to voice and be heard concerning his or her current and changing state of well-being. The dying patient has a right to be active, as long as possible, in decisions concerning care and treatment. Attending persons and relatives should not be overprotective of the patient or create a sense of unreality. To be cared for may be helpful and comforting; to be taken care of may be demeaning.

Guideline 6: Sharing and Planning for Changes

The dying person should be given the opportunity, when possible, to share in planning for changes that death will impose on the survivors. Attending persons should assist in making resources available for planning by the patient and for sharing concern for the relatives, both during the process of dying and after death. Such planning could include planning for the distribution of one's estate, discussing how decisions will be made in later stages of care if one becomes decisionally incapacitated, and sharing the concerns of relatives and their futures. Care should always be extended to the family and not just to the terminally ill patient, and this should include the grieving process. Families should not be cut off from care once the patient has died. Hospice programs have attempted to provide a place for families after the death of the patient, including grief counseling; acute-care institutions have not.

Guideline 7: Dying in a Familiar Environment

The dying person should be accorded a familiar environment, one with familiar things and familiar faces, or surroundings as nearly homelike as possible. It goes almost without saying that most people, if given a choice, would prefer to live out their last days in the familiar and often comfortable environs of their own homes, though there may be some variation in preference depending on ethnic group or religious persuasion. In any case, patient preferences should be honored as much as possible. Acute as well as terminally ill patients frequently prefer to be surrounded by persons and possessions that are familiar, not by strangers and strange circumstances. The familiar surroundings and faces help to relieve the psychosocial suffering encountered in the dying process and allow for free and uninhibited communication between the patient and family. Indeed, the home care of dying patients by hospice programs, widely practiced in the United States, has several advantages, including that of affording the patient greater opportunity to regain control over his or her life and death.

Terminal home care can often produce a remarkable closeness among the patient, relatives, and friends. Families can experience a greater sense of involvement in the care of the patient and sharing in the remaining days of their loved one than when a terminally ill patient is in a hospital or institution. This sharing can include, in diverse ways of expression and presence, in-depth listening and saying "good-bye." Not only are physical comfort and privacy realizable benefits from home or homelike environments, but it is more likely that a continuity with normal, everyday life can be maintained. Care delivered at home, for example, can be intensely personal and rewarding for all involved. Though home care may not always be the best course or even a possible course for all patients, the benefits and virtues that it can provide ought to be a goal of all terminal-care situations and a priority of any ethics of terminal care.

CONCLUSION

The various topics discussed in this chapter on the ethics of terminal care, especially the seven guidelines specifically offered, are not intended to foreclose discussion, but to stimulate it further. Effective and ethical care of terminally ill patients has grown substantially in the past 20 years in the United States, especially through the development of hospice programs and improvements in symptom and pain control. However, it is also a sober reality that most terminally ill patients are not receiving care that reasonably approaches the standards of good and proper care or what would fulfill an ethics of terminal care as outlined here. Fully effective care for terminally ill patients will entail changes in policies, practices, and systems of access and delivery. Flexible and innovative approaches must be developed. Training in caring for terminally ill patients should be a part of curricula in all medical and nursing schools. Additional and more advanced training should be more widely available. Research into the effectiveness of terminal care, including institution of improved standards of care, development of outcome measures, and research into improved substances and methods of use in pain and symptom control and prevention, are essential. These changes and continued developments could lead to greater and more humane care for all dying persons, which, by the definition of mortality, will include all human beings.

8

Ethical Issues in the Care of the Judgment Impaired

Lawrence Heintz

Judgment impairment is a matter of degree and comes in many forms. The individual who has total and permanent loss of judgment possesses a very different set of problems from one whose loss is partial or intermittent. Correspondingly, the moral questions that arise when we are dealing with the patient in a persistent vegetative state, for example, are very different from those presented by the confused or disoriented patient. We will be able to consider only some of a whole spectrum of moral questions that arise in this context: To what degree is this individual able to make health care decisions? If the individual is not able, who should make decisions and on what basis? What role do advance directives play? Who should become the surrogate decision makers, and what standards should such decision makers use in forming their decisions? But first let us remind ourselves of the scope or the magnitude of the population and issues that we are dealing with.

WHO IS INCLUDED IN THE "JUDGMENT IMPAIRED"?

The magnitude of the problem begins to be grasped once one recognizes that by the year 2000, 11.5% of Americans will be over 65, and estimates vary that from 10% to 18% of them will have clinically significant cognitive impairment. Also, there are two important progressions taking place (see Tables 1 and 2) in the aging of America—the number of elderly and the distribution of the elderly—that, when understood, reveal the ballooning nature of this problem.

Table 1
Share of U.S. Population over 64 Years of Age, 1900, 1940, 1960, 1975, and 2000

Year	Percentage
1900	4.0
1940	6.5
1960	9.0
1975	10.5
2000	11.5

Table 2
Distribution of U.S. Elderly Population by Age Group, 1950, 1975, and 2000

Age Groups	Percentage of Total Elderly		
	1950	*1975*	*2000*
65–74	71	62	54
75–84	25	30	34
85 or older	4	8	11

Source: National Institute on Aging. (1977). *Our future selves: A research plan toward understanding aging.* Washington, DC: National Institutes of Health.

Another way to gain a sense of the extent of the population that will be affected by the questions of this chapter is to realize that 80% of Americans die in hospitals and nursing homes. Most of this group will lose the ability to make decisions and ironically may be kept in that condition for an extended period due to capabilities of and advances in modern medicine (Buchanan & Brock, 1989; President's Commission for the Study of Ethical Problems in Medicine and Biomedical and Behavioral Research [President's Commission], 1983).

In the law, judgment impairment is discussed in terms of competence and incompetence. Judicial determinations of incompetence are infrequent and usually result in the appointment of a guardian or involuntary commitment of the subject. What is of special interest to us is the wider question of the decision-making capacity of the elderly. That capacity varies with the subject matter, is a matter of degree, often is intermittent, and can be greatly affected by the environment and the behavior of others, but its loss may be chronic. The other side of loss of capacity is the loss of autonomy. Out of respect for the right of self-determination, we must presume an individual's competence and place the burden on those who question it to make a case for their view (Beauchamp & Childress, 1994; Buchanan & Brock, 1989; Faden & Beauchamp, 1986; Freedman, 1981; Hofland, 1994; President's Commission, 1983; Roth, Meisel & Lidz, 1977; Venesy, 1994). We will use the following three cases to introduce a range of moral issues involved in cases where the question of competence is raised.

Case A

Mrs. S is a 66-year-old who is currently unresponsive to nearly all interaction and stimulation. She has been in the nursing home for 12 years after a long history of early-onset Alzheimer's disease. She has no other serious medical problems but is in need of total nursing and comfort care.

Case B

Mr. F, age 57, has suffered from a series of strokes that are related to a severe case of diabetes, has lost all vision, and is unable to care for himself. He lives in an extended-care facility and resists his weekly dialysis treatment. He is a proud individual who at one time was a leader in his immediate community and extended family. He rarely communicates with his caregivers or visitors, and over the 18 months in the nursing facility his visitors and support community have steadily dwindled. When he entered the nursing home, a family conference, in which his two brothers took the leadership role, determined that the dialysis treatment was to continue. His mother visits him three times a week, one sister visits once a month, and his two brothers no longer visit. They ask, "Why should we visit? He is no longer himself and rarely knows we are there." His mother now requests a discontinuance of the dialysis because of the continued resistance that the patient exhibits at each session. Mr. F no longer communicates with his physicians, nor does he respond to inquiries from the staff of the facility. His level of decisional capacity is undetermined due to the low level of cooperation with his caregivers. His mother believes that his mind is good but acknowledges that sometimes weeks go by without his acknowledging her efforts to communicate with him. Other family members do not respond to efforts to arrange a family conference.

Case C

Mr. P is an 87-year-old widower with no known family who has vascular disease in both legs, with gangrene developing in his right leg. He has refused recommendations for amputation on several occasions. The patient has a living will that has very general language but that includes statements to the effect that he wants no heroic measures, no cardiopulmonary resuscitation (CPR), no artificial feeding, and no surgery, but requests comfort care and pain relief. After a referral to a consulting surgeon, the patient signed a consent for right-leg amputation. One month after an unremarkable recovery, the attending physician and nursing staff now face the progressing vascular disease, which now includes gangrenous sores on the patient's remaining large toe. Since the previous surgery, the patient has shown little interest in anything around him and does not seem to understand the developing problem with his left foot when it is explained to him. A social worker, while reviewing the patient's chart, notices the living will and refers the case to the hospital's ethics committee.

Loss of decisional capacity may be due to one or more medical disorders, such as (*a*) degenerative neurological disorders (Alzheimer's, Parkinson's), (*b*) cerebrovascular accidents (stroke), (*c*) severe acute or chronic depression that may impair cognitive function, (*d*) temporary or permanent coma, (*e*) mental retardation, or (*f*) severe personality disorders. In addition, the last stages of many chronic illnesses are accompanied by a high incidence of judgment impairment. Long-term hospitalization and care are also often accompanied by loss of decisional capacity. The capabilities of contemporary medicine, such as ventilators and artificial feedings, often prolong the life of patients with conditions that compromise and even totally impair cognitive function. Some medications compromise cognitive function (steroids and some highly toxic drugs used in cancer therapy), and effective dosages of narcotics for pain management often compromise one's ability to communicate (Beauchamp & Childress, 1994; Buchanan & Brock, 1989; Faden & Beauchamp, 1986; Graber, Beasley, & Eaddy, 1985; Hofland, 1994; Jonson, Siegler, & Winslade, 1982; President's Commission, 1983; Winkler, 1983).

How are determinations of decisional capacity in the elderly made? Not surprisingly, most determinations of "incompetence" in the elderly are made informally, that is, without a psychiatric consultation and/or not through the legal system. The moral worries loom large here when we consider the problems that arise in formal, legal determinations of competence. Formal determinations of incompetence for decisions concerning finances and living arrangements often involve errors that fail to take into consideration the extent to which incompetence is intermittent or not permanent and varies with the decision, issue, or question at hand. Another error is that the diagnosis is sometimes confused with or precludes a determination of competence. A second problem is that a determination of incompetence results in a justification of total decision making by surrogate decision makers (Buchanan & Brock, 1989; Cranford & Doudera, 1984; Faden & Beauchamp, 1986; Freedman, 1981; Roth et al., 1977; Venesy, 1994). These are very complex and technical matters that go beyond the scope of these remarks.

WHO BECOMES THE DECISION MAKER FOR THE JUDGMENT IMPAIRED?

In the traditional progression of decision making, the presumption is that the family comes first. The individuals biologically closest or whomever the individual is most closely associated with are thought to be in the best position to reflect the wishes of the patient. Decision making is usually a shared process; rarely is it advisable that surrogates should operate in isolation. Understandably, physicians because of their expertise play an important role in shaping decisions. Patients and families rely on their advice, defer to their expertise, and often shift the burden to them (Beauchamp & Childress, 1994; Buchanan & Brock, 1989; Faden & Beauchamp, 1986; Hofland, 1994; King, 1991; President's Commission, 1983). This shifting of decision-making function is not confined to health care but is found in most professions where we consult experts (lawyers, accountants, bankers, brokers, and so on). Most often, shared decision making is highly desirable and itself can provide a kind of safeguard (short of procedural ones) that ensures accountability and detects conflicts of interest. It must be noted that there is a legislative movement in this country to require specified surrogate decision makers for all decisionally incapacitated persons. With the issue of decision making in mind, let us look at the three cases A, B, and C set out earlier.

In case A, the decision maker could be any of the following in order of involvement and/or availability in the case: family (spouse, adult children, parents, siblings), court-appointed guardian, or caregivers. In this sort of case, moral problems can arise when or if the decision maker's interests or concerns diverge from the views (if known) or the best interests of the patient. Such patients are particularly vulnerable because they and their care are totally dependent on the decisions of others whose interests may diverge from theirs. It is vital that all those involved in such cases be alert to the needs of the patient and the benefits and burdens of care and interventions provided, keeping consideration of the best interests of the patient clearly in mind.

In case B, the competence of the patient has never been formally determined, and the decision making has devolved for cultural reasons to the male siblings, who have become less engaged in the case. The family dynamics present numerous problems of decision-making authority and cloud assessments of the grounds being used for care decisions. Divided and/or noncooperative families add layers of moral questions to those already present in this case. But caregivers, by focusing on the standard of the best interest of the patient, which will be discussed later, can best guard against major moral lapses in this case. They must be ready to take steps to challenge the family decision makers by obtaining the services of a guardian through probate court.

Case C is one in which the physicians have by default become the decision makers and have followed a course that may have been based on suspect consent for surgery, given the patient's expressed wishes in his living will. The second amputation was prevented only by the intervention of institutional decision makers (an ethics committee). This case illustrates how the elderly who may have some impairment of judgment can be at great risk and are in need of advocates, whether within or outside the health care system. In such cases of conflict of judgment, the elderly patient is in need of an advocate. This case illustrates why physicians should not be decision makers in cases but rather use their expertise to make recommendations to others.

Challenge to the authority of the family should be limited to cases where informed and reasonable individuals would come to the assessment that the family decisions are clearly in conflict with the incompetent patient's best interest and there is a likelihood of serious harm. Another situation that would call for overriding a family is when the family's decision is in conflict with a clear, unambiguous advance directive and again the consequence would be serious harm or injury (Bandman, 1994; Buchanan & Brock, 1989; Faden & Beauchamp, 1986; Freedman, 1981; Hofland, 1994; President's Commission, 1983; Rubin, 1985).

The major challenge to the authority of the family comes from those who believe that where families waver, either doctors or judges should decide. But the professional decision makers are relied on far too uncritically for decisions that lie beyond their knowledge and expertise. Numerous studies have shown that the physician's knowledge of patients' wishes is greatly overestimated and that the family's ability to make reasonable decisions is underestimated. Also, a physician's medical expertise is confused with moral expertise when in fact physicians have no special moral credentials. It is not clear that the court has special moral credentials either. Additionally, the problem with decision making by the court is that such a process is very costly, cumbersome, and slow and ignores the special moral relationship between the patient and the family. Detailed criticism of the medicalization and/or judicialization of decision making is widespread in the literature (Beauchamp & Childress, 1994; Buchanan & Brock, 1989; Cranford & Doudera, 1984; Faden & Beauchamp, 1986; President's Commission, 1983; Sartorius, 1983).

All who are providing patient care when surrogate decision making is involved have a moral obligation to ensure the soundness of these decisions. In troublesome cases, one alternative that can protect family standing and at the same time place the decision making in an institutional context that can assure the quality of the decision making is the use of institutional ethics committees. Such committees can provide a decision-making process that (*a*) is public (open to caregivers and family), (*b*) is principled (explained and justified by explicit widely accepted principles), (*c*) invokes mechanisms to ensure impartiality, (*d*) is informed (has access to and utilizes expertise), and (*e*) is investigative but not adversarial. The family or anyone involved in the patient's care can initiate a referral to an ethics committee. Ethics committees through their independence and impartiality are great equalizers because of their ability to expose biases and unearth unarticulated assumptions of parties deeply involved in patient care, while at the same time they can challenge the family's decision-making authority short of invoking the legal system (Beauchamp & Childress, 1994; Buchanan & Brock, 1989; Cranford & Doudera, 1984; Gibson, 1994; Graber et al., 1985; Jonsen et al., 1982; President's Commission, 1983).

The more that is at stake, the greater the reason to broaden the review of surrogate decision matters. The dangers to the elderly judgment impaired, this most vulnerable of groups, may be the greatest when there is agreement between a family and the physician regarding a not-so-well-founded decision to withhold life-sustaining care or treatment. In cases where so much is at stake, it is all the more important to have some critical independent review or oversight. The possibility for error, or even abuse, here raises the question of whether all such cases ought to be reviewed by such committees or independent consultants.

I would urge much greater use of ethics committees as consultants to those who must make decisions for others. In the most comprehensive book on surrogate decision making, we read this assessment of such committees: "The chief virtue of institutional ethics committees is that they can provide some of the impartiality and critical scrutiny of judicial proceedings in a way that is less cumbersome, less expensive, less adversarial, and less invasive of the patient's and the family's privacy" (Buchanan & Brock, 1989, p. 150). A well-functioning ethics committee offers critical review from multiple perspectives and a forum for collaborative decisions on the most difficult of life-and-death matters. I fully concur with Cranford and Doudera, who believe: "Ethics committees present a challenge and an opportunity to physicians and nurses, health care administrators, lawyers, families, and others to take the initiative and to develop this means to insure that reasonable and fair decisions are made by those who should make them—patients, physicians, and families" (1984, p. 18). The major problem with ethics committees is their underutilization.

ON WHAT GROUNDS ARE THE DECISIONS FOR CARE BASED?

Advance Directives

In fear and/or anticipation of judgment impairment, roughly 15% of the current population has taken the initiative to execute some form of advance directive. An advance directive for health care is an instrument in which one expresses one's views about the sort and extent of health care services one wishes for oneself in the event one is unable to participate in those decisions at that time. For those facing this issue, the ancient admonition "know thyself" could not be more poignant. In an advance directive, one is expressing one's present views about the care one wishes to receive or not receive in some future state. The epistemological difficulties for such directives are formidable and may account for why many people do not get around to executing such directives and also for why most directives that are executed are so general or vague. Granted that one cannot with full confidence speak for one's future self, the question becomes this: "Am I now the best spokesperson for what questions will be faced for my care?" During the last three decades, a major shift has occurred on this question from "my doctor will know best" to "my doctor in consultation with my family will know best" to "I had best go on record to express my preferences." The public has come to see that the sorts of care so often delivered to severely compromised elderly patients are far more aggressive than they would wish for and that steps need to be taken to guard against this divergence between what is provided and what they would hope for. It is out of this problem that advance directives emerged (L. L. Emanuel, Barry, Stoeckle, Ettelson, & E. J. Emanuel, 1991; L. L. Emanuel & E. J. Emanuel, 1989; Heintz, 1988, 1997; High, 1993).

Let us first identify the major types and features of advance directives (see also chapter 7 for an instructive discussion of advance directives). I will then analyze a sample directive in detail in order to lay out their features, strengths, and difficulties. Advance directives have many labels and come in many overlapping forms. The most common labels are directions for care, living will, living will with proxy, advance directive for care, general durable power of attorney, and durable power of attorney for health care. There are two different functions that these instruments are meant to accomplish: first, to provide directions or an expression of one's views, and second, to identify and authorize an agent to speak for one. These functions are often combined, as in the sample discussed here and in most durable powers of attorney for health care. Many people have used a living-will form like that provided by the Society for the Right to Die, which I will use to illustrate the features of advance directives.

LIVING WILL DECLARATION

1. **To My Family, Doctors, and All Those Concerned with My Care**
2. I, _____, being of sound mind, make this
3. statement as a directive to be followed if for any reason I become unable to participate in
4. decisions regarding my medical care. I direct that life-sustaining procedures should be
5. withheld or withdrawn if I have an illness, disease, or injury, or experience extreme mental
6. deterioration, such that there is no reasonable expectation of recovering or regaining a
7. meaningful quality of life. These life-sustaining procedures that may be withheld or
8. withdrawn include, but are not limited to:
9.   SURGERY   ANTIBIOTICS   CARDIAC RESUSCITATION
10. RESPIRATORY SUPPORT   ARTIFICIALLY ADMINISTERED FEEDING AND FLUIDS
11. I further direct that treatment be limited to comfort measures only, even if they shorten my
12. life. *(You may delete any provision above by drawing a line through it and adding your*
13. *initials.)*
14. Other personal instructions:
15. These directions express my legal right to refuse treatment. Therefore, I expect my family,
16. doctors, and all those concerned with my care to regard themselves as legally and morally
17. bound to act in accord with my wishes, and in so doing to be free from any liability for
18. having followed my directions.
19. Signed _____ Date _____
20. Witness _____
21. Witness _____

PROXY DESIGNATION CLAUSE

22. *If you wish, you may use this section to designate someone to make treatment decisions if*
23. *you are unable to do so. Your Living Will Declaration will be in effect even if you have*
24. *not designated a proxy.*
25. I authorize the following person to implement my Living Will Declaration by accepting,
26. refusing, and/or making decisions about treatment and hospitalization:
27. Name _____
28. Address _____
29. If the person I have named above is unable to act on my behalf, I authorize the following
30. person to do so:
31. Name _____
32. Address _____
33. I have discussed my wishes with these persons and trust their judgment on my behalf.
34. Signed _____ Date _____
35. Witness _____ Witness _____

We see that two things must occur in order for the living will to be triggered. First, one must be unable to participate in decisions regarding medical care (lines 2–4), and second, a certain set of conditions must obtain (lines 4–7). The determination of the fulfillment of these conditions must be by others, and invariably it is one's physicians who must make the call whether "there is no reasonable expectation of recovering or regaining a meaningful quality of life." While considerable agreement has been reached about illness, disease, or injuries that produce conditions that are irreparable, irreversible, and/or terminal, there is less agreement about "meaningful quality of life." The patient's wishes may be stymied at this point if one's physician will not concur that these conditions have occurred or does not find them meaningful. In this event, the living will may have little influence in the clinical care decisions unless there is a proxy provision (lines 22–35) or family members, other care providers, or involved parties who actively and aggressively pursue the views expressed in the living will.

Clearly, another problem that faces one who signs a living will is how to identify which life-sustaining procedures in an unspecifiable future state of affairs one would want withdrawn or withheld. It is for this reason that lines 7–10 only give examples of the kind of interventions that might be at issue. Again, in this case it is most likely to be the physicians who are the ones placed in the position to make the recommendations and determinations. Much of the current literature suggests two ways to overcome the problems inherent here. They are (1) to name a proxy and (2) to give a much more detailed account of one's preferences. The most effective way to increase the likelihood that one's wishes will be followed is to have detailed discussions with one's physician (L. L. Emanuel et al., 1991; L. L. Emanuel & E. J. Emanuel, 1989; Heintz, 1988, 1997; High, 1993; Morrison, Olson, Mertz, & Meier, 1995).

A major shortcoming of living wills is that much of the legislation that recognizes them and offers protection from civil and criminal charges to those who adhere to them does not provide sanctions against those who do not follow them. Usually, such statutes only call upon physicians to transfer the patient to the care of another if they are unable to adhere to the patient's instructions. Rarely are such provisions for transfer of patients followed, nor does the course of care usually last long enough for the care to reflect the patient's wishes before death. Lines 14–17 serve the very important function to remind those who care for the patient that the living will is an expression of the patient's legal right to refuse treatment. Such paragraphs may be especially important if one has not designated a proxy or lacks a strong advocate. In cases where one does have an advocate, such paragraphs can be decisive in making the advance directive effective.

This living will also contains an optional Proxy Designation Clause. By doing so, it addresses the second function that was identified earlier, namely, identification of a decision maker for health care decisions. It is important to note that lines 22–34 when taken together do two things: (a) give instructions to the proxy and (b) authorize the proxy to implement those instructions but also to exercise his or her judgment (to go beyond the specific directions) on the signer's behalf. It is this feature that transforms a living will into a much more powerful instrument. This instrument is no longer a static text to be interpreted by others but rather one that enlists the full capabilities of the proxy to be an agent of the maker of the advance directive. The decision making goes beyond the patient and makes use of the mind of the proxy.

Such a living will with proxy is functionally equivalent to a durable power of attorney for health care (DPAHC). While the two types of documents may be recognized by different statutes in some states, and these statutes may diverge in their details and consequently have significant legal differences, they possess the same or equivalent moral force. A DPAHC may do nothing more than identify the authorized decision maker in the event of the incapacity of the patient to make health care decisions, or, like the living will, it may also provide an expression of the preferences of the principal.

The major difficulties with DPAHC are (1) the selection of an agent and (2) the continuing congruence of views between the principal and the agent. The person selected as the agent is very likely to be placed in the position of trying to decide whether to refuse physician-recommended life-sustaining interventions in situations that the principal has not discussed with him. If the agent is a close relative or loved one, the burden of the patient's illness and imminent loss is likely to be a very heavy one. The other major problem is that no matter who is selected, it is very likely that the principal and the agent will not communicate sufficiently about the decisions that will have to be made. On the other hand, if the communication is good, then the DPAHC is surely the best insurance that the patient's wishes regarding care will be followed.

Recent studies of advance directives reveal major problems with their effectiveness in ensuring that the patient's wishes will be followed in clinical circumstances. The major barriers to effectiveness are that the documents often are not available, recognized, or honored when medical decisions must be made. For advance directives to have effect, they must be placed in the right hands and in the right places so that they will be utilized. Since advance directives are a vehicle of communication, they are most likely to be successful if they are placed in the hands and, more important, in the consciousness of one's physician. This is best done in the physician's office, with copies placed in the patient's long-term-care facility and hospital medical records. But unless there is someone who reminds others of and asks about the availability of the advance directive, it may be overlooked or forgotten. As often as not, it may not be in the proper place in the chart, or the chart may not be properly flagged to indicate its presence. When patients transfer between facilities (from ambulatory to acute-care settings), there is an even greater danger that their advance directives will not play a role in clinical decision making. In a study that I am currently conducting on the efficacy of advance directives, I find that even when the advance directive is in its proper place in the medical chart and is noticed, it still has little or no impact on clinical practice because physicians seldom acknowledge that the patient has the conditions designated (lines 4–7) to trigger the advance directive. The best hope for such patients is to have a strong, assertive proxy or agent acting on their behalf (L. L. Emanuel, et al., 1991; L. L. Emanuel & E. J. Emanuel, 1989; Heintz, 1997; High, 1993; Morrison et al., 1995).

In case C at the outset of this chapter, the patient had a living will that had no impact on his care. Why was that? There could be many reasons, but one likely one is that the patient had no family and no advocate, and despite several refusals, the referrals to specialists and the recommendations for surgery kept coming. Eventually the patient gave in to the professional and institutional persistence and signed a "consent" for surgery. From the professional's perspective, the living will was not relevant because the patient was able to make the decision. It was merely a matter of convincing the patient that amputation was the appropriate course of treatment for a gangrenous foot. But was it the appropriate *care* for this patient who repeatedly refused amputation and had a living will stating "no surgery"? There are many points to make about this case (including questions about the validity of the surgical permit), but I believe that the heart of the matter is best seen as an instance of the widespread failure of health care professionals to recognize that living wills (and all advance directives) are not merely expressions of a patient's wishes, that is, *evidence of preferences*, but also are *performatives*. This distinction deserves its own paragraph.

It is vital to realize that advance directives are performative, not just evidentiary. They are the expression of a deliberate choice that has been made. When I say "I do" in certain contexts, I thereby "make someone my spouse." This "I do" is not merely evidence of a preference that I have, but is the consent to marry. It is the way I marry, the way I *perform* the act. Evidence of preferences can be direct or indirect; it can be inferential and does not have the same weight as an act or performance. In the case of an advance directive, we have a performance that contains the expression of preferences. The confusion is that among health professionals the document is seen as evidence of a person's wishes, and the performative force of it is overlooked. This existential, performative dimension of advance directives is too often ignored, and in doing so, we violate the patient. In case C the physician imposed an alien will, his will, on the patient and thereby treated a gangrenous foot (an object), not a person. The performative/evidentiary distinction is one that is well established in ethical and legal theory. There is reason to believe that the slow learning curve of health care professionals is finally being addressed on this topic, but I believe that it continues to play a key role in explaining the minimal impact of advance directives in clinical practice (Heintz, 1997; Morrison et al., 1995).

Substituted Judgment

In the absence of an advance directive that expresses one's wishes, the decision makers must find another basis for decision regarding care. In such cases, the decision maker attempts to determine what in his or her judgment would be the wishes of the patient. The question is asked: "What would the patient have decided in this situation?" The substitute decision maker seeks an accurate expression of the wishes, views, or judgment of the patient, which he or she then expresses for the incompetent individual. What is "substituted" in such cases is the *expression* or *exercise* of judgment rather than substituting one judgment for another. Without an advance directive, where would the wishes of the patient be found? It is here that one must rely on other, less formal expressions of the patient's views.

The range of expression of one's wishes can, at one extreme, amount to an oral advance directive before witnesses or, at the other extreme, to very indirect and indeterminate accounts about expressions of preferences. Letters, diaries, messages, and reports of formal or casual conversations with family, friends, clerics, and professionals (social workers, lawyers, health care providers) form the primary sources for this information. The credence that decision makers give to such information can range from full confidence to having little or no force. We all know of situations where a person says, "I would not want to be kept alive like that," but what status or significance such remarks will have when they are brought to the attention of those asked to exercise "substituted judgment" rightly will have everything to do with the context and the extent, gravity, depth, force, and consistency with the subject's value set about life that the collection of remarks (testimony) reflects. When assessing the strength of evidence for a reliable expression of the individual's views, we should consider the following: specificity of the preference expressed, self-reference as opposed to reference about others, the number of sources, the reliability of the sources, repetitions of the same view, and the intervals of time and the care with which the expressions were made. The objective of those who are utilizing the substituted-judgment standard is to discover the position that best expresses the subject's point of view. Given how much is at stake, those making such determinations need to do so with caution, care, and attention to detail (Beauchamp & Childress, 1994; Buchanan & Brock, 1989; King, 1991; President's Commission, 1983; Venesy, 1994).

Caution is always in order in assessing the sources of evidence. Families and friends, intentionally or not, may misrepresent or overstate the incompetent individual's views. More and more physicians and other caregivers are not well acquainted with the patient's values when he or she was competent, and this lack of independent evidence raises a shadow over the substituted-judgment standard. Given that families may have a serious conflict of interest that could distort their testimony, special care and institutional safeguards are needed. Short of the requirement that substituted judgment be exercised only by a judge or court-appointed guardian ad litem, which would produce a major bureaucratic hurdle in most contexts, carefully constituted, well-functioning hospital ethics committees may provide the appropriate institutional safeguards.

Best Interest

In the event that there is no basis on which to form a "substituted judgment," as would be the case with infants or those who have lacked competence since birth or for a very long time, or those for whom we lack a reliable basis to use the substituted-judgment standard for any other reason (including lack of information), decision makers invoke the "best-interest" standard. Decision makers face the problem of determining what the interests of the individual are and how to weigh the benefits and burdens of actions that affect that individual in terms of his or her interests. Some interests are especially germane in these contexts (e.g., avoiding death and pain), and many interventions (e.g., ventilator support, tube feedings, Foley catheters) provide both burdens and benefits. This standard is called patient centered because it is concerned with advancing the patient's present and future interests (Beauchamp & Childress, 1994; Buchanan & Brock, 1989; Griffin, 1986; King, 1991; President's Commission, 1983; Venesy, 1994).

The "best-interest" standard does not apply to cases of patients who have total and permanent loss of consciousness, for such patients have no interests. Decisions in such cases must either utilize the substituted-judgment standard or consider the interests of others (e.g., family members) and should not be confused with the standard of "best interests of the patient." The point here is that whatever the basis of the decision, when the burden that continued care may place on the family or other interested parties is the basis of the decision, it is not the standard of the interests of the patient that is being invoked.

Sometimes the substituted-judgment and best-interests standards cannot be sharply separated. Problems over which standard to apply are manifold and are found in court decisions as well as in the thinking of health professionals. In the Quinlan and Saikewicz cases, the courts held that substituted judgment was the standard to use in all cases of incompetents. However, they failed to realize that some incompetents have never been competent, and thus the substituted judgment would not apply, or, again, in many cases incompetents have never expressed their preferences prior to the onset of incompetence or may have expressed contradictory preferences, in which case only the best-interests standard would apply. The court's misapplication of the substituted-judgment standard could not be more dramatic and fundamental than is found in the Saikewicz case. Substituted judgment does not apply to Saikewicz since he was estimated to have a mental age of about "one" since birth and never possessed the conceptual capacity to form the relevant preferences, let alone express them. Yet we see in this case the court attempting to ascertain his preferences in order to protect his right of self-determination (Buchanan & Brock, 1989; President's Commission, 1983).

In the Spring case, in order to apply the substituted-judgment standard, the court stretched the standards of evidence or prior wishes. Spring's family could offer only anecdotal evidence that Mr. Spring would not want his care continued because he was used to a vigorous life and now was greatly restricted. An amicus curiae brief, while pointing out that the family's evidence was virtually nonexistent, remarked: "It is almost always true as people get older that their level of activity declines, and is often severely curtailed. It does not follow from this that such a person would prefer to cease living because of the curtailment of such activities" (Annas & Glantz, 1980, p. 389). Such dangerous speculation is too often engaged in about others with severe disabilities ("I would not want to go on living like that"). Here it is doubly disturbing since the court was actually confusing such thinking with the substituted-judgment standard rather than the implementation of the best-interests standard (Beauchamp & Childress, 1994; Buchanan & Brock, 1989; President's Commission, 1983).

In conclusion, here are some reminders and suggestions. Attention needs to be given to how we make determinations of incompetence. Who makes such decisions and what qualifies them to do so? What standards are being used? Are we being sensitive to the fact that competence is seldom an all-or-nothing matter but rather is decision relative and fluctuating? Is there consistency in the process, and do we have mechanisms in place to guard against abuse and error?

The use of advance directives needs to be encouraged as a method for the elderly to have their wishes regarding end-of-life care honored. A major educational effort is necessarily directed at the general public, caregivers of all sorts, and especially physicians in order both to increase execution of advance directives and to ensure their impact on clinical practice. Improvement of legislation may be needed to provide penalties for those who refuse to follow valid advance directives.

Much more attention needs to be given to developing institutional mechanisms in health care facilities to ensure that institutional policies actually are reflected in clinical practice. Much better use of existing policies and techniques for dealing with predictable crisis in the care of the elderly is long overdue. Timely discussion of such orders as do not resuscitate (DNR), do not hospitalize, do not tube feed, and do not administer antibiotics and careful and timely attention to existing living wills and advance directives are vital to ethical decision making in the care of the judgment-impaired elderly. The medical records of the elderly are full of failures by health care professionals to discuss and address these long-established ways to deal with predictable problems in a timely manner. As is so often the case in moral matters, the problem is not so much that of not knowing what to do or what ought to be done, but of lacking the will to do it.

9

Ethical Issues in Mental Health Care

Martha Holstein and David McCurdy

ETHICAL ISSUES AT THE INTERSECTION OF MENTAL HEALTH AND AGING

With few exceptions—ethics and dementia, competency and decisional capacity, guardianship, and adult protective services—the intersection of mental health, aging, and ethics has received little attention. More broadly, considerations of ethics and mental health have focused on distributional questions, for example, priority setting for insured mental health benefits (Boyle & Callahan, 1995; Sabin & Daniels, 1994) or the ethical implications of diagnostic classifications (Sadler, Wiggins, & Schwartz, 1994), without regard to the possible relevance of age. Recently, efforts to understand the ethical implications of managed care have touched upon mental health services for older people (Wetle, 1993).

This chapter will move in other directions. It opens by describing a specific way of thinking about ethics, mental health, and aging. This perspective is broadly social in orientation and focuses on issues that transcend individual decision making. Thus the chapter's second section will address the historical context in which many of these social problems arose. Turning next to practical issues, the chapter will identify ethically sensitive issues in mental health care for the elderly. Next, it will raise and suggest answers to the question, what ought to be the ends of mental health care for the elderly? In conclusion, it will develop recommendations for mental health care grounded in normative ends. This chapter will not address questions that are well covered elsewhere, such as issues of competency or guardianship (see *Generations*, suppl. 1990, for an overview of these themes).

ETHICS, AGING, AND MENTAL HEALTH

To reflect about mental health, ethics, and aging is also to ask, what is the territory for such reflection? For the past decade, as ethicists have considered aging and gerontologists and geriatricians have deepened their interest in and knowledge about biomedical ethics, ethics has tended to focus on bracketed moments when individuals must make decisions. In this thinking, ethics became a "decision-procedure for resolving conflict-of-choice situations" (Hauerwas & Burrell, 1977, p. 8). Moral issues remained invisible until a quandary arose. A person with dementia, for example, regularly forgot to turn off the stove or took off in the car and got lost. Caregivers appropriately worried about safety: should they take away the car keys or insist that mother can no longer live alone? This "dilemma," generally framed in terms of autonomy versus beneficence, obscures other moral aspects of the person's unique situation. She must reshape the ongoing course of her life in radically different settings and in changed circumstances. The car keys and the stove are elemental issues of safety, but only one aspect of the patient/caregiver moral encounter. Attention to "safety" is not limited to physical safety; it has to be tested against other goals (Collopy, 1995) and other moral responsibilities, such as supporting continuities for the sake of self-preservation. Are there ways to facilitate the patient's ability to live according to old habits and ways of life while also protecting her from endangerment?

Support for such self-maintenance activities for the person with mental or physical diminishment is a central ethical concern. A sense of self, the ability to answer the question "who am I?", is foundational and therefore prior to autonomy. This good relies on knowing our beliefs and values and thus what we consider good or bad, worth doing or not doing, what has meaning and importance, and what is trivial and secondary (C. Taylor, 1989). This understanding of the self means that we do not act simply according to preferences. A deeply evaluative dimension often resting on unarticulated moral sources is central to this conception of the self (ten Have, 1994).

Thus choices about specifics occur within a broad framework of meaning, and the mix of beliefs, values, and sources constituting this framework is simultaneously embedded in culture. This interplay between particularity—that which gives each of us our integrity and personal identity—and culture underscores the relationships among context, notions of self, and personal and social meanings. We can, for example, exercise real autonomy only when we can make choices within the realm of what matters. Viewed in this light, many of the options that society offers older people do not constitute real choices. If this observation is correct, it can have considerable influence on the state of one's mental health. Imagine living in a world in which the choices we faced were, in essence, meaningless to us; the choice between beef and pork is not a choice to the vegetarian.

Even the person with dementia has the need to struggle as much as possible to maintain connections with a sense of self. What kind of self remains? What can others do to preserve or enhance that self? For the person with dementia, traditional notions of personhood, in which moral agency and continuity are central features, may need revision. We would like to offer Tom Kitwood's (1997) definition of personhood. Kitwood, a social and moral psychologist from Bradford, England, suggests that "personhood . . . is a standing or status that is bestowed upon one human being, by others, in the context of relationship and social being. It implies recognition, respect, and trust. Both the according of personhood, and the failure to do so, have consequences that are empirically testable" (p. 8). While this definition barely does justice to Kitwood's rich notions and practical suggestions for its enhancement, it does remind us that dementia does not remove the sufferer from the ranks of being a person. While it may be more difficult for him or her to articulate and act upon internal moral beliefs, we can still engage with him or her and show our continued commitment to him or her as a person. One moral responsibility, then, is to show respect, to encourage dignity, and to help demented elders find ways to enact what they believe are their deepest moral values. For example, might others support an elder's failing memory by sharing their own recollections of the elder and events in his life?

To live a life defined as good for the person with dementia and for people with less disabling mental and physical impairments thus requires enabling circumstances. This conception of morality is necessarily expansive. It means, for example, recognizing disabling conditions in society, seeking to rectify them, and doing what is possible to facilitate an older person's ability to live in meaningful ways, however threatened he or she is by internal or external changes. Quandary ethics and its decontextualized understandings, in contrast, generally take background conditions for granted, particularly the existing social, economic, or cultural framework in which quandaries arise. Although it grapples with distributional questions, it generally fails to take seriously other challenges to justice and human well-being—marginality, cultural imperialism, and powerlessness, to name just a few—that can easily affect the mental well-being of older people (Young, 1990).

Addressing mental health, aging, and ethics in the fullest sense requires attention to these more expansive concerns. It means doing so not only in traditional distributional terms—that is, assessing the extent, type, and distribution of health care services appropriate for the elderly—but also in terms of other conditions that sharpen and broaden conceptions of justice. Yet even distributional questions, which gained particular attention following proposals for age-based rationing of health care, have never been adequately addressed. As a community, we have effectively limited discussions about distributional issues where the elderly are concerned. Thus the discussion here will indicate that these distributional questions—both on micro and macro levels—remain open and are particularly important in mental health care for older people.

In the view of ethics we propose, dignity is also a critical grounding both for ethics and for mental health. Dignity is not obtainable in isolation since it requires that we see ourselves as commanding the respect of those around us (C. Taylor, 1989); therefore it transcends autonomy. It recognizes a crowded moral universe of others to whom the elder wants to be accountable and from whom he or she wants due regard. This way of understanding morality means entering the often "messy," not easily articulated, but rich moral world of elders, their families, and communities. At a most fundamental level, it asks us to come to know their world in intimate detail, for only then can we know what confers dignity and how we can help preserve it as they face an often painful confrontation with late life. Caring, justice, mutuality, and reciprocity interact to support dignity.

Thus ethical reflection must attend to how people act toward one another in the quotidian world of everyday encounters. It asks what is important to and for someone and in what ways; it asks how to conduct our relations with other people; and it encourages critical awareness of what one approves and disapproves, and why. This understanding encompasses individual relationships, group interactions, and broader social responsiveness. Each of these situations has a moral valence.

In matters of mental health and illness, attention has normally centered on competency determinations and legal remedies for the person unable to care for himself or herself. A standard question, for example, is how to respond ethically to self-neglect (as determined by norms that may differ from the client's). The sources of self-neglect, however, may be rooted in the anomie of meaninglessness or depression. What then, in this view, do we owe people—other than a pharmacological fix—that addresses grief or depression or meaninglessness while it also preserves dignity? What social remedies are available to rectify the loss of dignity or the absence of meaningful choices? What interactive qualities of family and other caregiving relationships affect the behavioral manifestations of dementia or other forms of mental illness? What cultural conditions arouse feelings of social devaluation or stigma or, alternatively, heighten an elder's sense of belonging and responsibility? The view of ethics we propose moves questions that had once been contained in the social service or public policy arena into the ethical arena.

Given this enlarged definition of the ethical terrain, the very question of the definition of need becomes both significant and ethical in nature. Who defines need and on what terms is fundamentally an ethical question. An enlarged view of ethics also takes seriously social values about aging and old age. Neither society's definition of need nor its priorities are ethically neutral. They provide the subtext that shapes how key actors respond to older people, to their mental health needs, and to the conditions that often provoke mental changes. Ethical issues, on a social level, then arise at the level of needs definition and action. Can or ought need, for example, to be addressed on the individual level rather than focusing on the social conditions that often helped create need in the first place? For mental health professionals, this question means thinking about the breadth of their mandate with patients and families—to cure or ameliorate mental illness or to shape notions of the good life and speak to its enactment (this issue is further discussed later). As the historian Michael Ignatieff (1986) pointed out, at the heart of responsible political argument is the question of which needs can be met by politics, that is, socially, and which cannot. "Much of politics is ... an effort to define need collectively" (D. Stone, 1988, p. 81). In the area of mental health, answers to questions such as what needs ought to compel attention and who decides do not command universal agreement. For Ignatieff, "A theory of human needs has to be premised on some set of choices about what humans need in order to be human: not what they need to be happy or free, since these are subsidiary goals, but what they need in order to realize the full extent of their potential" (p. 15). These needs include love, respect, honor, dignity, and solidarity with others. We cite Ignatieff's generous vision that situates need within a larger theory of human good both as indicative of the value-based nature of needs definition and as a contrast to the impoverished notions of need that have configured social responses to the elderly, especially elders with mental impairments.

On the one hand, this chapter cannot address each element in the ethical terrain just described; on the other hand, it will address some questions not raised so far, such as the ethical responsibility of the individual elder in relation to his or her mental health. The chapter will focus primarily, however, on those issues that relate to questions of access, the amelioration of the social conditions and cultural devaluation that contribute to the incidence of suboptimal mental health in older people. The reminder, however, that ethical behavior toward and with the older person afflicted with mental disabilities transcends decision making should be kept in view as one engages in services for and with that person. Whatever helps an individual to maintain a sense of self, to be able to give an account of meaning, and to feel a sense of social connectedness and solidarity is a moral action and should not be discounted.

MENTAL HEALTH AND AGING: HISTORICAL BACKGROUND

Historically, American society has had ambivalent responses toward its aged members. On the one hand, older people have generally been favored as "deserving"; thus the state attempted, however modestly, to provide some care for older people in need. At the same time, the medical profession and the broader society had few expectations of these elders. These low social expectations shaped conceptions of what constituted "normal" mental health. Well into the second half of this century, these attitudes blurred the line between health and disease and camouflaged signs of mental distress or illness. Even "senile dementia" was often taken to be consistent with old age.

This assumption—that serious decline in mental status accompanied old age— and its consequences show how normative premises influence definitions of normality and pathology. Because they influence distributional schemata, these premises are insistently ethical in nature. Conditions defined as inevitable or expected consequences of old age could not simultaneously ground a "need" since "treatment" for an inevitable condition was, on its face, absurd. The situation placed older people with mental impairments in the proverbial "no-care zone." Families, who bore the brunt of daily care for older people with mental and physical disabilities, remained largely invisible. Society presumed their caregiving.

Older people who either needed more care than their families could provide or had no families had few options. For much of the nineteenth century, the almshouse brought together the poor of all ages, the mentally and physically disabled, and vagrants of all sorts; it provided little more than a bed and some food. The "deservingness" of the aged did not translate into better care. Later in the century, many older people were rediagnosed and transferred to state mental hospitals to take advantage of state financing. Older patients rarely received treatment; once they were admitted and labeled as having "organic brain syndrome," they were abandoned as these low-budget state hospitals provided whatever minimal care they could to those they believed had a chance for recovery (Hartwell, 1943, p. 138). As historian Gerald Grob (1983) noted, "The role of caretaker for individuals who were socially marginal and who lacked either resources or families (or both) was frowned upon by a specialty [psychiatry] that defined its mission in medical and scientific terms" (p. 143). Nascent nursing homes (or homes for the aged) emerged in the nineteenth century to care for individuals of certain religious or racial backgrounds but provided little or no medical care.

More recently, the community mental health movement and the 1987 Omnibus Budget Reconciliation Act (OBRA) mandate to provide mental health services to older people in nursing homes have provided the structure and the regulatory backing for the care of older people with mental impairments. Yet their impact has not been great. For reasons to be described in the next section, older people have not been regular users of community mental health services, and psychiatry has not been a visible presence in the nursing home. Pharmacological interventions are easier to provide than group therapy or individual psychotherapy (Binney & Swan, 1991; H. G. Koenig, George, & Schneider, 1994). Part of the reason may lie in social attitudes toward aging, old age, and mental illness that the aged and their families, and even practitioners, internalized. It is to these social attitudes and their ethical implications that we now turn.

SOCIAL ATTITUDES TOWARD OLD AGE AND MENTAL ILLNESS

Many elders and their families (Kraft, 1991) share the shame that society typically attaches to individuals who publicly display signs of mental illness. Such stigma not only accentuates the distress caused by the illness itself (Sievertsen & Brown, 1996; Hiatt & Dell, 1993), but also reinforces an unwillingness to seek treatment, especially if that treatment is available only with public assistance. "Deliberate attempts to make the use of welfare services unpleasant or degrading" may compound the shame and can embarrass both patients and families (Scallet & Havel, 1995, p. 89). As Ignatieff (1986) suggests, welfare services meet important instrumental needs; they are to be judged morally, however, by the interactions they foster and the dignity they uphold.

In addition, the erroneous belief that "mental health decline is inevitable with aging"—a living remnant of past misconceptions—reflects a widespread tendency to "pathologize" old age (Osgood, 1995; Wykle & Musil, 1993). Attributing mental discomfort to old age itself may induce patients, family members, and even practitioners unconsciously to raise their threshold of symptom identification and deny that any "real" problem exists. The result may be a resigned passivity affecting all parties involved, including professionals (Ahmed & Takeshita, 1996–1997; George, 1993). These dynamics have important ethical implications. They lead families—and elders themselves—to jeopardize the elder's well-being by delaying efforts to seek treatment. They block professionals' recognition of specific and treatable medical problems and thus undermine the medical prevention or amelioration of harms to patients. In the process, they perpetuate familial and social conditions that impede elders' flourishing.

The devaluation of old age and the belief that old age itself is the cause of mental symptoms may be concealed in such ostensibly objective calculations as cost-benefit analysis and quality-adjusted life years (QALYs), which often ground resource-allocation strategies. These measures inevitably reflect someone's or some group's values about what constitutes a mental health "benefit" to aging persons, what "quality" of mental health is expectable and acceptable, and how long that benefit or life quality should last to be deemed affordable and reimbursable. Judgments based on these measures are not value neutral—in fact, they tend to devalue old age—yet they affect services targeted at promotion and prevention and the treatment of mental illness itself. These judgments deserve ethical scrutiny because they are not merely "medical" or "economic," but philosophical and ethical in nature. They reflect a tacit moral weighing of individual and societal interests, an assessment of the value (or disvalue) of life itself in later years, and an interpretation of the meaning and worth of mental health as one good among others. Such observations redirect attention to needs identification: who will make these important value-laden decisions, and on what basis?

It is difficult to gauge fully the depth and effects of societal attitudes toward mental illness in aging persons. If professionals and others perceive that the mental health needs of elders represent a potential drain on society's resources and also believe that the aged get only minimal and fleeting benefits from such services, then the incentive to invest time, resources, and emotional energy will be minimal. Indeed, until quite recently the mental health problems of the old interested few providers (Finkel, 1993). Provider fears about mental illness itself, or the effort involved in "managing" it, have sometimes contributed to this reality and exacerbated elders' access problems in the process. Families seeking to place a cognitively impaired loved one with a history of mental illness, for example, may find few facilities willing to accept the patient as a new resident, even if symptoms of the illness are not currently evident. Fortunately, if also ironically, economic pressures have recently led some nursing homes to reevaluate this reluctance (Sievertsen & Brown, 1996). As in the past, care seems to follow funding.

Similarly, a history of mental illness can affect access to health insurance; it can precipitate the cancellation or denial of coverage just when older persons may wish not only to continue existing policies but also to acquire supplemental coverage (Hiatt & Dell, 1993). What societal attitudes might lie beneath the continuing permissibility of such "actuarial" denials of access? While it has become fashionable to blame "managed care" for the limited resources available to treat mental illness or support preventive efforts (Sharpe, 1997), one can ask whether managed care (or the insurance industry generally) is actually the scapegoat societally assigned to enact implicit values of cost containment and treatment limitation that we as a society are reluctant to acknowledge openly (Sabin, 1995).

Each of the problem areas discussed in this section exerts a subtle influence on society's response to mental health needs in the elderly, whether at the level of resource allocation or in individual cases where the tendency to discount signs of distress has social roots. Further, this brief examination of background conditions shows how socially shaped beliefs and values can influence determinations of what constitutes a need to which society will respond. Mental illness, for example, becomes a social problem only if decision makers consider the behaviors manifested as sufficiently deviant—by some standard—to warrant interventions. For much of American history, the view that older people had limited capacities and potentialities for self-realization and participation in family and institutional life was held almost universally. This view, which in some measure persists today, generally meant that serious mental conditions of the elderly received little attention.

For these reasons, ethical analysis that focuses almost exclusively on distributional problems puts the proverbial cart before the horse. Before one can decide a distributional formula, one must decide what goods will be distributed. Yet that cannot be done fairly without a deep understanding of social attitudes toward the aged and the conditions deemed worthy of attention. Prejudicial perspectives preemptively limit the range of goods considered available for distribution. This problem may be compared to the problems associated with organ transplantation. While a good system exists for determining how available organs will be distributed to individuals on the national transplant list, the issue of how people make it to the list in the first place is clouded by tacit social valuations of who will be a "good" recipient. The background conditions are rarely the subject of ethical analysis.

FACTORS RELATED TO MENTAL HEALTH AND MENTAL ILLNESS

Taking these background conditions seriously requires attention to factors that influence the experience of mental wellness or illness. On the most basic level, psychological well-being—feelings of comfort, high self-esteem, belief in one's own dignity, self-respect, solidarity—is no less important in old age than at any other stage of one's life. In old age, however, threats to such well-being are so frequent and pervasive that they may be taken for granted. These threats emerge from many directions simultaneously. Despite the general success of the Social Security program in lifting older adults from poverty, many individuals, especially women of color, still hover very close to the poverty line. Low socioeconomic status is an important contributing factor in the development of late-life mental illness and may be the thread that links gender, race, ethnicity, and mental illness (Wykle & Musil, 1993). A long-term chronic illness such as Alzheimer's disease is not only devastating in itself but can easily push a once-comfortable family into poverty. Ill health, among the strongest predictors of psychological distress, can easily reinforce the threats to well-being that economic fears instill. As such, ill health contributes to lower life satisfaction and psychological symptomatology (Levin & Tobin, 1995). Many of these factors reinforce one another; that is, female gender, low socioeconomic status, poor physical health, and stressful life events tend to interact, to the detriment of an individual's mental health. Other contingent features of old age also negatively influence feelings of well-being. Among them are widowhood, troubled relationships with spouses or children, and lack of social contacts. These factors can result in transient depression or more lasting mental impairments. Ignoring these problems and again focusing too single-mindedly on distributional questions will only assure the continuation of many sources of mental health problems in the elderly.

Other cultural sources of discomfort and disease are less visible but nonetheless potent. In a society that values doing over being, stresses productivity, and expects people to meet middle-aged functional norms well into old age, the older person can easily feel devalued if he or she cannot live up to these norms (Fahey & Holstein, 1993). Emphasizing the productive capacities of older people, for example, requires a dual ethical analysis. Most advocates of this approach have focused on its benefits. These benefits, however, must be set against serious threats that this new cultural ideal poses, especially for older women (see Holstein, 1999).

What, then, are the most salient ethical implications of this broad survey of the underlying factors that connect mental illness and old age, and how do they relate to decisions about levels of intervention? First, ethical analysis should begin with the most comprehensive understanding possible of the conditions known to be associated with mental health and its converse. While we, as a society, may opt to respond only at the individual and "repair" levels—if we respond at all—it is still essential to probe for the underlying conditions that may provoke the onset of disabling mental conditions. Once a detailed understanding emerges of the factors that contribute to mental illness in old age, the next question is whether society has any moral obligation to improve those conditions susceptible to amelioration.

Some of these conditions, as described in the preceding section, are broadly cultural and social. Other factors are associated with the ways mental illness manifests itself in old age; these factors, in turn, affect the nature of the mental health services that should be offered to older people. A common feature of these factors is their tendency to hinder prompt and accurate recognition of the illness itself. Without adequate diagnosis, appropriate treatment does not follow. Recognizing problems is the first step in assuring that services—even basic services—are available. It is to concerns about recognition and associated issues that we now turn.

RECOGNITION, RESPONSE, AND ACCESS IN SPECIFIC CIRCUMSTANCES

Recognizing a mental health problem is critical to obtaining or providing timely and effective responses to the problem. Societal recognition of problems, as previously noted, is also crucial in assuring access to care. Striving, both as individuals—practitioners, family members, and elders themselves—and as a society, to maximize recognition of genuine problems, provide appropriate access to care, and thus relieve suffering and minimize harm to the elders affected is a pivotal, shared moral responsibility. Achieving this goal is more easily said than done. Problems arising in the interaction of physical and mental symptoms, in developing mental illness in old age or growing old with mental illness, and in addressing elder depression, anxiety, and substance abuse all highlight issues associated with recognition.

Physical ailments, for example, may render mental health problems invisible or may distract health practitioners from attending to the patient's psychological distress (Gurian & Goisman, 1993; Wykle & Musil, 1993). Biomedicine tends to focus on physical symptoms; consequently, it looks for physical rather than "psychological" causes of mental problems, thereby reinforcing problems of recognition. Reimbursement, in turn, depends on identification. If mental health problems often appear in physical disguise or if mental health problems result in physical symptoms, then it is the obligation of physicians, other providers, and ultimately the medical research and education communities to recognize these interactions so that harm to patients is prevented or at least mitigated.

In addition to the often direct relationship between physical problems and mental conditions, medications used to treat coexisting illnesses can exacerbate the effects of physical illnesses on mental disorders and vice versa. These interactions may be undesirable, unpredictable, and quite different from patterns in younger people (Ahmed & Takeshita, 1996–1997). Both patient and practitioner may miss the cognitive, emotional, and physical signs of these untoward drug interactions, which are often worsened by an elder's self-medicating habits. Such failures of recognition can result in unintended harm to patients.

While inevitably physicians and other practitioners will sometimes fail to recognize and respond appropriately to the mental health problems of older patients, when such failures affect a particular patient group disproportionately, they constitute not only a harm but also an injustice. If failures to provide optimal care can stem from inaccurate and biased societal assumptions about age and old people, then it is true that societal ageism also affects practitioners, who are, after all, embedded in a larger cultural milieu that tends to devalue old age (Osgood, 1995). When one source of both harm and injustice can thus be located in the larger culture, questions must be raised about the obligation to respond at the cultural level.

Many older adults experience not only psychological discomfort but specific forms of mental illness (here we refer to conditions other than dementia). Some have grappled with such conditions on and off throughout their lives; some become mentally ill only in old age. In contrast to care for psychological well-being, care for mental illness most often falls within the purview of biomedicine, where older people encounter problems of access and appropriate care comparable to problems of younger people. As noted earlier, their own internal resistances to mental health care and external resistances from their families and the mental health profession often compound such problems.

Diagnostic gray areas for both late-onset and continuing mental health problems, whatever their cause, contribute to important ethical problems associated with problem recognition. Elders are more likely than younger people to experience one or more symptoms of mental illness that substantially affect their quality of life without qualifying as full-blown mental illnesses by *DSM-IV* criteria (American Psychiatric Association, 1994). Sometimes the symptoms are secondary to Alzheimer's disease or another dementing condition; for example, patients with early dementia may display paranoia and other cognitive and behavioral symptoms. These symptoms, often resulting in physical violence toward others, can pose particularly difficult management problems for spouses and other family caregivers. For these caregivers, medical and payer acknowledgment of these dementia-related symptoms as a form of mental illness is critical (Sievertsen & Brown, 1996); access to reimbursable psychiatric treatment hinges on the validation provided by such acknowledgments.

Depression and anxiety—either as late-onset or as continuing conditions—also frequently manifest themselves as discrete symptoms rather than disorders that fully meet *DSM-IV* diagnostic criteria (Wykle & Musil, 1993; George, 1993; Gurian & Goisman, 1993). The frequent admixture of depressive or anxiety symptoms enumerated in *DSM-IV* with symptoms of physical illness and cognitive impairment raises questions about the appropriateness for older patients of *DSM-IV* criteria (George, 1993; Ahmed & Takeshita, 1996–1997; Gurian & Goisman, 1993). Perhaps it is time to reconsider the "age-fairness" (George,

1993, p. 37) of these criteria, not only in order to secure just reimbursement for age-appropriate treatment but also to reeducate clinicians who use *DSM-IV* criteria as a primary guide in recognizing depression and anxiety symptoms. This distinctive clinical presentation in elders can intensify the tendency of both practitioners and patients not to recognize these mental health problems.

Suicide is a particular risk associated with depression in elders. The suicide rate for older persons in the United States is nearly double that of the population at large, with older men at greatest risk. Few suicidal elders seek mental health treatment, yet three-quarters of those who do commit suicide "are likely to have seen a physician or other primary health care provider in the last month of life" (Ahmed & Takeshita, 1996–1997, p. 19). If this figure points to a widespread failure to recognize clinical signs of suicidality, the depression that is a prime risk factor for suicide also goes widely unrecognized: "only one-sixth" of elders affected by depression "are properly diagnosed and treated" (Ahmed & Takeshita, 1996–1997, p. 48). In addressing suicidality, the obligation to improve clinical recognition derives not so much from the effort to prevent or remove impairments to the elder's quality of life, but primarily from the prevention of avoidable premature death that, tragically, could result from a normally treatable condition. It might also be worth asking whether any unspoken societal attitudes and values play a role in the massive failure of recognition that untreated depression and the high rate of elder suicide represent.

The abuse of alcohol and other substances by elders often goes unrecognized (Atkinson, Ganzini, & Bernstein, 1992), in part because these disorders inspire persistent denial by the patient and even those close to the patient. Thus a primary need is to promote awareness of the signs of substance-abuse disorders among elders and counteract the tendency to deny their existence. Often a second need is to help others avoid blaming the elder in the mistaken belief that a failure of character and "will power" is the primary cause of the substance-abuse problem. Instead, education and counseling or support-group participation are often needed and usually helpful. The demonstrated benefits to substance-abuse patients, including elders, of following a spiritual recovery program suggest the further obligation to cultivate among all concerned—perhaps especially providers and payers—awareness and acceptance of these programs and their potential benefits (H. G. Koenig, 1995).

Ethically, our consideration of the recognition and access issues arising in elder depression, anxiety, and substance abuse suggests two overriding aims that should guide our societal and medical approach to mental disorders generally. We should seek proactively to reduce the incidence of such disorders and their symptoms, and we should strive to minimize their debilitating effects when they do occur. In so doing, we will act not only to prevent or remove specific harms, but also to relieve elders' suffering and even to increase their freedom, which can be severely constricted by the suffering and debility that mental illness inflicts.

GOALS, STRATEGIES, AND SOCIETY'S OPTIONS

The answers to several fundamental questions will influence perceptions about mental health and older people and the distributional issues that inevitably arise in their care. First, what goals should mental health care serve? Second, how do interventions relate to outcomes? Third, how much or what kind of care should society provide (Sabin & Daniels, 1994)? Each of these questions has contestable answers. For older people, mental health care can focus on any of three ends: helping to make well those already suffering from mental illnesses or impairments of various kinds; developing and implementing strategies that might help older people avoid mental illnesses; and striving for improved mental health and therefore enhanced potential for happiness. The first approach is circumscribed; the second and third approaches are more expansive, focusing not on the absence of mental disease but on the individual's ability to function in desirably positive ways, that is, to experience a subjective sense of well-being that is also socially validated. At their most expansive, these approaches can direct attention to identifiable prevention and enhancement strategies, especially for conditions that are provoked by the contingent features associated with old age. This view asks about the nature and extent of society's obligation to ameliorate conditions that contribute to disease. As such, it moves toward questions about culture, society, economics, and family, to name just a few variables, each beyond the biomedical system of care. Yet that system has tended to be the best-supported and the most available locus of care; thus older people are most apt to receive care in their role as patients or clients.

The prevailing, though not hegemonic, view is that mental health services for the old, as for other age groups, have as their primary obligation the treatment of mental illness and, to some extent, "problems in living," however defined. Despite this bias, strong arguments for the more expansive view are readily available. For example, Browning (1991) observes:

Psychiatry cannot focus properly on mental illness unless it has positive images of mental health (which must in part be elaborated philosophically) as well as more general images of the good person and the good society.... [P]sychiatry can have no defensible grounds on which to address problems in living unless it attends to larger issues of social philosophy. Dealing with problems in living entails removing illness or developmental impediments; it also involves investigating with the client certain positive images of how to live—images that will inevitably entail ideas about the good person and the good society. (p. 7)

This view can consider psychiatry as a foundation for promoting social change and social reform (Drane, 1991). More modestly, it can "survey and test images of the good person and good society" as the substructure for working with individuals who are either mentally ill or experiencing "problems in living"

(Browning, 1991, p. 7). These images, as the historical review has suggested, are necessarily value laden. It is possible, however, to face these value dimensions openly. If psychiatry does not do so, it has little recourse except retreat to the biomedical model and its reductionist views. A biological conceptualization of mental illness can, as observed earlier, result in the psychological abandonment of patients who face situational problems.

Medical understandings and medically managed treatment of mental illness constitute the biomedical model that has dominated care of the mentally ill for many years. The medicalization of old age, although a more recent development, is an undeniable if somewhat less pervasive reality. Because it typically "treats" problems that already exist, the medical approach favors what some have termed "illness care" as contrasted with health care. In the illness care approach, health has typically meant the absence of disease, and treatment of pathology has generally received more attention than prevention of illness or disease. The promotion of health or wellness, except on the explicitly individual level, has typically received even less attention.

In our view, the ethics of mental health and aging must place prevention and promotion on individual, social, and cultural levels at the center of its concern. To suggest a concept of mental health is to identify the goods at the intersection of aging and mental health that we as persons and as a society should enact and promote. Such a positive concept attempts to go beyond the biomedical model, which too often confines itself to identifying the evils (illness or pathology) to be avoided or mitigated. Thus in what follows we explore various ideas of mental health and suggest our own working concept, examine the prevention of mental illness and the promotion of mental health, and suggest approaches to prevention and promotion in light of our understandings of mental health and mental illness.

CONCEPTS OF MENTAL HEALTH

Because health is a complex concept, efforts to "define" mental health can be diffuse and ambiguous. Moreover, formal definitions are one thing; operational usage is another. In practice, mental health has often been construed minimally as the absence of mental illness. In the prevailing biomedical model, a second distinction has existed between health as the absence of illness and health as the absence of disease. In this view, illness is a condition of, and is suffered by, persons, while disease is properly a process affecting a bodily organ (Hill, 1996)—normally, in the case of diseases constituting mental illness, the brain. Operationally, the biomedical model has tended to focus on disease, which is itself a polysemous concept. Disease definitions are themselves shaped by normative notions of human functioning. As nineteenth-century thinking about health and disease in old age revealed, if one has low expectations for functional capacities in old age, a condition will not be viewed as a disease.

Given the definitional difficulties, one might be tempted to abandon the hope of constructing a broadly acceptable concept of mental health as a positive good. It is nonetheless important to make the attempt. Historically, in the biomedical model it is concepts of *disease* that have served to define what is worthy of societal attention and action. Disease concepts have, in effect, defined a range of evils to be avoided or at least mitigated through strenuous societal, professional, and (often) personal efforts. Ideas of disease do not, however, delineate a range of goods to be sought and promoted, nor do they create space for societal means to join or even replace medical measures in serving and promoting the human good of which mental health is a key dimension. Still less have disease concepts addressed *attitudes* of society and its members that may affect the mental health of elders (Osgood, 1995; Ignatieff, 1986).

Alternatively, in recent years and largely as a result of the mid-twentieth-century community mental health movement (Anderson, 1990), mental health has often been viewed as a positive goal to be pursued, a "state of being well" (Hill, 1996, p. 785) according to some understanding of "wellness." Indeed, the term " 'positive' mental health," elaborated in a 1958 study by the Joint Commission on Mental Illness and Health, grows out of the community mental health perspective (Sherman, 1993). Unlike the biomedical model, which focused on disease as a biological entity, the community mental health movement has operated from the conviction that psychosocial and spiritual factors played a significant role in both the attainment of mental health and the prevention of mental illness. In this operational model, relationships, societal supports and norms, and religion all play a vital part in promoting and maintaining mental health. Moreover, the focus of intervention moves from merely supporting an individual's day-to-day survival, as is the tendency of the illness care model, to concern for the genuine well-being of a person living in some psychosocial context (Kivnick, 1993).

Mental health or wellness in this model has been variously described. Like health generally, mental health may be an indispensable precondition of "a full and satisfying life" (Hill, 1996 p. 788) and thus an instrumental good enabling persons to "thrive, not merely survive" (Sherman, 1993, p. 43). More specifically, mental health is often assessed by such measures as "subjective well-being" or "psychological well-being," constructs deemed capable of individual self-rated assessment with the use of appropriate research instruments (Levin & Tobin, 1995). Some seek to use both "positive" and "negative" assessment categories that blend biomedical and psychosocial perspectives. Lebowitz and Niederehe (1992) propose a conceptually rich definition of health: statistical normality, the "relation of individual functioning to group or species norms," the "controllability or treatability of disordered states," and "ideals of positive functioning." Thus mental health, no mere "absence of mental disorder," entails a person's ability to function in "desirably positive ways" (p. 7). This mixed concept fails, unfortunately, to incorporate a straightforwardly psychosocial dimension, although its authors recognize inadequacies in the biomedical model. Sherman's (1993) concept of "adaptivity" as "efficacious functioning" of the person in his or her context blends subjective and observable criteria (in contrast to measures of "life satisfaction" alone), yet is not tied to a normative understanding of how people "should" age in a mentally healthy way.

Taken together, the concepts of adaptivity, positive mental health, and " 'everyday' mental health" (Kivnick, 1993, p. 15) portray a vision of the thriving elder and identify resources and attitudes that facilitate its realization. Positive mental health incorporates concepts of self-esteem, personal growth, and self-integration while recognizing that values and commitments beyond the self—"family, nation, culture, and religious belief"—are vital to "a sense of self in later life" (Sherman, 1993, p. 44). Everyday mental health points to the identification and optimization of each elder's strengths and functioning in a context of potential "resources." It is a corrective to the frequent overemphasis on deficits and losses and the tendency to decontextualize and isolate aging persons unduly. Indeed, these strengths and resources assist elders in "compensating for the weaknesses and deficits" that are an undeniable fact of their life (Kivnick, 1993, p. 15).

The vision of everyday mental health as "vital involvement" (Kivnick, 1993, p. 15), an expression of the potential of the "human spirit" (Kivnick, 1993, p. 13), may seem too optimistic and indeed may not fit all elders and their contexts equally well. Nevertheless, in focusing on the human spirit and the social resources that support it, this perspective recognizes not only elders' needs for meaning and their capacity to discover or create meaning, but also the importance of culture and religion in supporting such vitality of spirit. As part of the "territory" of ethics described earlier, continuity of self and security in one's meaning system are foundational for older people, as for others.

Thus achieving everyday mental health is not simply an individual accomplishment. It needs cultural and communal support if its internal strengths are to flourish. In later life, cultivating these strengths is, if anything, more important than ever. "As physical strengths diminish, and external supports fade away, internal strength and health become increasingly important to every elder's ongoing integrity" (Kivnick, 1993, p. 16). Thus "change or loss in one area is responded to in a compensatory manner in another area" (G. Cohen, 1993, p. 48).

Unfortunately, in modern society the social supports that undergird such integrity are in particular jeopardy. Traditional societies have generally accorded elders significant roles in relation to "the sacred aspect of culture" (Gutmann, 1992, p. 86). Meeting the society's needs through participation in these roles has also supported the relational, emotional, and spiritual well-being of the elders themselves by providing "social status; respect, often verging on fear and awe; the assurance of social security from obligated kinfolk; and the sense of connection to a benevolent spiritual order" (Gutmann, 1992, p. 86). Such role-related benefits to the elder also ward off or neutralize psychological and spiritual perils that threaten the aging person, such as self-absorbed distortions of normal narcissism that react to the losses and vulnerabilities of aging with "hypochondria, egocentricity, fussily obsessive rituals, hypersensitivity to minor slights,'' or reactive depression (Gutmann, 1992, p. 87).

Modern cultures generally weaken the traditional structures that had previously supported and buffered elders psychologically and spiritually. For example, opportunities to participate in respected roles and mediate the sacred are typically diminished or absent. The resulting "deculturation" both "deprives the aged of congenial, development-sponsoring social circumstances" and "depletes their intrapsychic domain" (Gutmann, 1992, p. 94). It does so, in part, by depriving elders of significant obligations and responsibilities, not only to but for their communities. Concepts of reciprocity and the ability to enact such concepts in practice are often at the center of a person's self-evaluation, the sense that he or she is or is not a good person leading a good life. A culture that has no significant place for its elders denies them this fundamental moral value.

Ironically, the very modernity whose technology has lengthened life and improved elders' physical health more than many had predicted has simultaneously eroded or even destroyed crucial psychosocial and spiritual supports that promote (and, equally important, maintain) elders' everyday mental health. The ethics of preventing mental illness and promoting mental health must therefore consider not only the remedies and preventive measures supplied by biomedicine, but also the essential contributions of culture, community, and religion to maintaining and enhancing well-being in later life.

PREVENTING, PROMOTING, AND MAINTAINING

Preventive medicine commonly speaks of primary and secondary prevention. *Primary prevention* seeks to "prevent the onset of a disease." *Secondary prevention* "aims to identify an established disease in a presymptomatic stage in order to cure or prevent its progression" (Rubenstein, 1996–1997, p. 48). While some primary preventive measures (e.g., those aimed at preventing hypertension or diminishing certain cancer risk factors) are quite effective, medical prevention in mental health is more likely to be secondary prevention (e.g., medication to prevent the recurrence of depression).

Efforts at prevention assume that research has identified a potentially preventable condition, assessed its prevalence and morbidity, and identified potentially effective interventions. Controlled tests determine an intervention's efficacy prior to implementation in "real-world" settings where human factors such as noncompliance or incomprehension complicate the intervention's effectiveness. Last but not least, the intervention's effectiveness is weighed against its cost (Rubenstein, 1996–1997). Such a process has become a major approach in cost-benefit and cost-effectiveness analyses, which in turn have shaped distributional systems, with significant if unintended impacts on elders.

Thus it is particularly relevant that a consensus of expert panels has singled out depression as a mental health problem that is medically "preventable" (Rubenstein, 1996–1997). Clearly, depression meets the prevention criteria just outlined in that it "affects almost a third of the elderly population, is often not detected, can be effectively treated, and causes preventable suffering and even suicide." As a result, when the expert panels recommended preventive measures for inclusion in "periodic healthcare provider visits," the sole mental health intervention explicitly suggested (besides attention to "memory problems" and "cognitive impairment") was preventive screening for depression (Rubenstein, 1996–1997, p. 51).

Especially because elders who commit suicide usually visit primary-care physicians shortly before their deaths, this preventive recommendation deserves applause as far as it goes. One may ask, however, if this narrow recommendation meets the provider community's responsibility for proactively assessing elders' mental health status. On the other hand, a lack of sound data identifying other "preventable" mental disorders and symptoms or supporting the effectiveness of proposed interventions renders the limited mental health recommendations understandable. In light of the recognized impact of mental disorders and symptoms on the aged (Wykle & Musil, 1993; Ahmed & Takeshita, 1996–1997; Gurian & Goisman, 1993), the need to fund and undertake new studies that rigorously consider these questions is apparent.

More problematic, perhaps, is the reality that optimal preventive care in geriatric medicine is multidisciplinary and comprehensive, addressing psychosocial as well as medical aspects of the patient's health. Such a thorough approach is "time-consuming" and "usually poorly reimbursed" and thus unlikely to be undertaken frequently (Kavesh, 1996–1997, p. 56). Unfortunately, it is also true that predominantly psychosocial preventive programs are seldom evaluated adequately, and their conceptual bases have tended to lack cohesion (Stacey-Konnert, 1993). Often, for example, preventive programs whose stated aims espouse the ideals of promoting independent living and "empowering" older persons fail to address such aims in their day-to-day implementation plans (Stacey-Konnert, 1993). Moreover, such programs, along with much of the research on mental health as "life satisfaction" or "psychological well-being" (Levin & Tobin, 1995, p. 31) may fail to address the spiritual or religious life of the person as a dimension of, and a resource for, psychosocial prevention.

In the absence of a greater number of demonstrated medical preventive interventions, can and should predominantly nonmedical, psychosocial preventive interventions assume a greater role in supporting the mental health of elders? Calls to assess and draw on the aging person's existing strengths, on inner as well as contextual resources, recognize implicitly that "mental health" is more than a medical or medically achievable good. The fact that society is more likely to support medical interventions through insurance reimbursement, however, tends to reinforce the higher status accorded these interventions.

If we are to take seriously the social responsibility to recognize and use an elder's strengths, then society must also give more attention to thinking about and describing the moral status of the elderly. Western culture, which lacks collective meaning systems and so contributes to the experience of "deculturalization," can offer little guidance about what it means to grow old (T. R. Cole, 1997). This conversation is foundational to calls to draw on the elder's own strengths. Thus, families and communities have a moral responsibility to recognize and elicit these strengths, both as resources for elders' well-being and as barriers against needless deterioration of their mental health. Further, Gutmann's (1992) observations about the devastating effects of "deculturation" on the older population would argue for the ethical desirability of cultural and communal interventions, such as efforts to restore or create anew significant roles and responsibilities for elders in their communities.

These psychosocially, spiritually, and culturally oriented efforts are more than preventive. To label them in this way understates their meaning and begs the question of an ethical responsibility to promote the mental health of elders. Clearly, "prevention" connotes avoidance of the negative, that is, illness or disease or "symptoms," without directly addressing the enhancement of mental health. We contend that just as in some sports "the best defense is a good offense," in mental health the best prevention is the active promotion of mental well-being.

If mental health promotion is limited to the biomedical framework, however, significant questions of funding and reimbursement quickly arise: Should insurers, employers, or governments pay for measures intended to optimize mental health or well-being? Do such measures belong in the insurable rubric of "medical necessity" (Sabin & Daniels, 1994)? These questions specifically concern those patients and families who face persistent severe mental illness, especially since societal commitments to foster mental well-being in the heyday of the community mental health movement often diverted resources from the chronically ill (Michels, 1995; Grob, 1983). These problems are integral to most analyses of priority setting for mental health services: who shall be treated—the worst off, those who will benefit most from treatment, or others—and for what conditions (see Boyle & Callahan, 1995, for a full treatment of priority setting in mental health).

While such questions have their place, they reveal the limits of the framework within which they are raised. Thinking about prevention and promotion tends to assume that "health," that is, most often, the absence of disease, is an end in itself and is a direct outcome of actions aimed at fostering it (or at avoiding illness). This focus overlooks the possibility that "mental health" may be more a by-product of an entire way of living within a given context than a product of goal-driven activity explicitly aimed at health or at illness avoidance. The latter view directs attention to deeper sources of mental disabilities rather than locating them entirely within the individual. This limited framework, focused on achieving mental health or avoiding mental illness, may unwittingly contribute to an unhealthy self-preoccupation (Gutmann, 1992) that undermines a legitimate sense of the elder's continuing ability and responsibility to contribute something worthwhile to others and to the community. Both elders and others in the community may, and we argue should, seek to internalize this understanding if elders are to assume (or reassume) a role that is optimal both for themselves and for others.

American society, dominated by a philosophy of liberal individualism and its rights-based claims, has a limited language with which to think about a "public philosophy on the meaning of aging" (D. Callahan, 1987, p. 32). Such a philosophy can provide a conceptual grounding for societal thinking about aging; the public discussion required to develop societal consensus about the philosophy could also challenge the attitudes of all generations, including elders themselves, in positive ways. Optimally, this process would serve two important ends. It would enhance elders' interior sense that their lives had meaning and elevate the significance of their lives in the eyes of the society around them (J. J. Callahan, 1988). Thus elders would receive social appreciation as they met the ethical responsibility to value their own lives and live accordingly (Sapp, 1995), together with their responsibility to contribute to the greater good. Moreover, by attending to society's attitudes toward elders, the development of a public philosophy on the meaning of aging would also address those needs of elders that cannot be met simply by the bureaucratic social mechanisms of the welfare state, no matter how efficient and supportive. Needs for belonging, dignity, and respect—to name a few such needs—can be met only in family and community, that is, through interpersonal relationships that no governmental provision can supply, let alone mandate (Ignatieff, 1986).

These larger notions of self and self-in-society relate directly to mental health. Once what moderns term mental well-being emerged from life in community, especially from contact with what the community holds sacred. Elders often had a genuine responsibility to mediate that sacrality and the community's wisdom; as a result, they had significant roles within religious or spiritual communities. With the increasing desacralization of society, elders rarely have these important communal roles that once played such an instrumental part in their continued well-being. The community mental health movement recognized religious communities as a resource and attempted to develop working relationships with those communities and their leaders for the sake of community members' mental health (Anderson, 1990). Thus religious communities assumed a real if limited role in promoting individuals' mental health and sometimes in providing mental health services. More important, they played, and can continue to play, a significant secondary-prevention role in helping those with chronic mental illness to maintain a level of relative well-being and avoid recurrences.

Perhaps most important, however, even in a more secular (or at least non-traditionally religious or spiritual) age, religious communities can be a place where elders can still give of themselves to others. In the end, the best sort of mental health or well-being appears to be a product of living for other goals and purposes in life (Anderson, 1990), perhaps especially those that involve elders and others in causes that transcend self-interest and draw them out of potential self-absorption into the service of values that elevate and fulfill them.

BALANCING THE IDEAL AND THE PRACTICAL: NORMATIVE GOALS FOR MENTAL HEALTH AND AGING

As the previous discussion has made clear, a robust normative vision for mental health and aging takes seriously the cultural, social, and other limits that older people experience in their efforts to lead personally meaningful and socially significant lives. To the extent possible, a broad social strategy is a critical vector in facilitating these ends. At one step removed from this large social vision, prevention is the desirable approach for those conditions for which we understand, at least at some basic level, the "causes." The stronger the evidence about causation, the more compelling the case for intervention; the case becomes even more compelling if the roots are socially remedial. In contrast, providing services to elders who are already impaired is more manageable; it directs attention to the more commonly addressed distributional questions: how much of which services shall be provided if the resources come from a commonly held resource pool? What justifications will ground any particular distribution? How can the state or private providers make these decisions? How do decision makers weigh and, if possible, reconcile the moral claims of different individuals and groups all contending for what are perceived to be scarce social resources? Do the elderly have any special claims on social resources, especially if society is at least partially responsible for their plight? What services should society make available to older people with mental disease? Does it matter if the mental disease is progressive and irreversible, such as multi-infarct dementia or dementia of the Alzheimer's type? In the latter case, even if the dementia is irreversible, does society have other obligations to these patients?

The last questions lead to the underlying concern touched upon throughout this chapter: what is the relationship of an individual person with a mental illness to the society in which he or she lives? Is the etiology of mental illness located within the individual, perhaps biologically or genetically based? Is the etiology of mental illness interactional (individual and environment), or is it largely contextual? What would it mean to think about mental illness in biopsychosocial terms? How can we prevent mental illness and enrich the experience of old age? Responses to these prior questions guide interventional decisions but also direct attention to underlying conditions.

These issues, however, do not exhaust the ethical problems at the intersection of mental health and aging. Both prevention and intervention require thinking about underlying or foundational moral demands that we should make on any mental health policies or services. They also raise questions about "worthiness." Can people be held blameless if their illness has its roots in chronic alcoholism or other socially disvalued activities? Who should decide what services are offered to whom?

To answer these questions requires the as-yet-unavailable public conversation about aging in society. Mental wellness, perhaps more than any other aspect of old age, cannot be divorced from society and culture. To take up mental wellness as a goal means to think seriously about collective meaning systems and a public philosophy. The hardest task then will be to balance the most desirable approach with the one that might be possible within the sociopolitical context in which we now live. That task truly lies ahead of us.

10

Ethical Issues in Personal Safety

Georgia J. Anetzberger

To live is to be at risk. It is impossible for any of us always to be perfectly safe so that harm will not happen and injury or anguish will not result. It matters little whether we are with family and friends, with strangers, or alone. It matters little whether we are at home or in another type of setting. The possibility of harm is everywhere. Each of us can try to mitigate the likelihood of harm and its effects. We can seek protection through various means, from surrogate decision-making authority in case of mental incapacity to special law enforcement for fear of crime. However, every form of protection carries with it its own set of consequences, sometimes limiting our personal freedom, sometimes creating injustices for other persons.

This chapter addresses the ethics of personal safety. The contents are arranged around five major areas of risk for older adults:

- Mistreatment by others
- Self-neglect
- Fear of crime
- Risk at home
- Risk in institutions

Although each area of risk is addressed separately, they have a unifying theme. All of us live with risk, but it is more commonplace and complicated for older people. Because they are more likely to be frail and impaired or vulnerable in other ways, older people are more likely to be dependent upon others for care. Under these circumstances, ethical dilemmas around personal safety arise in at least two ways. First, they occur in the pull between beneficence and autonomy, because it is difficult to provide care and not erode some personal freedom. Second, they result from the distribution of protections, because it is difficult to offer scarce resources to some without simultaneously depriving others.

The ethics of personal safety is a relatively new subject of study. The literature base on it is small. Paradigms for resolving ethical dilemmas on personal safety are few. The primary work has been done in the fields of elder abuse and institutional care, but even here there are only a handful of related scholarly discussions and strategies for decision making. Moreover, what exists is recent and largely untested.

Most of the work on the ethics of personal safety has been done in the United States. Although Great Britain and a few other countries, principally those in Western Europe, have expressed an interest in issues of personal safety during the past decade, this has been mainly an American domain of study and model development. Where significant work has been done elsewhere or cross-culturally, it will be presented. Otherwise, this chapter reflects American concerns and approaches.

Each chapter section has a similar organization. It begins with the description of an older person facing the risk area under consideration. The case situation is used at various times during the subsequent discussion on risk dynamics, ethical issues and dilemmas, and existing frameworks for ethical decision making to further illustrate key constructs. After all five risk areas have been examined, the chapter concludes with recommendations on what is needed to improve policy, practice, and research on the ethics of personal safety as well as projections about what the twenty-first century might hold for protecting older people and preserving their well-being.

MISTREATMENT BY OTHERS

Wilda and Thomas's Story

Wilda was blind and nearly deaf. Although arthritis and hypertension posed additional difficulties, she enjoyed reasonably good health. At age 85, she had outlived two husbands and currently resided with her only child, 57-year-old Thomas, in a second-floor inner-city apartment. The bottom floor housed a grocery of sorts on one side and a small bar on the other. Both offered staples for the household. Wilda could manage the stairs and get food at the grocery; Thomas spent most of his day drinking at the bar.

Alcoholism was a long-term problem for Thomas. His excessive drinking began in the armed forces. It became addictive following a divorce and period of unemployment that never ended. Years ago Thomas gave up looking for work, accepted public assistance, and grudgingly came to live with his mother. It was not the arrangement he preferred. However, it was cheaper than living alone, and someone had to be on hand to help when blindness and other disabilities prevented Wilda from effectively navigating her way in the world.

The household generally had an uneasy tension about it. When he was home, Thomas tended to station himself in the living room by the front window, trying to remain distant from Wilda and her constant demands. For her part, Wilda did what she could around the house and called out for Thomas when she needed help. Thomas regarded Wilda's requests as incessant nagging. Sometimes he ignored them, even to the extent of leaving the house. Other times he became enraged and lashed out at Wilda both verbally and physically. Although tirades had been going on for years, twice recently they had resulted in injury—once bruises and a bloody nose, the other time a broken arm.

Ethical Dilemmas: Comparing Elder Abuse and Other Forms of Family Violence

In some ways, the ethical dilemmas surrounding elder mistreatment by others (henceforth referred to as elder abuse) are the same as those surrounding other forms of family violence. In other ways, they are different. Some similar dilemmas include the following:

- Should health and social service professionals be required to report family violence when reporting is seen as an abridgment of patient confidentiality or may erode hard-won rapport established with the patient?
- Is family violence a private matter, or by its very nature is it subject to public scrutiny?
- Should family violence be reframed when an ethnic or religious group defines particular behavior otherwise?
- Should perpetrators be treated as criminals or persons with problems?
- Do individuals have the right to elect to remain in violent relationships? Does this right of self-determination change when society is asked to bear related health care and other costs?
- Do victims have a right to expect quick and consistent response to calls for help, even when they refuse to follow through with recommended protective measures?

Elder-abuse dilemmas differ from those for other forms of family violence. They differ from those surrounding violence against younger adults, including spouses, because age is more likely to bring with it chronic illness and disabilities. The results are dependency, need for care, and diminished opportunities for self-sufficiency or escape from the current situation based more upon physical than psychological incapacity. However, it is important not to overgeneralize the diseases and disabilities associated with old age. Most older people are not functionally incapacitated, and few suffer from Alzheimer's disease or other forms of cognitive impairment (R. A. Kane & R. L. Kane, 1987; Office of Technology Assessment, 1990). The tendency of American society to infantilize older people can result in the acceptance of this negative image by elders themselves and their consequent adoption of childlike behavior as a kind of self-fulfilling prophecy (Utech & Garrett, 1992).

Moreover, the distinctions between victim and perpetrator as well as independent and dependent are often blurred in elder abuse. There are many documented instances of violence going in both directions in these situations (e.g., Steinmetz, 1981, 1988; Coyne, 1991; Paveza et al., 1992). Typically, dual-directional abuse happens when the "victim" has dementia or other cognitive impairment with violent behavioral manifestations and the "perpetrator" is the primary or only caregiver with few coping skills or sources of social support. Similarly, several studies have found that at least with regard to physical abuse, perpetrators are more likely to be financially and otherwise dependent upon the elder than vice versa (e.g., Pillemer, 1986; Anetzberger, 1987). The introductory story illustrates the blurred dependency often characteristic of elder abuse. Thomas is financially and socially dependent on Wilda, but she is physically dependent on him.

Elder-abuse dilemmas also differ from those surrounding violence against children, because older persons who have not been adjudicated legally incompetent are categorically adults, with all the rights and responsibilities accorded adults in American society. This includes the right to pursue unpopular and even unhealthy or risky lifestyles. In addition, the caregiver role for parents with young children is clearer than that for adult children with elderly parents needing assistance. For example, it is understood that all infants need physical help and guidance from their parents. In contrast, the care requirements of disabled elderly parents by their adult children are neither culturally prescribed nor certain. Therefore, child care and its antithesis, child abuse, are less subject to ambiguity and uncertainty both legally and morally than elder care and elder abuse. Finally, the disturbing or troublesome behaviors of children that can contribute to child abuse are seen as transitory, with the expectation that children will outgrow them in normal development (Straus, Gelles, & Steinmetz, 1980; Frodi, 1981). The same perception does not apply to older people in elder-care situations, where disturbing behaviors, such as those exhibited by Wilda, represent deterioration and increasing difficulty over time (Korbin, Anetzberger, & Eckert, 1989).

Ethical Dilemmas in Elder-Abuse Roles

Ethical dilemmas in elder abuse can be analyzed by intervention role. Ten roles are particularly important to understanding and addressing this problem:

- Victim: experiences elder abuse
- Perpetrator: inflicts elder abuse
- Family, friend, or neighbor: witnesses elder abuse or its effects
- Reporter: detects elder abuse and describes it to authorities

- Investigator: assesses reported elder abuse and determines the need for services
- Service provider: offers assistance in correcting or discontinuing elder abuse
- Program administrator: manages services aimed at preventing or treating elder abuse
- Community planner: develops program and community education initiatives to address elder abuse
- Legislator: enacts public policy related to elder abuse
- Researcher: conducts studies to better understand elder abuse and effective strategies to impact it

The first three intervention roles are held by persons closely associated to particular abuse situations, the remainder by persons with professional responsibility for addressing or studying elder abuse. Each role has inherent ethical dilemmas that reflect its unique perspective on elder abuse. Illustrations of these ethical dilemmas by intervention role follow:

- Victim: If authorities find out about my situation, what will happen to me? Will they blame me for causing the problem? Find me mentally ill or incompetent? Remove me from my home? What will the authorities do to the perpetrator, who also represents family to me? What are my responsibilities to that person?
- Perpetrator: Doesn't the elder have an obligation to help me out with housing and spending money, since I'm unemployed and likely to inherit her estate anyway? Isn't it better to tie the elder in a chair than to have her wander out of the house and maybe get hurt?
- Family, friend, or neighbor: Does the abusing family's right to privacy take precedence over my responsibility as a neighbor to help? When should I act to protect others from the possibility of the perpetrator exploiting elders whom he befriends?
- Reporter: Should I report an elder-abuse situation when I don't believe that reporting will make any positive difference in it? Should I report if this places the elder at greater risk or labels someone as an elder-abuse perpetrator?
- Investigator: How honest am I with the victim as to the purpose of my visit? How much contact do I initiate with family and neighbors of the victim in an attempt to gain information?
- Service provider: What separates establishing rapport with the victim in an effort to offer service from cajoling her into compliance with my service plan? Is it appropriate for me to abandon a victim who refuses protective intervention?
- Program administrator: What are the implications of offering elder-abuse programming when scarce funding limits it to short-term crisis intervention without provision for follow-up services? How much emphasis should be placed on use of the criminal code in elder-abuse situations?
- Community planner: Should community education on elder abuse be initiated when insufficient resources exist locally for addressing the problem? What is the relative importance of case finding and crisis intervention to case prevention?

- Legislator: Should elder-abuse laws be enacted without adequate accompanying appropriations? Should protective-services laws cover all adults or only elderly ones? Does this decision in any way reinforce ageism in American society?
- Researcher: What should I do if a respondent acknowledges elder abuse? Will reporting the situation to authorities compromise my role and integrity as a researcher?

Mandatory Elder-Abuse Reporting as an Ethical Issue

Probably no ethical issue in elder abuse has engendered more controversy and discussion than mandatory reporting (e.g., Faulkner, 1982; J. J. Regan, 1990; Kapp, 1995a; Capezuti et al., 1997). The controversy surrounding mandatory reporting begins with the vague definitions of elder abuse usually associated with these laws, which do not provide a clear basis for abuse identification (J. C. Callahan, 1988; R. S. Daniels, Baumhover, & Clark-Daniels, 1989). Without this, there is concern that reporting may result in the inappropriate labeling of persons or situations as abusive, with consequent stigma or even criminal sanction wrongly applied (J. J. Callahan, 1982; Blanton, 1989). Beyond this, reporters worry about the following issues in mandatory reporting:

- Abridging patient confidentiality (Thobaben, 1989)
- Jeopardizing the relationship established with the patient (Coyne, Petenza & Berbig, 1996)
- Referring patients to agencies in which they have little confidence or that are ill equipped to provide adequate follow-up (Ambrogia & London, 1985)
- Liabilities accompanying the reporting of patients who deny that the injuries were caused by another person's actions or failure to act (Clark-Daniels, Daniels, & Baumhover, 1990)
- Reporting when there is a difference of opinion among professional colleagues on whether or not the situation should be reported or what kind of response is appropriate with ambiguous symptoms (Wetle & Fulmer, 1995)

Mandatory reporting became commonplace following the introduction of H.R. 7551 in the 96th Congress, which encouraged states to modify their adult-protective-services and elder-abuse laws and procedures to include required reporting by health officials and others in order to be compliant with the anticipated new federal law's provisions (Cravedi, 1986), which stated that the federal government would "provide assistance to States which provided for the reporting of known and suspected instances of elder abuse, neglect, and exploitation" (U.S. House Select Committee on Aging, 1981, p. 126). Today nearly all states have enacted laws that require health and social service professionals to report known or suspected situations of elder abuse (Tatara, 1995). The vast majority of states also have enacted these laws without accompanying appropriations, thereby often effectively limiting interventions to reporting and investigation (Quinn & Tomita, 1997). As a result, the variety of services required to address elder abuse situations typically is not available through public agencies charged with handling abuse reports (Capezuti et al., 1997; Jones, 1994; Meagher, 1993).

Legislators argue that the importance of mandatory reporting lies in case finding (J. J. Regan, 1990). Even if resources are not presently available to adequately address every reported abuse situation, case discovery provides a foundation from which to advocate for increased funding for protective services (Salend, Kane, Satz, & Pynoos, 1984).

An alternative perspective is offered by Crystal (1986), who argues that instead of increasing resources for older people, elder-abuse legislation has had the effect of drawing revenues away from other deserving service programs. Actually, revenues for adult protective services have decreased as elder-abuse reports have increased. In 1986, the National Aging Resource Center on Elder Abuse documented 117,000 elder-abuse reports nationwide. By 1991, reporting had reached 227,000, a 94% increase (Tatara, 1993). In contrast, the percentage of state budgets for adult protective services declined from 6.6% in 1980 to 4.7% in 1985 to 3.9% in 1989, a 41% decrease (U.S. House Select Committee on Aging, 1990).

It is interesting to note that in an effort to evaluate the effectiveness of mandatory elder-abuse reporting, the U.S. General Accounting Office (1991) surveyed 40 officials in state units on aging and adult-protective-services agencies. The results suggested that a high level of public and professional awareness was more effective for identifying abuse victims than mandatory reporting. In addition, in-home services were seen as more effective than mandatory reporting for both preventing and treating elder abuse.

D. A. Gilbert (1986) analyzed mandatory elder-abuse reporting laws from ethical and health professional perspectives. She concluded that mandatory reporting contradicts the current trend in health care that emphasizes patient autonomy. Therefore, voluntary reporting laws that promote respect for individual wishes are preferred over mandatory reporting laws. In addition, Gilbert argues:

- It is more important to obtain patient consent based upon an assumption of competence than it is to stop harm through abuse reporting.
- It is more important to protect patient confidentiality than it is to report abuse, since elder abuse is not a threat to the general public.
- It is inappropriate to report elder abuse without an adequate intervention system in place to address it; otherwise, reporting simply creates false expectations and offers no necessary benefit to abuse victims.

Several others offer guidance on when, or if, to report elder abuse, notwithstanding the mandate of reporting laws. For example, Matlaw and Mayer (1986) recommend reporting only when it will produce the most benefit for the parties involved, especially the victim. This requires assessment of the positive and negative effects that reporting will have on the elder-abuse victim. Fulmer and

O'Malley (1987) find that if the potential harm caused by reporting is great and the benefits marginal, then the situation probably should not be reported.

Assessing the effect of reporting may include evaluating the performance of agencies charged with handling elder-abuse reports (Fulmer & Anetzberger, 1995; Stein, 1991). There is some evidence to suggest that the reporter's satisfaction with authorities charged with report investigation varies inversely with the number of situations reported (Clark-Daniels et al., 1990). The result may be a reluctance on the part of victims and professionals to report further elder-abuse situations (R. S. Daniels et al., 1989). One way to overcome this barrier to reporting is for professionals to maintain a good working relationship with protective-services workers and address reporting problems directly (Anetzberger et al., 1993). Another way is to promote the establishment of public agency quality-assurance and inspection systems (Manthorpe, 1993). Too often now there is little emphasis on either quality-assurance or inspection systems in public agencies. Quality assurance means the formation of performance standards, peer-review panels, and staff training on quality improvement. Inspection systems means regular oversight by state authorities and community advisory councils. Both require an openness to scrutiny and willingness to undertake needed change.

Anetzberger has developed a hierarchy of principles for adult protective services that reflects an emphasis on individual autonomy (Anetzberger & Miller, 1995). From the most to the least important considerations for intervening on behalf of abused elders, they are the following:

1. Freedom over safety
2. Self-determination
3. Participation in decision making
4. Least restrictive alternative
5. Primacy of the adult
6. Confidentiality
7. Benefit of doubt
8. Do no harm
9. Avoidance of blame
10. Maintenance of the family

These principles can be useful to the adult-protective-services worker investigating Wilda's abuse, described earlier in the chapter. Respecting Wilda's wish for privacy (principle 5), the worker will restrict contact with family and neighbors to that absolutely essential for determining the extent of endangerment and Wilda's need for protective services. The focus of intervention will be on preventing further harm (principle 8), so long as actions taken reflect Wilda's choices and decisions (principle 2), even if that means that she continues to live in an abusive relationship with Thomas (principle 1).

In discussing the abuse with Wilda, the adult-protective-services worker learns that Wilda would ask Thomas to leave if he were not financially dependent on her. This means that the worker must try to help Thomas become self-sufficient. Possible interventions include alcoholism treatment, housing assistance, and job training and placement. As these are being explored, Thomas can benefit from counseling aimed at redirecting his aggression and frustration more appropriately and productively.

The adult-protective-services worker must establish rapport and work with both Wilda and Thomas, recognizing and emphasizing their strengths as a family (principle 10) and avoiding blame of either one as contributing to abuse occurrence (principle 9). Also, since Wilda would be less demanding of Thomas with assistance available from other sources (principle 4), the worker can help make service arrangements, including telephone reassurance and housekeeping, so long as Wilda has participated in all decisions about their selection and delivery (principle 3).

Lehmann (1992) offers an approach to evaluating clinical decisions about abuse against women using Kitchener's model of ethical justification. Like Anetzberger's, Kitchener's model is hierarchically tiered. When individuals cannot resolve ethical dilemmas at a lower level, they can engage in ethical reasoning at higher, more abstract levels. The lowest level, intuitive, focuses on ordinary moral sense and the facts of the situation. The second level, critical-evaluative, considers ethical principles, notably autonomy, nonmaleficence, beneficence, justice, and fidelity. The highest level, ethical theory, is concerned with universality and balancing achieved in ethical decision making.

Kitchener's hierarchy suggests that autonomy does not denote unlimited freedom. Applied to Wilda and Thomas, this means that Thomas does not have the right to cause Wilda physical harm and thereby jeopardize her safety and well-being. Reporting the abuse situation is desirable because of the possible benefits intervention would bring to either or both Wilda and Thomas. If Wilda refuses assistance, her right of refusal will need to be respected, because she is competent. As Quinn (1985, p. 24) reminds us, the greatest ethical challenge to practitioners in the field of elder abuse is presented by "the competent elder adult who is being abused or neglected and refuses intervention." However, reporting the abuse situation allows for the option of accepting or refusing services in a way that failure to report cannot.

SELF-NEGLECT

Anna's Story

Anna had always been considered "slow" and a loner. Sheltered by protective parents who themselves were regarded as "eccentric," she attended school only a few years before the taunting of other children convinced her parents that she would be better off at home. There Anna remained throughout her adult years. Her parents taught her to perform household tasks and garden. They also were virtually her only social contacts, since she had no friends and was never gainfully employed. On those occasions when her parents became ill, Anna provided the care that they required, rarely leaving their sides and never accepting help. When they died, she remained in the family home. By this time she was in her 60s. Her needs were few, and most of these she could manage herself from gardening, keeping guinea hens and a goat, and selling collected aluminum cans and other discarded items. Her occasional journeys into town were made on an old bicycle until a collision with an automobile left her with a single leg and limited motion in her right arm.

Anna's fortunes changed after the accident. Because she could no longer collect items for sale, she had no money, and bills went unpaid. Gardening became a monumental undertaking, with failure evident in the scant produce yield. Too quickly the house needed repairs that were impossible. With the only bathroom on the second floor, Anna began using jars and cans for waste. The discontinued utilities posed minor inconvenience until winter came, with its subzero temperatures and eventual accumulation of over 100 inches of snow. Isolated in her frigid house, Anna burned broken furniture in the fireplace and huddled close in blankets for warmth. The neighbors became concerned when they failed to see any trace of her after a major storm and contacted the sheriff, who arranged for her to stay the winter at the county home following hospital treatment for frostbite.

Characteristics of Self-Neglecting Elders

Anna's story is familiar to adult-protective-services workers who handle cases of self-neglect on a daily basis. Specifics vary, but the general circumstances of personal dysfunction and risk are the same everywhere. Actually, Anna's story is a composite of three situations of self-neglect encountered in nonmetropolitan areas of Ohio. Like others, it has seven characteristic elements (Fabian & Rathbone-McCuan, 1992; Vinton, 1992; Longres, 1993; Dubin, Lelong, & Smith, 1988; Duke, 1991; Lachs, Berkman, Fulmer, & Horwitz, 1994; Lustbader, 1996):

- lives alone,
- is socially isolated,
- is mentally impaired,
- has medical or physical health problems,
- is unable to self-care,
- fails to recognize her functional limitations, and
- experiences a life-threatening incident.

Each of these elements potentially raises ethical issues or poses ethical dilemmas with respect to intervention in Anna's life. For example:

- Living alone: Is society more responsible for protecting those who have no family or other informal support? Do individuals have a social responsibility to elect living arrangements that reflect their level of functioning, even when these are contrary to their personal preferences?
- Social isolation: Should lifestyle choices take precedence over community standards for housing and the environment? When does living on the social periphery become social deviance and dysfunction?
- Mental impairment: What are the appropriate measures when mental impairment erodes ability to make informed decisions? What happens when mental impairment is intermittent or relevant only to certain areas of functioning?
- Medical or physical health problems: Does failure to comply with traditional medical practice signal the need for protective services? What happens when the medical prognosis is little more optimistic than present circumstances?
- Self-care incapacity: Whose standards of self-care apply? Can individuals expect to elect different standards of self-care in different situations or life stages?
- Failure to recognize limitations: Should self-awareness be an individual expectation under all circumstances? What is society's responsibility for identifying individual problems and suggesting potential remedies?
- Life-threatening incident: Does imminent danger justify involuntary intervention? Can individuals freely choose substantial risk?

Controversies Surrounding Self-Neglect

No form of elder abuse receives more public and professional involvement than self-neglect (including self-abuse). This is evident in at least three ways: (1) the higher reporting of self-neglect over other abuse forms (Tatara, 1996), (2) the breadth of agencies encountering self-neglect situations (Fiegener, Fiegener, & Meszaros, 1989), and (3) the importance placed on handling self-neglect cases in protective practice (Duke, 1991; Rathbone-McCuan & Whalen, 1992; Anetzberger, 1996).

Likewise, no form of elder abuse is more subject to ethical debate than self-neglect. This is not a new phenomenon. Rather, self-neglect has been the focus of controversy for decades. Some of this controversy emerges from inquiry into the evolution of protective services (Anetzberger, 1996). Protective practice defined itself in the 1960s to be a range of services with potential use of legal authority aimed at preventing or remedying neglect or exploitation experienced by adults whose reduced mental or physical capabilities meant that they could not protect themselves (G. Horowitz & Estes, 1971; Blenkner, Bloom, Nielson, & Weber, 1974). The target population of early protective practice was not unlike the self-neglecting elder of today, although the population was not so labeled.

Growth in protective services, primarily as a result of funding from the 1974 passage of Title XX of the Social Security Act, was closely followed by widespread disenchantment with the practice. Disenchantment centered on the belief that protective services often abridged individual liberties (Horstman, 1975; Hobbs, 1976). The controversy over protective services during this period was described by Ferguson (1978, p. 40) as social value conflicts:

Adult protective services touches the fundamental issues of the extent to which our society actually means human beings have a right to make choices about themselves and their own lives and the extent to which we, as a society, will allow a person to choose his or her own time and place of death. The issues of how altruistic our society is and how nurturing we are to the vulnerable, powerless, and infirm persons in our midst are also joined.

Value Conflict: Freedom versus Safety

Value conflicts surrounding protective practice and self-neglect continue today. Although several dilemmas are discussed in the literature, none is more addressed than that between freedom and safety (Collins, 1982; Cutler & Tisdale, 1992; Anetzberger & Miller, 1995; Mixson, 1996). Reflecting the ethical dilemmas of autonomy versus beneficence, this tension is most acutely experienced by both the older person and the practitioner when endangerment is greatest. Applied to Anna, it becomes a matter of continued residence at home, no matter what the consequences. More specifically, should Anna's wish to remain at home be respected, even with the risk of hypothermia? Or, recognizing her mental and social limitations, should Anna be placed in a protective setting against her wishes, at least for the duration of winter?

To respect Anna's wish to remain at home may suggest respect for self-determination in the extreme to many practitioners. Few would argue that older people should be able to make even socially unpopular and physically unhealthy decisions, so long as others are not denied rights in the process and so long as the decisions are freely and knowingly made (Kapp & Bigot, 1985; Kaufman & Becker, 1996). Certainly allowing Anna to remain at home does not seem to deny others their rights. More problematic is the issue of Anna's decision-making capacity. What are the implications of being "slow" in making informed choices about health and safety? Who is to determine the nature and extent of "slowness" for Anna? What are the effects of long-term social isolation and an "eccentric" upbringing on the ability to receive help from strangers? Who is to judge the appropriateness of help offered?

Autonomy can be a hollow concept when older people lack the ability, information, or background for decision making (Potter & Jameton, 1986; Hayes & Spring, 1988). For example, Anna's developmental disabilities and lack of knowledge about individual rights meant that she was ill prepared to resist the sheriff's placement of her into the county home, even though she would have preferred returning to her own home after hospitalization instead. The history of services to older people suggests that too often they reflect misguided paternalism at best (E. S. Cohen, 1988) and ageism, intrusion, or even abuse at worst (Faulkner, 1982; Potter & Jameton, 1986). The erosion of autonomy is especially common for older people like Anna, who are poor or devoid of a socially acceptable lifestyle (Traxler, 1986).

The value conflict of freedom versus safety has fostered varying perspectives. Some perspectives differ historically: certain eras have promoted complete abandonment, other eras strong intervention (J. S. D. Regan, 1985). Other perspectives differ by professional discipline or philosophical orientation. In a national study on group concern about involuntary protective services, Duke (1993) found that social workers, physicians, and the general public were the most interested in protecting vulnerable older people's health and safety. In contrast, attorneys, advocates for the aged or disabled, and representatives of civil liberties organizations were the most fearful about the use of involuntary protection, seeing it as a violation of adult rights or erosion of due-process protections.

Resolving the Conflict

Few writers offer actual guidance in dealing with freedom versus safety as a value conflict surrounding interventions on behalf of self-neglecting elders. Unfortunately, even those who do typically provide suggestions that are vague and abstract, such as having a basic foundation of beliefs for practice (Hayes & Spring, 1988) or clearly articulating the meaning of "doing good" in individual situations (McLaughlin, 1988). For some, the source of both comes from professional codes of ethics (Burstein, 1988; Mixson, 1995). For others, it is a framework of ethical assessment to examine the use of influence in protective practice (Abramson, 1991). Some writers on protective interventions suggest that practitioners ask themselves if they would deal with situations the same were clients in their 20s or 30s rather than in old age, or were they refusing help on religious grounds rather than for other reasons (Callender, 1982; Potter & Jameton, 1986). Other writers refocus the value conflict from resistant clients to resistant or inadequate service systems (J. J. Callahan, 1988; Collopy & Bial, 1994). Finally, still other writers propose the creation of protocols for decision making. E. S. Cohen (1996), for instance, offers a protocol with six elements to protect elders with diminished mental capacity.

Realities of Protective Practice

Most self-neglecting elders are resistant to protective investigation, even more than elders mistreated by others (Longres, 1994). Still, few actually refuse services (Duke, 1993). It is perhaps ironic that service refusal and service acceptance both can have severe consequences in the exercise of freedom for protective clientele. For example, Anetzberger (1995) found that clients of voluntary service agencies who are vulnerable and noncompliant with treatment plans may be reported to authorities more often than those who are vulnerable and compliant with treatment plans. Moreover, Sengstock, Hwalek, and Petrone (1989) found that even service acceptance may result in the application of restrictive forms of intervention, like institutional placement, supervision/reassurance services, and police visits.

FEAR OF CRIME

George's Story

It was true that the neighborhood had changed. Freshly painted houses had been replaced by houses with boarded windows and vacant lots. The corner store was less a hangout for children coming home from school than for young men peddling drugs. Fences were decorated with graffiti, and abandoned cars dotted the streets. Most of the neighbors that George had known so well during his working years had left the city long ago for sprawling suburbs or the rural landscape beyond. Only a few remained, all old like himself and many increasingly isolated in their homes as the ravages of age and illness took their toll. George was one of the few "old-timers" still able to get around fairly well. At age 90 he had outlived his wife and his only son. Somewhat unsteady on his feet and nearly deaf, he managed to walk to a nearby restaurant for lunch every day and board a bus for banking and grocery shopping every week.

George was not actually afraid of living in the neighborhood, only very cautious, especially after two teenage boys had mugged him a year ago. One pushed him down on the pavement, while the other took his wallet and kicked him in the side. The broken rib and bruises were painful, but they failed to deter him from his routine. Money could be replaced, and injuries could heal. The desire to remain independent and do what he wanted provided George all the incentive he required to eventually overcome the crime. More upsetting to George had been the recent torture of a neighbor's cat. Doused with gasoline and set on fire, the cat died, leaving its owner deeply depressed and inconsolable. The incident also left George feeling at odds with life around him, which he no longer seemed to understand very well.

Image and Reality

It is often said that older people, like George, are particularly vulnerable to crime. This image is fostered in the mass media, which headline and sensationalize incidents of crime against the elderly. It is perpetuated by advocates for the aged, who, each decade, highlight this problem in the White House Conference on Aging recommendations for social change. It is even echoed among older people themselves, who in public opinion polls regularly identify crime as a major personal concern.

The origins of the image are found in the distorted and stereotypic portrayal of older people as retired, sick, incapable, and institutionalized that was reinforced during the 1970s (L. Harris & Associates, 1975; Achenbaum, 1978). Once the major issues of poverty and lack of health care had been successfully addressed through federal public policy initiatives in the 1960s, attention afterward turned to other problems requiring action. In this context, interest in crime against the elderly emerged out of concern about the environment of older people and especially was related to research findings on the impact of public housing in the lives of elderly residents (Sherman, Newman, Nelson, & Van Buren, 1975; Lawton & Yaffe, 1980).

The decade of the 1970s was a period of considerable activity concerning crime and the elderly (G. E. Finley, 1983). It surpassed all preceding and subsequent decades in research, publications, and demonstration projects on the subject. It was the pivotal decade for shaping both our image and understanding of older crime victims. In its aftermath, the importance of this problem as an area for investigation and intervention was diminished and remains so today, two decades later.

The spectacular rise and fall of crime as an area of interest in gerontology reflects the discrepancy between the image and the reality of crime in the lives of older people. Initially the image of crime against the elderly suggested that older people were more likely to be victims of crime than other age groups. Robert Butler presented this image as late as 1975 in his Pulitzer Prize–winning book *Why Survive? Being Old in America* when he remarked, "Old people are victims of violent crime more than any other age group" (p. 300). However, U.S. Department of Justice crime statistics indicated otherwise, causing concerns to narrow and focus on older people as frequent victims of only certain types of crime, such as fraud and shoplifting. Similarly, the early image of older crime victims suggested that they experienced the effects of crime to a greater degree than did younger persons. In the classic work on this subject, Goldsmith and Goldsmith (1976, p. 2) write, "One reason for focusing special attention on crime against the elderly is the differential impact of crime and increased vulnerability of the elderly. There are physical, economic, and environmental factors associated with aging that increase vulnerability to criminal attack and that magnify the impact of victimization." Research showed the effects of crime on older crime victims to be no greater than on younger ones, curtailing widespread interest in crime and the elderly among policymakers and practitioners (F. L. Cook, Skogan, T. D. Cook, & Antunes, 1978; Quay, Johnson, & McClelland, 1980).

Reality contradicts the traditional image of crime against the elderly in nearly every regard. According to Bachman (1992) of the U.S. Bureau of Justice Statistics:

- Older people (those age 65 or over) are the least likely age group to experience crime.
- Even personal larceny (such as pocket picking and purse snatching) occurs as often among younger persons as older ones.
- Crime against the elderly peaked in the mid-1970s and has declined ever since. Violent crime in 1990 was 61% lower than in 1974, theft 22% lower than in 1976.
- Older victims are more likely to report all forms of crime to the police compared to younger victims.

In addition, various studies reveal that the physical, psychological, and financial consequences of victimization are no greater for older people than they are for other age groups (F. L. Cook et al., 1978; Quay et al., 1980). These facts, however, do not negate the seriousness of crime affecting individual older persons or the vulnerability of the elderly in general under certain circumstances. For example, older robbery victims are more likely to face multiple offenders and those armed with guns (Bachman, 1992).

One aspect of crime against the elderly seemed to remain intact after fact was separated from fiction: namely, fear of crime was greater for older people than for any other age group. In summarizing the literature on this subject, G. E. Finley (1983, p. 31) found that age was irrationally related to fear of criminal victimization in that it "bears no relationship to the reality of potential victimization." The effect of this fear for the elderly may be restriction of activity and social isolation (Lebowitz, 1978). In contrast to these conclusions, recent reviews of previous research on fear of crime among adults suggest that the prevalence of fear among older people has been overestimated (LaGrange & Ferraro, 1987). In this light, a national survey of adults age 18 years or over found no significant correlation between fear of crime and age. Irrational fear was more related to sex (women scored higher) than any other factor (Ferraro, LaGrange, & McReady, 1990).

Policy and Programming

The public response to the criminal victimization of older people and their fear of crime has been multifaceted. Particular emphasis has been placed on crime prevention, including training programs, self-defense courses, and installation of locks and other safety devices. In addition, various locales have organized "neighborhood watch" to spot crime or "crime stoppers" to report information on it. Some law-enforcement agencies have specially trained police units to serve older people or have enhanced monitoring of high-crime areas using special equipment or personnel. Victim-compensation laws offer restitution to victims in many states. Emergency shelters or financial assistance are available in select communities to deal with the immediate needs of victims in the wake of crime. Victim-assistance programs, a few of which have elderly specialists, provide support in navigating through the criminal justice system.

Finally, some state laws require a greater penalty for crimes committed against older people (Boston, Nitzberg, & Kravitz, 1979; Roberts, 1990; J. L. Simmons, 1993; Kapp, 1995b).

Historically, certain national associations and federal agencies have assumed leadership roles in addressing crime against older people, notably the American Association of Retired Persons, the Law Enforcement Assistance Administration, and the Administration on Aging (Gelfand, 1988). Recently the Administration on Aging, in partnership with the U.S. Attorney General, announced new programming authorized by Public Law 103–322 to improve the safety and security of the elderly, including crime-prevention activities, victim services, and community policing (Torres-Gil, 1994). Although much of this programming is not new, it does represent renewed activity around the problem.

Ethical Issues

Many ethical dilemmas emerge from this discussion on the image and reality of crime against the elderly. Perhaps the most important ones relate to responsible journalism and social advocacy. They include the following:

- To what extent is journalism ensuring readership by exaggerating the problem or accurately reporting facts?
- Should advocates for the elderly focus only on issues substantiated through research, or should they also respond to those issues that ignite public interest and activity?
- Does emphasizing crime against the elderly perpetuate the stereotypic portrayal of older people as vulnerable and incapacitated, or does it foster social action around the broad needs of this age group for safety and security?
- Do more severe penalties for crime against the elderly represent social justice or ageism?
- If a more accurate portrayal of crime and the elderly is provided, will the behavior of older people change and increased victimization occur?
- Do special crime-prevention programs for the elderly help reduce the incidence of crime or inappropriately divert resources away from younger age groups more likely to experience crime?
- By developing housing for the elderly, are we segregating this population or creating safe homes for them?
- Are special protections for the elderly justified by the status of older people in society, or do they serve to discourage self-defense by this age group?

Almost none of these ethical dilemmas have been discussed in the gerontologic literature. Therefore, paradigms for resolving them have not been developed. Any general approach requires the following:

- Assessment of related facts, norms, values, and opinions
- Deliberation on moral options and their possible consequences
- Decision and justification for a course of action
- Evaluation of the decision by considering alternative possible actions under similar circumstances

Additionally, since moral principles provide guidance for ethical decision making, it is important to identify those central to the dilemmas in question. For ethics and aging, four are usually considered dominant: autonomy, beneficence, nonmaleficence, and distributive justice. Yet "the 'correct answer' to an ethical dilemma may be less a matter of agreeing on an abstract set of principles than it is a matter of showing a commitment to free and open communication" (Moody, 1992, p. 38). Given the infancy of moral discourse around crime and the elderly, free and open communication, or "communicative ethics" as described by Habermas (1990), is an understandable goal.

RISK AT HOME

Catherine's Story

Catherine lived alone in the house that she and her husband had occupied for nearly all of their married life. In it she had raised two daughters and accomplished the various housekeeping tasks expected of a woman in her childbearing years at midcentury. The house had more memories than even 50 years of residence would suggest. To Catherine, who she was as a person and life at 755 Sturges Avenue were synonymous. She could not imagine the existence of one without the other. This attachment to home was apparent from the beginning. When Catherine and her husband first bought the house, she would walk around touching the woodwork, surveying the rooms, and smelling the lilacs that brought color to the backyard each spring. She regarded her new house with both reverence and awe. In old age, these feelings remained, coupled with those of comfort and familiarity.

The reality of life at 755 Sturges Avenue had changed over time. The house posed daily challenges for Catherine, now widowed and with daughters out of town and neighbors as old as she. When she was in her 20s, it did not matter to her that the bath and bedrooms were on the second floor. At age 78 with severe arthritis, it did. Earlier, too, it was unimportant that the house required constant tending, both with regard to cleaning and yardwork. After two heart attacks and frequent shortness of breath, keeping up with these tasks was difficult at best.

However, both daughters worried more about Catherine's increasing cognitive deficits than they did about her physical limitations. Catherine was beginning to be forgetful, leaving the oven on unlit and keys in the outside doors. They believed that it was time for Catherine to move into a protective setting, perhaps assisted living, where others were around to offer supervision and assistance when needed. Catherine refused to go. She did not want to "hang around with old people. It's too depressing." She felt that she could manage on her own if only someone, possibly a college student, moved in with her to help once in a while. But mostly Catherine just did not want to leave her home, saying, "It means everything to me."

The Importance of Autonomy

Autonomy is widely regarded as the most important ethical concept in American culture (Gaylin, 1994). It is seen as the basis of human dignity and essential for moral discourse. The ability to act as one wishes (so long as the autonomy of others is not compromised) and to do so without coercion or interference also is fundamental to adult relationships and professional practice.

Many believe that autonomy should never be compromised without strong moral justification, and then only reluctantly and after considerable deliberation (Hogstel & Gaul, 1991). Those in control are thought to be particularly obligated to refrain from undue coercion and interference. In this regard, Abramson (1985a) argues that there are only three circumstances under which it is morally justified to curtail autonomy (when the individual's actions do not cause harm to others): (1) the individual lacks the capacity to make informed decisions or understand their consequences, (2) the implications of the decisions are far-reaching and irreversible, and (3) temporary interference ensures future autonomy. Even under these circumstances, however, the motivations for curtailing autonomy must be carefully scrutinized along with the qualifications of the decision makers and the caliber of the information upon which the decisions are based. Applying Abramson's arguments to Catherine's situation results in a set of questions, each one of which should be satisfactorily answered before decisions are made about Catherine's living arrangements:

- Are Catherine's cognitive deficits so severe that she is incapable of making reasonable decisions or understanding the consequences of decisions made?
- What are the implications for Catherine of not changing her living arrangements? How likely is irreparable harm? Will alternative living arrangements serve to increase Catherine's independence in ways not possible at 755 Sturges Avenue?
- Why do the daughters want Catherine to change her living arrangements? Does this personally benefit them in any way?
- How knowledgeable are the daughters with regard to Catherine's functional abilities, care needs, and values? How informed are they about local housing and services for disabled older persons, including the availability and adequacy of these resources?

Threats to Autonomy in the Home

With Americans living longer, the number of older persons having disabilities has grown. This has led to increased concern about their risk in the home. In this regard, there is a tendency to underestimate their potential autonomy because of prejudice and stereotypes (E. S. Cohen, 1988). For example, in a study on the images of aging conducted on behalf of the American Association of Retired Persons, most surveyed Americans of all ages estimated that poverty, poor health, and loneliness were serious problems for people over age 65, even though they are not (Speas & Obenshain, 1995). Perceptions such as these suggest a greater degree of incapacity and need for assistance on the part of older persons than actually exists. Likewise, there are occasions when the passivity to authority of the current generation of older persons undermines their ability to maintain self-determination once it is threatened (Purtilo, 1991).

Threats to autonomy are not uncommon in the lives of disabled older persons. Sometimes the threats are subtle, as when family members exaggerate information (Coy, 1989) or professionals use knowledge or technology to gain authority (Guccione, 1988). Other times the threats are obvious, as when families or professionals simply substitute their own values or goals for those of the disabled older person (Collopy & Bial, 1994).

Families are the primary source of assistance in old age (Horowitz & Dobrof, 1982; E. M. Brody, 1985; Stone, Cafferata, & Sangl, 1987). Their help emanates out of gratitude, remorse, or love (Selig, Tomlinson, & Hickey, 1991). Professionals supplement or substitute for family care. The basis for their support comes out of personal commitment, investment in the job, or agency mission. Factors associated with families and professionals shape the exercise of autonomy in caring for disabled older persons at home (Young, 1990). For families, the factors include available caregiving resources, personal relations, and intergenerational issues. For professionals, they include home care reimbursement, worker availability, and public policy regulation. Resource shortages or diminished capacity for relations for both families and professionals may serve to curtail autonomy.

Techniques for Preserving Autonomy at Home

The dilemmas families and professionals face in preserving the autonomy of disabled older persons are widely acknowledged (Job & Anema, 1988; Collopy, Dubler, & Zuckerman, 1990; Hogstel & Gaul, 1991; Rooney, 1997). Suggestions for resolving the dilemmas generally take the form of better understanding the individual or framing the issues, consultation with a supervisor or ethicist, or use of case conferences or interdisciplinary team meetings.

Values histories enable families and professionals to better understand the individual (Davis, 1992). They do this by explaining underlying life values and personal perspectives across a whole range of care issues. The National Values

History Project developed and tested a values history inventory that has been widely disseminated and translated into many languages (Gibson, 1990). It is divided into several sections and includes questions on attitudes regarding independence, control, personal relations, and illness and dying.

Values mapping is a relative of values histories. It, too, can be used to better understand the individual. Values mapping is based on a set of questions that consider the decision-making process and self-reported values that respondents find relevant to long-term-care alternatives. In applying values mapping to a sample of older persons, family members or friends, and professionals involved in long-term-care decision-making, McCullough, Wilson, Teasdale, Kolpakchi, and Skelly (1993) found that the top-ranked values for older persons related to environment, self-identity, and relationship; for family members and friends, care, security, and psychological well-being; and for professionals, care, physical health, and the link between relationship and psychological well-being. The differences in value rank between older people and family members are illustrated in the situation of Catherine and her daughters.

Framing the issues can mean adopting a structure for decision making or emphasizing certain ethical principles over others in determining a course of action. T. F. Johnson (1995b) suggests that there are perhaps three basic steps in ethical decision making: information gathering, deliberation, and negotiation. This means dealing with ethical problems by being sensitive to the situation, assessing the facts and underlying values, taking time to deliberate, justifying any chosen action, and evaluating the choice after it is made. Fitting (1986) emphasizes a cost-benefit analysis that weighs the potential consequences of choices made against alternative actions. Applied to Catherine, staying in her own home may expose her to gas asphyxiation (from leaving the oven on unlit), but placing her in assisted living against her wishes may expose her to mental anguish. A practical alternative might simply be substituting a microwave oven for the gas one and removing this source of risk, with Catherine's consent, of course, since to the extent that she is able, Catherine must decide her own destiny (Haddad, 1989; Collopy et al., 1990).

For professionals, the process of assessment and deliberation is aided by the use of professional codes or ethics committees (Davis, 1992; M. M. Hughes, 1995) and agency or community guidelines for ethical decision making. For example, the *Code for Nurses* of the American Nurses' Association (1985) includes respect for human dignity and individual uniqueness as well as safeguarding privacy. An Ethics and Aging Committee was formed in Lake County, Ohio, as a result of a series of roundtable discussions on ethical issues faced by professionals and caregivers working with older persons. Committee functions include case consultation, education, and resource development. Agency guidelines for ethical home care are represented in the policies and procedures for ethical decision making developed by the Home Health Assembly of New Jersey (Iozzio, 1992). They arose when it was recognized that the application of ethical principles should not be restricted to crisis intervention, but, instead, should be integral to all health care delivery for any given agency. Finally, a set of community guidelines on ethics and the care of people with Alzheimer's disease was the product of a nine-month dialogue series at Fairhill Center for Aging in Cleveland, Ohio. An interdisciplinary group of practitioners and ethicists developed the guidelines as a consensus statement for ideal care, addressing such common issues as diagnostic disclosure, driving, and behavior control (Post & Whitehouse, 1995).

Two final references for ethical decision making should be mentioned. Listings of clients' rights provide a basis for action that underscores the primacy of self-determination as a guiding principle and autonomy as the underlying concept. Sabatino (1990) offers rights of home care clients, and Bookin (1992), those of community-dwelling disabled older persons in general. In addition, Whitbeck (1996) suggests using principles of design practice in engineering for ethical decision making. In this model, solving actual moral problems focuses more on devising possible responses than on simply choosing the "best" one. Since there may be no best solution or no solution at all, design practice allows its user to solve problems creatively and practically through four defined stages: considering the uncertainty of the situation, developing possible solutions, acting under time constraints, and recognizing the dynamic character of possible solutions.

However, the existence of professional codes, ethics committees, agency guidelines, clients' rights, and the principles of design practice does not guarantee their use. For example, a study of social workers found that 74% had not consulted the profession's code of ethics for decision making during the preceding year. Even among those who did, the code represented the first reference choice for only 9% of the respondents. Most elected to use their own personal values or informal discussions with coworkers for decision making (Klosterman, 1994). Likewise, research by R. A. Kane and her associates (1993) concluded that in resolving ethical dilemmas, social work case managers most often rely on discussions with supervisors (68%) or colleagues (39%). These approaches were used more often than ethics committees (2%), reference to rules (2%), training (4%), or even case conferences (17%).

Emphasizing certain ethical principles over others in home care decision making is frequently discussed in the literature on ethics and aging. Dubler (1990), for instance, recommends using the concept of accommodation rather than autonomy in guiding ethical decision making. Accommodation requires mediating between the older person's wishes, the competing interests of others, and the reality of existing services. Moody (1992) emphasizes dignity and self-respect as ethical principles over autonomy. Accordingly, families and professionals become more concerned with negotiated than informed consent, and tools for ethical decision making focus on communication, bargaining, and empowerment.

RISK IN INSTITUTIONS

Virginia's Story

Virginia was over 100 years old when she entered Spruce Hill Nursing Home. Coming there was not what she wanted. However, rather than upset her daughter and son-in-law, she agreed to go. Both in their 70s, they found it tiring to travel between Florida and Ohio, supervising and arranging Virginia's home care while still having a life of their own. On the other hand, Virginia enjoyed good health. She had no problems with any of her vital functions—no heart disease, respiratory difficulties, or the like. However, two broken hips had limited her mobility, and Alzheimer's disease had left her often confused and forgetful. Because she was friendly and compliant with the wishes of others, Virginia quickly became a favorite of the staff at Spruce Hill Nursing Home. As she wheeled through the facility, they would stop their work and talk to her. Virginia's smile and soft voice were a welcome contrast to many other residents.

Spruce Hill Nursing Home had a reputation for quality care. It was a reputation its administrator sought to preserve. Therefore, when Virginia fell out of her wheelchair and suffered internal injuries, and nursing staff failed to notify either the physician or the family about the incident, the administrator decided to let the matter pass. Even when Virginia died from the injuries, he dismissed the incident as an unfortunate accident, not reflective of overall conditions of care at Spruce Hill Nursing Home. A subsequent investigation by the Long Term Care Ombudsman Program uncovered that the head nurse had recorded contact with the family about the incident, and the family had agreed that medical attention was not necessary. In fact, no family member had been contacted. Moreover, Virginia had been alone at the time of the incident, and no one discovered her lying on the floor until a hour or two later—enough time for the blood on her arm to dry from a scratch suffered in the fall. Virginia had called for help following the fall, but no one came. She did not persist in calling, because she did not want to "bother staff, when obviously they were busy with others."

Ethical Dilemmas Associated with Risk

The ethical dilemmas surrounding risk in institutions are different from those surrounding risk at home. At home, risk management is a personal or family affair. In institutional settings, it is the responsibility of strangers, typically administrators and professional or paraprofessional service providers. Success in risk management within institutional settings is measured by the degree to which the resident remains protected (e.g., does not wander off), receives adequate care (e.g., does not suffer dehydration or medical neglect), retains worldly goods (e.g., is not robbed), incurs no injury (e.g., is not hit), and exercises individual rights (e.g., is not unnecessarily restrained).

The expectations attached to institutional care are high, especially those associated with nursing homes. Having gone through the anguish of placing a relative in a nursing home, families expect compassionate care, comparable to that offered at home. If they also pay for the care themselves, then their expectations tend to border on the ideal. Likewise, federal and state regulators and long-term-care ombudsmen demand that nursing homes offer high standards of service and environmental conditions, predicated on the vulnerability and needs of the residents along with the belief that with public payment comes strict requirements and tough scrutiny. It is commonly said that nursing homes are the second most regulated industry in the country, after nuclear power plants. They are certainly expected to safeguard their residents (Kapp & Bigot, 1985). The dilemmas associated with fulfilling this expectation, however, are many.

Minimally, nursing homes are expected to provide residents with appropriate care and safety and still be reasonably priced, respect individual rights, and admit those in need of residential care no matter what their idiosyncratic behavior or service requirements are. However, it is not easy to contain costs and have well-qualified, trained, and supervised staff. But without such staff, quality care is threatened and the possibility of resident abuse increases. It is not easy for residents to move about freely within the facility, given their mental and physical limitations and the concern about accident or misfortune. But without such movement, the autonomy of residents is diminished and individual rights are compromised. It is not easy to admit as residents persons with psychiatric or substance-abuse problems, since they may intimidate other persons or may require so much attention from staff that the care and security of other residents are eroded. But not admitting these residents is suggestive of discrimination and does not offer equal access to care for all those persons who need it.

Virginia's story illustrates some of these dilemmas. First, she was not restrained. Rather, she had free movement throughout the facility, despite her physical and mental disabilities. When she fell, it represented the kind of risk associated with such freedom of movement. Second, Virginia's accident was not quickly discovered, and when it was, the accident was not appropriately reported. Training and supervision issues are evident here as well as the likelihood that protocols were not established for dealing with various mishaps.

Resident Abuse

One aspect of risk for nursing-home residents is possible mistreatment. Awareness of resident abuse, neglect, and exploitation by staff has a long history, with public concern about the problem culminating during the 1970s. In 1970, Ralph Nader called for an "old people's liberation movement" when an investigation of nursing-home conditions uncovered instances of fatal food contamination and drug experimentation on residents (Townsend, 1971). A few years later Stannard (1973) reported incidents in which nurses and aides punished residents who were aggressive or defecated on the floor by violently shaking, threatening, or throwing water on them. However, it was Mendelson in 1974 who shocked the nation with an exposé of fraud, corruption, and deceit at every level of the nursing-home industry. Her book *Tender Loving Greed* described conditions of resident risk ranging from inadequate equipment to stolen checks and personal property. The following year Gubrium (1975) found life at Murray Manor just as horrible, with the sedation of residents who disrupted staff routine and the staff inaccurately charting records to make them appear less negligent and uncaring. During the same period, the U.S. Senate Special Committee on Aging conducted hearings on fraud and abuse in nursing homes, and the General Accounting Office investigated the theft of residents' personal funds (Halamandaris, 1983). Besides research, citizen inquiry, and public hearings, the 1970s acknowledged resident abuse through popular literature, such as works by Simone de Beauvoir (1972) and May Sarton (1973).

There have been only a few recent investigations on the nature and scope of resident abuse. In the aftermath of public hearings on the subject, the U.S. House Select Committee on Aging (1986) estimated that 15% of nursing-home residents are physically abused, 35% are medically neglected, and 40% are psychologically abused. In addition, many more are denied individual rights, including 25% freedom of movement, 45% privacy, and 75% opportunity to complain. MacNamara (1988) offers a record of resident abuse following 10 years as chief administrator for an organization serving 2,000 institutionalized persons. The record includes numerous instances of physical and psychological abuse, such as hairpulling, cold showers, avoidance, and screaming at close range. Pillemer and Moore (1989) surveyed nurses and aides from 31 East Coast nursing homes and discovered 10% admitting to physical abuse and 40% to psychological abuse the previous year. Sengstock, McFarland, and Hwalek (1990) identify the various abuse forms found in institutional settings, then urge that special attention be given to the use of restraints and problems with identifying the abuser. Meddaugh (1993) discusses how resident abuse can be covert, as when isolation or labeling is employed. Payne and Cikovic (1995) analyze 488 incidents of elder abuse reported to Medicaid Fraud Control Units throughout the nation and find that 84% committed by nursing-home staff represent physical abuse and 9% represent sexual assault. Finally, D. K. Harris and Benson (1996) survey nursing-home employees in six nursing homes and find that 4% report stealing something from a resident in the past year and 10% say that they saw their employees steal from residents during that period.

Major correlates to resident abuse have emerged from the research of Pillemer and Moore (1989) and the U.S. Department of Health and Human Services (1990b). They include job frustration, high stress, lack of empathy for the aged, viewing residents as childlike, and belligerent residents.

There are numerous ethical dilemmas surrounding resident abuse. Besides those already discussed, they include the following:

- As an employee who observes resident abuse: should I report, if by reporting my coworkers shun me and no longer come to my aid when needed?
- As a family member who suspects resident abuse: should I complain, if by complaining my relative could be subjected to retaliation?
- As an administrator faced with an employee accused of being abusive to a resident with dementia: should I believe the resident, when there are no injuries or other signs of abuse, and when the resident has a long history of belligerent and aggressive behavior herself against staff? If I do not believe the resident and abuse has occurred, will she ever feel comfortable coming forward and reporting further instances of abuse? If I believe the resident and discipline the employee, the discipline becomes a part of the documented work history of this employee and may adversely affect future job opportunities, although this is the only allegation of abuse ever made against the individual in three years of employment at the facility?

The image of nursing homes has improved from the "human warehouses" of the 1970s. Today nursing homes are seen as part of the continuum of long-term care (Evans & Welge, 1991). They represent important service options in the community, along with adult day care, home care, and protective services (Kart & Dunkle, 1995). Nonetheless, the public remains hesitant in its praise of nursing-home care. Certainly the continuing high incidence of abuse in these settings and the difficulty of protecting residents against its occurrence despite federal and state laws help to justify this cautionary attitude (Clough, 1996; Hirschel, 1996).

Restraints

Nursing homes have a long history of using physical restraints, like mittens and Posey restraints, to control the movement of residents (Covert, Rodrigues, & Solomon, 1977). Restraints were thought to decrease the likelihood of residents falling or wandering off. They also enable staff to engage in other work activities without having to spend time overseeing the movements of specific residents. However, restraints can cause long-term problems as a result of residents remaining in the same place for extended periods. These problems can include incontinence, decubitus ulcers, and agitation (Lofgren, MacPherson, Granieri, Myllenbeck, & Sprafka, 1989; Tinetti, Liu, Marottoli, & Ginter, 1991).

Ethical dilemmas associated with restraint use in many nursing homes pit the principle of beneficence against the principle of autonomy (Brower, 1992). Staff typically employ restraints for the benefit and protection of the resident along with others who might be victimized by the potential annoying or violent behavior of that person (S. H. Johnson, 1990). Although most residents who are restrained suffer from dementia, many advocates of nursing-home reform express concern that restraints diminish resident independence and self-determination, fostering dependence and mental anguish (E. Wilson, 1986).

Nursing-home reform has resulted in decreased use of physical restraints. Perhaps more important, there is a growing opinion that their wholesale application is abusive and unacceptable (Romano, 1994). Nevertheless, some recent studies indicate that restraints remain fairly common in nursing homes, and those with the lowest quality of care have the highest number of residents in restraints (Health Care Financing Administration, 1988; Archea, Whittington, & Strasser, 1995).

As some forms of restraints, like straightjackets, have nearly disappeared from nursing homes, new forms have emerged (Office of Technology Assessment, 1992). These include "chemical" restraints, like psychoactive drugs (R. A. Kane, 1993a), and "institutional" restraints, like tightly scheduled daily activities (Lidz & Arnold, 1990). Among the fastest growing are locked special care units for persons with Alzheimer's disease. Their use is not without controversy (M. G. Simmons, 1990). For example, Noyes and Silva (1993) argue that locked units are essential for those with diminished mental capacities at risk of harm from wandering. Because cognitive impairment limits their ability to choose autonomy, interference with their freedom of movement is justified. Beitler (1990) disagrees, stating that locked units abridge civil liberties. Anyway, other means exist to address wandering. Among the means frequently cited in the literature are providing alternative activities for residents or alerting staff to be watchful of those persons likely to wander (Rader, 1987; Blakeslee, Goldman, & Papougenis, 1990).

Environmental Hazards

Another aspect of risk for nursing-home residents surrounds the living environment. Wet and slippery floors and chairs without supportive sides can be dangerous for residents who are unsteady on their feet and prone to falling. Inadequate air conditioning and ventilation can affect the health and well-being of residents with respiratory problems. Insufficient smoke detectors and improper evacuation procedures can result in resident injury or even death in the event of the outbreak of a fire. Minimizing all of these environmental hazards rests on ensuring appropriate facility design, operations, and oversight. Ethical dilemmas can surface when potential hazards are addressed, however, because they usually require the expenditure of funds, deployment of staff, management control, and activity prioritization. For instance:

- Regulations require clean floors and an odor-free atmosphere. Yet maintaining cleanliness and controlling odors mean frequently washing and buffing floors, which can crowd hallways and present slippery conditions, at least temporarily.
- Central air conditioning is important for temperature control during hot weather. It is also costly, diverting resources from staffing and service areas. Moreover, it is sometimes not appreciated by those residents who complain of "constantly being cold and chilled."

- In an effort to prevent fires, nursing homes have installed sprinkler systems, smoke detectors, and extinguishers. In addition, escape procedures are displayed conspicuously on every floor of the facility. All this detracts from the "homelike" atmosphere desired by residents and families and sought by potential admissions.

Environmental hazards are not uncommon in nursing homes. Among the nine major complaint categories handled by the Long Term Care Ombudsman Program are those that consider environmental hazards, such as administration and building, sanitation, or laundry (Berry, 1990). Together they account for about 25% of complaints received (Paton, Huber, & Netting, 1994). Similarly, the U.S. General Accounting Office (1987) found that 41% of skilled and 34% of intermediate care facilities were not in compliance with one or more requirements likely to affect resident health and safety across three consecutive inspections by regulatory agents.

Techniques for Preserving Autonomy in Institutions

Autonomy is the most fundamental issue for nursing-home residents. In a survey of 135 cognitively intact residents in 45 facilities, the majority emphasized the importance of personal autonomy in all areas of their lives except visitors (R. A. Kane, Freeman, Caplan, Aroskar, & Urv-Wong, 1990). Perhaps because it is so easily compromised in institutional settings, the preservation of autonomy is at the heart of ethical decision making there (Wetle, 1985; Collopy, 1988; Caplan, 1990; Hofland & David, 1990; Brower, 1992; Agich, 1993).

Autonomy in the face of personal risk is such a critical concern for nursing homes that several techniques have evolved to deal with related ethical dilemmas. They range from informal practices to formal ethics committees. K. F. Crawford (1994) surveyed members of the American College of Health Care Administrators and found that of 161 respondents, 77% had written policies to address ethical questions, 55% had ethics committees, 48% conducted consultation and case review, 17% offered in-service ethics training or the like, and 3% held ethics rounds. The establishment of policies and procedures regarding safety provides an alternative to dealing with problems on an ad hoc basis. They delineate practices the facility considers ethically acceptable and set forth value priorities for staff (Collopy, 1994).

Ethics committees in nursing homes began in the early 1970s. Today they are fairly common (Brown, Miles, & Aroskar, 1987) and similarly structured. Nearly all are interdisciplinary, meet regularly, and most frequently discuss issues of advance directives (Lippy, 1995). The benefits of ethics committees for facilities are many, including substituting the judgment of many professionals for that of a single one and reducing legal liability through an established form of conflict resolution (Barthalis, 1995). However, ethics committees have their costs, especially the time required to establish and sustain them. For ethics committees to be successful, they require clear purpose, goals, and role within the facility (American Association of Retired Persons [AARP], 1990); members committed to self-education (Gibson & Kushner, 1986); and formal operating procedures (Abramson, 1985b; Kimboko & Jewell, 1994).

Resident councils also can help resolve ethical dilemmas. At Andrew House in New Britain, Connecticut, the resident council formed 12 committees to influence facility policies and procedures. One of these was concerned with safety issues. The committees helped residents identify issues of collective concern and have a voice in facility operations (Molis, 1992). The potential benefits of resident councils extend beyond successful issue identification and problem resolution. Various studies have shown that measures, like resident councils, that promote personal choice, control, and independence for residents also increase their well-being and decrease their dependency (Schulz, 1976; P. Beck, 1982; Weinstein & Khanna, 1986; McDermott, 1989).

Staff training and education in ethics are important and need to be relevant if they are to be accepted (R. A. Kane, 1994; Spencer, 1996). At the Benjamin Rose Institute in Cleveland, Ohio, staff from all programmatic divisions were recently surveyed about ethical issues of interest to them in the performance of their jobs. The institute is a voluntary, nonsectarian agency established in 1908 to serve older adults. One of its divisions is Kethley House, a skilled 184-bed nursing home. Staff at Kethley House prioritized issues related to discrimination and inequality, end-of-life decision making, and economic and social justice. The resulting two-day ethics seminar addressed these issues through group discussion and case analysis. The seminar began with ethicists from local universities and hospitals providing an overview on ethics and aging. Afterwards, session participants met in small groups and used suggested frameworks for ethical decision making to decide how they would handle various scenarios involving nursing-home residents.

Resident rights are highlighted in the federal Omnibus Budget Reconciliation Act of 1987. The act asserts that residents of nursing homes are autonomous, independent individuals. As such, they have certain rights, like freedom of choice and the right to privacy, that the facility must protect and promote. With rights, however, comes resident responsibility for the risks and other costs of exercising rights. When facility staff and residents differ in their assessment of a situation and have concern about its consequences, they can call in a long-term-care ombudsman or state agency representative to act as a third-party mediator for handling conflict, including its application in working through ethical dilemmas (S. S. Hunt, 1989). Mediation is not exclusive to ombudsman and state agency representatives, however. In 1994, the American Bar Association Commission on Legal Problems of the Elderly began a three-year funded effort to bring education to 25 nursing homes in Maryland, Virginia, and the District of Columbia. The project trained staff to be mediators and then used the mediation model to resolve care disputes over a 20-month test period. The model is not without its own ethical dilemmas, nonetheless, including those related to an imbalance of power among conflicting parties, time constraints for model application, resident capacity for decision making, and resident difficulty in communications due to sensory or cognitive impairment (Wood & Karp, 1994).

CONCLUSION

The ethics of personal safety provides a rich arena for future research. Many research questions were identified earlier in this chapter as ethical issues or dilemmas. They bear answering before we enter the twenty-first century and a new generation of older Americans.

Unfortunately, most of the questions will not be answered. Typically policies and programs are instituted and not evaluated, or if evaluated, continued no matter what the results of investigation are. Historically this has characterized interventions that promote personal safety for older people. The effectiveness is largely unknown for approaches ranging from elder-abuse laws to ombudsman programming (Wolf, 1995). Moreover, areas that have been researched, such as adult protective services, have generated uncertainty about the viability of these approaches for resolving ethical dilemmas, in this instance, both reducing risk and protecting individual rights. Yet such findings have not necessarily served to stem the development of these interventions, once the momentum for expansion begins, as evidenced by the spread of adult protective services nationwide with enactment of Title XX of the Social Security Act, despite findings from the Benjamin Rose Institute and other research centers suggesting that adult protective services may result in increased institutionalization or even death for older people (Blenkner et al., 1974). Not only should more emphasis be placed on model development, testing and refinement before broad dissemination of results, but the results themselves must be given greater credibility, even when they prove unexpected and undesirable. This suggests the need for greater exchange between the foundations and other sources that support innovation and the governments and other organizations that institutionalize those that prove effective.

The twentieth century will be regarded as a test period for model development in the care and treatment of older people. It was during the twentieth century that persons age 60 or above grew significantly in both numbers and proportion of the total population (U.S. Senate Special Committee on Aging et al., 1991). It was also during this time that problems confronting older people received serious public attention, resulting in a panorama of related policies, programs, and paradigms for understanding and action (Lammers, 1983; Dunkle, 1984; Binstock, 1995; Hudson, 1997).

Issues of personal safety illustrate twentieth-century model testing. During this century the public came to regard older people as a group at risk of harm without special protection. Therefore, policies and programs promoting protection tended to be universal in scope, applying to all older people and not just those vulnerable as a result of disabilities or the frailty of advanced old age. This quality came to characterize most elder-abuse laws and penalties for crime against older people. Although they brought broad acceptance and use, universal policies and programs were seen to have negative consequences. For example, the freedom of those older people not at risk could be compromised, as when mandatory reporting provisions of elder-abuse laws violate individual privacy and family sanctity needlessly. In addition, the same needs of other groups could be ignored, as occurred with penalties for crimes against youths and other age groups at greater risk than older people. Finally, the absurdity of equally targeting with special protection an incapacitated 90-year-old and a vigorous 60-year-old ultimately could erode public concern for the aged as a whole. This is suggested in the growing media portrayal of older people as pampered and selfish (L. Smith, 1989; Samuelson, 1990).

Along with universal policies and programs, the twentieth-century approach to addressing problems of older people included use of government regulation as a kind of panacea to foster preferred practice and compassionate care. For issues of personal safety, this characteristic is evident in the increasing emphasis on licensing health care workers, registering instances of abuse, and imposing strict facility standards on residential long-term care in the belief that harm will happen without specific high expectations, strong oversight, and swift sanctions.

It may be that government regulation has reduced risk for older people. However, it certainly has not eliminated risk, as evidenced, for instance, by the large number of complaints about abuse and residential care received by the Long Term Care Ombudsman Program (*Report from the Secretary's Task Force on Elder Abuse*, 1992; Watson, Cesario, Ziemba, & McGovern, 1993). Moreover, regulation too often is not adequately enforced, due to a lack of funding or alternative bureaucratic priorities. Yet, once established, regulation creates a perception that a problem is solved, and the public can turn its attention to other issues. Regulation also poses various dilemmas for those affected, including the diversion of resources toward regulatory compliance and away from service provision, promotion of uniformity at the expense of individual differences in care and treatment, and increased scarcity of resources as those who will not comply with regulation drop out of professional or business practice. Finally, regulation can infringe on the individual rights of others with no guarantee of protecting older people. Registries, for example, charge aides and other health care workers with abuse or neglect without due process, thorough investigation, fair hearing, or ability to appeal allegations (Hegland, 1992). Better alternatives can be found in measures to attract and retain the most suited workers to health care, such as improved screening and hiring practices, wages and benefits, and training (especially in the areas of stress and conflict management).

There are two primary reasons for universality and regulation as twentieth-century approaches to policy and programming affecting older people. First, older people were considered categorically different from other age groups. In part, they were seen as incapable and childlike and therefore needing special protection (Fischer, 1978; Achenbaum, 1978; Covey, 1988; Featherstone & Hepworth, 1990). In part, too, they were regarded as having contributed to the progress of society and therefore deserving special protection (Hudson, 1989). Second, the growth of government, particularly at the federal level beginning in the 1930s, provided the foundation for public policy and program expansion. This growth especially favored groups, like the aged, with media appeal, high voting records, and established advocacy organizations, able to lend support to issues of concern (Elman, 1995; T. F. Johnson, 1995a).

Approaches to personal safety for older adults will change in the twenty-first century. The baby boomers have dominated culture and society during every decade of their lifetime (Mills, 1987; Strauss & Howe, 1991). They will dominate the early decades after the millennium in their old age as well. The social dominance of baby boomers suggests that in the future, advanced age will be regarded as part of mainstream American culture (Russell, 1995). Policy and programming for older Americans as a special population will be less necessary, and given the number of baby boomers, resources will not be available to support such programming. In addition, a generation emphasizing individualism and independence, like the baby boomers (Russell, 1993), is unlikely to tolerate the paternalistic approach to protection that often characterized twentieth-century interventions (J. J. Regan, 1981; Moody, 1992). Finally, the baby boomers' distrust of authority should be reflected in decreased government regulation.

We are beginning to see each of these trends unfold as the oldest of the baby boomers reach their half-century birthday. In the late 1990s, controversy looms with regard to the status and treatment of older people. Special provisions for this age group are questioned (N. Daniels, 1988; L. Smith, 1989; Morris, 1994; Howe, 1995; Hudson, 1997). Government is criticized for its erosion of individual initiative and intrusion into private enterprise, and Congress is positioned for radical change, with a thrust on deregulation and shifting responsibility to the lowest level (Toffler & Toffler, 1995; Stacks, 1995–1996).

With increasing emphasis on personal planning and responsibility, the twenty-first century is likely to regulate programs more by consumer demand than government decree. Older people will be expected to prepare for their own incapacity and ensure that those given responsibility for care or surrogate decision making are appropriate and adequately prepared for the task. There will be recognized differences between incapacitated and capacitated persons of all ages, including older people, with maltreatment of the former falling under protective-services law and maltreatment of the latter addressed through the criminal code. Use of guidelines for ethical decision making will be common, and only issues outside their domain will require exploration by ethics committees and case consult teams, which will be routinely established in health and social service organizations of all kinds. Community and even national forums will emerge as a popular vehicle for establishing guidance in new areas of ethical concern. Cleveland's Community Dialogue Series on Elder Abuse and Ethics (Anetzberger, Dayton, & McMonagle, 1997) and Canada's National Workshop on Ethical Dilemmas in Abuse and Neglect Cases Involving Older Adults (Spencer, 1995) represent early forum models around ethical decision making and issues of personal safety. Finally, public policy will better ensure autonomy and choice for disabled older people. This will include freedom from coercion by family members and others who would seek the placement of disabled older persons in protective settings against their will as well as from the sometimes subtle restraints used in nursing homes that attempt to manage resident behavior by routinizing it. When disabled older persons are no longer able to exercise choice through informed consent, surrogate decision makers increasingly will be asked to justify decisions made on their behalf through substituted judgment that is documented.

11

Ethical Issues in Nonfamily Care

Phyllis B. Mitzen and Arlene Gruber

> The test of a people is how it behaves toward the old.
> —Abraham Joshua Heschel

> Your work is a partnership. Let them [the older person] do what they can do. Help them to stay independent. They are already depressed because they can't do what they did before.... We are there to help them, to get them to help themselves.
> —Interview with home care aide

We all have an intrinsic desire to remain independent. This notion is tied to a belief that taking care of oneself, in one's own home, with one's own social support system, is the ideal. When disabilities occur, we must turn to others to help us maintain that ideal state. Whether or not independence can be maintained will be determined by the availability of family, friends, or outsiders in the form of paid professional help.

Professionalization of personal care for the elderly is a relatively new phenomenon brought about by a number of factors. Improved living conditions and medical advances in the twentieth century have resulted in a rectangularization of survival curves reflecting a general increase in life expectancy. There are more elderly people who are living longer. Another fact of life in the 1990s is that families are smaller (in 1900, mothers bore an average of 3.9 children; the current estimate is about 1.8), leaving fewer people to care for the disabled parent or surviving spouse. Finally, women, traditionally the primary family caregivers, have entered the work force. Although they continue to be the primary informal caregivers, they and their elderly parents depend more and more on the formal, paid interventions of professionals and paraprofessionals.

The professionals referred to are social workers, nurses, and geriatric care managers. The social worker provides mental health services and locates resources to address the family's needs. The nurse provides health education, access to medical care, and primary nursing services. Both are represented in the new and growing field of geriatric care or case management, in which they may provide the professional services outlined here. They also design care plans to meet the needs of the clients and may serve in a gatekeeping role for governmental and managed-care programs. They may also replace or supplement some of the functions provided by family members, such as checking up on the older person, maintaining communication with family members, and sometimes benign but essential tasks such as picking up needed groceries or accompanying the older person to the doctor. Paraprofessionals, home care workers, aides (certified and not), housekeepers, and homemakers provide most of the formal in-home care to frail, disabled older adults. We will be using "home care aide," a generic term that was coined by the Home Care Aide Association of America in 1995, in an attempt to bring clarity, consistency, and standards to this new and growing area of health care.

This chapter addresses ethics questions that arise in the provision of social support to the homebound elderly, with emphasis on the care provided by home care aides. Social support includes two types of interventions: concrete services (the provision of physical assistance and resources) and emotional support. In everyday life, a relationship that provides social support is characterized by mutual attraction, liking, and respect; an affirmation of shared values and outlooks; and an interdependent sharing of advice, assistance, and resources (S. J. Miller, 1986). We usually think of the individual as receiving social support from family members and friends, but there is also the expectation that social support should be provided by professionals and paraprofessionals when it is no longer forthcoming from families and friends.

Because concrete services such as shopping, bathing, and cooking have to do with the performance of specific learnable tasks, they can often be provided in an identical manner by family members, friends, professionals, and paraprofessionals. This is not the case, however, with the provision of emotional support. In personal relationships, emotional support (listening, advising, and the like) is characterized by *mutual* attraction; *shared* values and outlooks; and *interdependent* sharing of advice, assistance, and resources. In professional and paraprofessional relationships, it is characterized by empathic, interested, caring, *skilled*, and *objective* responses to the client's need to discuss thoughts and feelings about his life, interests, concerns, and problems. One of the goals is the client's better understanding of, accepting, and adjusting to his or her present situation. Absent from this professional/paraprofessional relationship with the client are attraction to personal qualities, mutuality, and interdependence. Unfortunately, the skilled and objective nature of the professional and paraprofessional/client relationship is sometimes misconstrued by homebound clients, paraprofessionals, and professionals alike.

It may be confusing to use the same term "emotional support" when speaking of behaviors emanating from two entirely different types of relationships: personal and professional. For the purpose of clarity in this discussion, therefore, *personal emotional support* will refer to empathic, caring exchanges given and received in relationships characterized by mutuality, liking, and interdependence, and *professional emotional support* will refer to empathic, caring, but objective responses given in professional/paraprofessional ones.

We will look at social support, personal emotional support, and professional emotional support in the context of rights, responsibilities, and the many relationships that exist in professional caregiving. These relationships are infused with the often competing values of all interested parties, including the client, the professionals and paraprofessionals, the agencies, and the funding source, that lead to miscommunication, misunderstandings of roles, and misinterpretation of expectations between client, family, worker, agency, and funding source. A greater understanding of these relationships will enhance the care of the elderly in their homes.

PUBLIC POLICY

It is not farfetched to say that the relationship between an older person and her or his home care aide is affected by public policy. Public policy both reflects and shapes societal attitudes and has significantly influenced the growth and direction of the home care industry. In 1990, government payment sources accounted for 78% of known home care spending. By the year 2000, the government's share for home care is expected to reach almost 90% of total expenditures (MacAdam, 1993).

The philosophy behind legislation establishing social supports determines how monies are allocated and programs are designed. In one model, the consumer pays directly for these basic and often personal services. In this case, the contract is between the purchaser of the services and the provider, and the purchaser can hire and fire at will. In the model in which the payer is a third party such as a government source, insurance, or a managed-care arrangement, public or corporate policy influences these contracts. It is difficult to determine if the consumer is the older person or the payer. The values of consumer choice and customer-driven services are often called into question in the provision of publicly supported programs. This reflects a desire on the part of various constituencies (funders, advocates, and others) to retain the autonomy of the consumer, recognizing that the element of choice in formal caregiving or social support impacts on relationships between the home care aide and the older person.

Publicly funded social support services for the elderly are primarily designed to keep people out of nursing homes or institutional care. There is a belief that the aging model undermines autonomy, with agency-based services and professionally designed care plans making the assumption that being vulnerable also means being unable to make decisions. Elias Cohen (1992, p. 50) describes aging services as a system based on an assumption that "disability in old age is a slippery slope toward inevitable decline and an ignominious end, and worse, the end of mastery." Cohen coined the term "elderly mystique," in which, much like the feminine mystique, he claims that we have created the perception that the elderly want to be protected, have designed and deliver services based on that assumption, and have made some very limiting conjectures about the vulnerability of people, their needs, and their desire for autonomy. If language and semantics tell us anything, one needs to look at the terms we use to define the social support providers in aging service. Aging clients have "case managers," someone managing their case, and "home care aides," someone taking care of them in the home.

Aging services are often contrasted to services designed for the disabilities community, which are reported to come from a strength and productivity model. The disabilities model is based on an acceptance of risk taking and uncertainty and encourages independent action on the part of the participants. It was developed to help young people with disabilities to become independent from their families and to lead productive lives, often away from their homes of origin. Disabled (younger) clients have "counselors," implying a coaching role, and "personal care attendants" or "independent providers" (IPs), implying the client's control over the care received. That control starts with an assumption that the client can hire, train, supervise, and fire the workers. Supports are sometimes built into the system to help the consumer learn the skills necessary to accomplish these tasks and to play these roles, along with training for the IP. Goals for these services include involvement and engagement, which give life meaning and go beyond survival and the limited aim of staying out of an institution. Consumers report a high degree of satisfaction with the IPs. On the other hand, some people in the disabilities community express frustration that care management is limited and that for some people in the program, recruiting, hiring, training, and firing IPs is a burden, not a freedom.

While there is a high degree of consumer satisfaction, there is also the potential for abuse of this system. Workers can intimidate consumers into signing bogus time sheets, case managers may authorize payment and leave the client on his or her own to find an IP who is never found, and physical or emotional abuse can occur, with the consumer fearful of losing the help on which he is dependent. One cannot ignore the economic implications in each of these models. Aging services, which are agency based, appear to be more expensive on a per unit basis. In addition to administrative costs that also include training and supervision, there are usually employee benefits, although meager, and an opportunity for collective bargaining, which theoretically increases the workers' ability to bargain for living wages. The disabilities approach often provides vouchers paid directly to the clients, who pay the IPs. The IPs are rarely trained, but are "people off the streets," according to one rehabilitation counselor. While the workers' direct wages in both programs may be similar, the independent-provider model appears to be less expensive and therefore more attractive to legislators. This may be an illusion.

In some states, when people with disabilities turn 60, they are given a choice as to whether they want to remain with their IP or to move into the aging system with its agency model. Most choose to remain with their independent provider. This may be due to their desire to retain their freedom, or it may be due to the relationship they have with their IPs. The point is that they have a choice between program models. That choice disappears once they choose to go into the aging services. Younger people with disabilities must select an IP. Older people with disabilities must select a home care agency that sends out one of its workers. Neither group has a choice of model.

RELATIONSHIP ISSUES

Although policy may dictate the type of relationship that will exist between home care aides and the homebound elderly, once the relationship is established, other issues emerge. The majority of homebound elderly have experienced close social support relationships with family members and friends. It is therefore difficult for them to adjust to the role of "social support client." Although many transition well and develop excellent relationships with their home care aides, it is not unusual for some elderly people to have expectations that cannot be met by the servicing agency or by the home care aides. Some elderly people want their home care aides to take the place of family and friends, expecting the type of relationship that has a basis in mutuality. Some go to the opposite extreme and treat their home care aides as servants. This latter situation is often exacerbated by the issues of race, class, and culture. Misunderstandings regarding the nature of the relationship prevent appropriate personal bounding, a "central feature of home care" (Eustis & Fischer, 1992), resulting in less than optimal intervention. Using a fictional Mrs. Smith as an example, we will explore some of these relationship issues.

Mrs. Smith is an 89-year-old widow who has lived at Hillside, a subsidized senior housing program, for two years. Prior to moving there, she resided in a nursing home for over a year after being hospitalized with a broken hip. Her assets were used to pay for her nursing-home care until the funds ran out. The nursing home then helped her to apply for Medicaid. She has one daughter and son-in-law who recently moved to Arizona for health reasons. The daughter has visited a few times and phones often. The Department on Aging in Mrs. Smith's state started a new program that actively attempts to bring people out of nursing homes. Mrs. Smith's doctor agreed that with assistance, she could manage. The case manager from the local Area Agency on Aging helped Mrs. Smith find a subsidized apartment, relocate, secure public entitlements, and set up a care plan for the services Mrs. Smith required: housekeeping and laundry, shopping, meal preparation, and bathing. Her worker comes three times per week for four hours each visit.

Expectations of Mutuality

Mrs. Smith misses the caring attention she received from her daughter and son-in-law. Carla, her home care aide, is a kind, friendly person who responds empathically to Mrs. Smith. She manages to get her work done while listening to Mrs. Smith talk about her interests and concerns. Mrs. Smith waits at the door for Carla and is sad to see her leave. She has told Carla that she is beginning to look upon her as another daughter; Carla is accepting gifts and invitations to stay for dinner and watches television with her, among other activities.

This scenario could move in another direction. Mrs. Smith tells Carla that she thinks of her as another daughter and is persistent in her attempts to form a personal relationship. Carla understands that Mrs. Smith should be able to talk about her problems and concerns, but she feels overwhelmed by Mrs. Smith's emotional needs. Carla found herself in this type of situation before and asked to be taken off the case. She is considering doing that now.

This expectation for the provision of personal emotional support by agency staff raises some interesting and difficult issues. Eustis and Fischer (1992) ask if "socializing" should be included as a purpose for the paid visit; if it is, will training for intimate but bounded relationships be a reimbursable cost, and as a matter of public policy, is the client owed a good relationship with a publicly paid caregiver?

Home Care Aides as Servants: Maternalism

Imagine that Mrs. Smith is Caucasian, and that her home care aide, Carla Jones, is African American. The fact that most paraprofessional work is performed by minority women often sets up expectations that the home care aide is a "servant," a situation exacerbated when the client or the employer is not a minority. Judith Rollins (1985), in her analysis of domestic service, coined the word "maternalism," likening this form of relationship to the paternalism historically found in the landowner's (or slaveholder's) obligations of protection and guidance in return for a servant's work, loyalty, and obedience. Aspects of its feudal and ancient history are evident in the "maternalism" exhibited by older middle-class (or formally middle-class) women toward their home care aides. It is not uncommon for home care aides to be referred to as "the girl," regardless of age, or for the aides to refer to themselves as girl: "I am her favorite girl."

Maternalism can also be found in agency practices. Education that implies that a person has little knowledge by not treating the home care aide as an adult learner, by infantilizing workers in the way directions are given, and by assuming that workers do not need support and supervision in negotiating boundaries all reinforce negative roles and undermine the workers' ability to define and maintain a social care relationship.

Control

Control issues may emanate from the maternalistic view of the worker as servant. There may be a struggle between the worker who needs to position herself as a professional and the client who needs to view her as a servant. For example, Carla, who wears her own white uniform, tries to establish clear expectations with her client based on the care plan and is detached but businesslike in going about her established routine, which she clearly spells out. She once was fired because she did not meet the "servant" expectation of her client.

Control can also be exercised in more benign behaviors. Mrs. Smith is fond of Carla and regularly tells her friends in the building about her "girl." She doesn't trust the substitutes sent out by Ms. Jones's social services agency when her regular worker takes a day off and has accused the replacements of stealing small items. She recently told the agency she didn't want them to send anyone else, implying that she doesn't trust African Americans when she said, "Carla is OK, though." Ms. Jones is paid the minimum wage for the hours she works, plus three "training hours" per quarter that she is required to attend. She supports her two children who are in high school and a granddaughter who lives with her. At times, Mrs. Smith allows Carla to leave early to tend to a family problem or to rest from her difficult work schedule. If the agency supervisor should call to talk to Ms. Jones, Mrs. Smith occasionally lies for her, saying, "Carla is at the store" or "Carla is cleaning the bathroom and can't come to the phone right now." Sometimes clients lie for fear that they will lose their worker on whom they are dependent. In many cases, however, clients "give" something to their workers, in the form of time off, for which the worker is paid by the agency (and the taxpayers). In a sense, both client and worker are exercising control over what is a quasi–employee/employer relationship. This type of collusion between home care aides and clients clearly crosses the relationship boundaries and is not uncommon.

Invisibility

On the other hand, Rollins (1985) discusses the invisibility of domestic workers and cites examples of families talking about highly personal matters as if the worker weren't there. Home care aides come to the older person's home to do tasks that the older person is no longer able to do for herself or himself. In fact, the older person may resent that she or he must now rely on someone else to do very basic functions such as shopping, cleaning, and cooking. These "activities of daily living" and "instrumental activities of daily living" are things one does not think about when one is strong and healthy; one just does them. When a person cannot do these tasks any longer, she or he may just want the task done without the burden of having to rely on an "actual someone" to do it. The older person may ignore the aide when she comes, allow threatening pets to run loose, or the like. While these manifestations may have root causes in the older person's state of mind (depression, anger at the losses she or he has suffered, resentment or embarrassment that she or he can no longer do things for herself or himself), this invisibility of the aide may also translate into a larger societal invisibility, where home care aides are not valued, and their work is seen as not important or as work that can be done by "anyone."

Cultural Issues

Cultural issues create some interesting problems in the way care plans are determined. Who provides the services and relationships between the participants giving and receiving the services all are issues for examination. This is especially true when there is a language barrier.

There are often barriers to access at the direct-service level. Agencies may not recruit and train workers from different cultures, and they may shun "hard" cases. Home care aides may be resentful or just insensitive to the cultural needs of their clients. Case managers and counselors who are gatekeepers to the programs often lack knowledge and/or understanding of the various groups they are assessing, may not speak the language, or worse, may be culturally insensitive. This puts them in a position of relying on family or friends to help them make "objective" decisions regarding the clients' plans of care.

Let's say that Mrs. Smith (née Solovey) came to the United States only 4 years ago to be reunited with her daughter, who had immigrated here 25 years ago. Her English is limited to what she needs to know to shop for her grocery items. The nursing home she entered had both residents and staff who spoke her language; however, she was anxious to leave the nursing home to join her two friends from the old country who live also at Hillcrest. When the case manager from the local agency did an assessment to determine her eligibility for services, Mrs. Smith requested and was given a home care aide, Wanda, who speaks her language.

Shared Culture

In home care, there is a normal delicate triangular balance between the client, the home care worker, and the agency (or agent). The worker has a formal contractual relationship with the agency to provide services to the client. She may have worked for that agency for a number of years and feels loyalty toward it. The agency has a contractual relationship with the client to provide services through the worker(s) and a contractual relationship with the worker to provide work, oversight, and payment. The client has a need that must be met, an entitlement to services, and an obligation to meet expectations of the agency (allow the worker in the house, pay any copayments, and the like). In the provision of care to ethnic populations, this balance may subtly shift.

It is not unusual for an alliance to form between the home care aide and the client when the caregiver is of the same cultural and class background as the care recipient. A "them versus us" mentality emerges, placing the worker in an ambivalent position, brought closer into the circle of family life and becoming absorbed into the system, almost as a family member. "Intimate geography," that is, parents living in the same building as their children, is common in many ethnic communities, due either to cultural or economic factors. This often makes it even more difficult for the home care worker to escape from being brought into the family circle. This is similar to the situation discussed under "Expectations of Mutuality," but here the pressures can be more intense because there is the expectation that *all* values are shared.

Family Caregivers

Hiring a willing family member is an easy way for case managers to meet a client's needs, especially when the case manager does not speak the client's language and cannot guarantee that the agencies from which the client must choose will have a worker who can speak her or his language. It is, however, a situation fraught with danger and raises challenging issues.

Mrs. Solovey's niece, Sima, was out of work, and since she could communicate with her aunt, the agency hired her to provide home care services. After several weeks, Sima took a part-time job at the local pharmacy. She continued to provide services to her aunt, but could not always promise exactly what time she would come because her schedule changed each week. Sometimes she came two or three times during the day, not staying long enough to do all of the jobs, but promising to come back the next day. At other times, she came later in the evening and just visited. Each week, Mrs. Solovey signed her pay voucher and sent it to the agency.

At first glance, it does not appear as if an example of family caregiving belongs here. However, in this situation, Sima has two roles: informal caregiving niece and paid, formal caregiver. Although she is performing very "informally," she is receiving a "formal" paycheck.

These are examples of just how complex the provision of social support is. It is not simply the performance of tasks; it is also the caring responses given to the vulnerable homebound elderly. "Caring responses" not only refers to those given by professionals and paraprofessionals, it also refers to those given by society through public policies and those given by agencies through their programs.

A great deal of responsibility for the successful implementation of policies and programs that allow the homebound elderly to maintain their independence falls on the shoulders of home care aides. Much of this success depends upon the nature of the relationship between the home care aide and the client, a relationship that is not yet fully understood and defined. In order for this understanding to occur, society and the providing agencies must clearly define their relationship with and responsibilities to the homebound elderly, which will help with the much-needed clarification of society's and the agencies' relationship with and responsibilities to home care aides. A discussion of social support in the context of rights and responsibilities may provide the needed groundwork.

SOCIAL SUPPORT: RIGHTS AND RESPONSIBILITIES

We begin with a brief explication of the terms "need" and "right." Although rights language in and of itself does not adequately address the complex issues found in the provision of home care services, it cannot be avoided when clients, agencies, and staff are attempting to determine the legitimacy of certain claims, requests, and demands. Rights language, however, will be tempered with the language of relationships and responsibilities.

A need is defined as a necessity, a lack of something that is required, or a condition in which there is a deficiency of something required. However, "The absence of certain things does not create a need unless this absence ought not to exist. Need-statements presuppose norms or standards" (Blustein, 1982, p. 19), and norms and standards suggest the existence of certain societal values. A need is often the foundation for a right.

A right is a legitimate claim to something along with the legitimate demand that others provide that something even if the specific "others" cannot be identified. "One of the chief purposes of morality in general, and certainly of conceptions of rights, and of basic rights above all, is indeed to provide some minimal protection against utter helplessness to those too weak to protect themselves. . . . Basic rights, then, are everyone's minimum reasonable demands upon the rest of humanity" (Shue, 1980, p. 119). They are the preconditions to being able to enjoy other rights and pursue other values.

Since sustenance is often listed as a basic need and right, let us look again at Mrs. Smith in the context of her not being able to shop for herself or do a great deal of cooking. She may have a right (a legitimate claim) to expect services from her family members and friends if her relationships with them have justifiably led her to believe that they can be counted on. Does Mrs. Smith have the right to expect her neighbors (those who are not her friends) to shop or prepare meals for her, and do those neighbors have the responsibility to do so just because Mrs. Smith has a need? Her neighbors may respond to Mrs. Smith's vulnerability by choosing to act altruistically although they may themselves have limited resources, or they may not respond if they are already responding charitably to others in need. Shopping or providing meals could, therefore, present too much of a hardship for any or all of them (family, friends, neighbors) because of relationship issues or because of a lack of time, energy, or resources. They would, however, still be expected to do the best they could regarding Mrs. Smith because of the human responsibility to respond to a basic need of a vulnerable person. They would most likely attempt to locate alternative resources, for example, a community agency.

Using needs and rights language, the absence of sustenance should not exist because this absence will prevent Mrs. Smith from meeting societally accepted standards of well-being, from exercising other rights, and from pursuing other values. As components of individual well-being, society values, among other things, life, health, and the pursuit of individual life plans. In addition to her very life's being at risk, if Mrs. Smith is malnourished and, therefore, unhealthy, she will not have the energy to enjoy activities that she values and that bring meaning to her life.

Making a case for Mrs. Smith's need and right to the provision of shopping and meal-preparation services does not appear to be difficult. From an ethics standpoint, someone or some entity in society is legitimately expected to address the issue of sustenance. But a case has only been made here for the provision of one type of social support service, not the provision of social support generally with its multitude of interventions, for example, housing, transportation, housekeeping, and personal and professional emotional support. The services needed for the provision of food may be a "minimum reasonable demand upon the rest of humanity" (Shue, 1980, pp. 18–19), but can the same be said about all social support?

Ought the absence of social support not to exist? Again, social support is defined as those concrete and professional emotional support services provided to the homebound elderly that enable them to maintain their independence. Would its absence prevent Mrs. Smith from meeting societally accepted standards of well-being? Yes, since society values independence, the taking care of oneself or being taken care of in one's own home, as a component of well-being. There are, however, social support services such as housing, transportation, and professional emotional support that must be examined individually to determine the status of each as a legitimate need and/or right. We will not attempt to legitimize countless concrete services, but will focus on the need for and right to emotional support, both personal and professional.

Personal Emotional Support

Personal emotional support is the empathic, caring exchanges given and received in relationships characterized by mutuality, liking, and interdependence. Throughout all stages of the life span, personal emotional support contributes to the individual's growth and well-being. Having a caring person to listen and be available for confiding in is important for the enhancement of life satisfaction and morale. The loss or absence of this type of relationship can result in emotional isolation, loneliness, depression, grief, and anxiety (Dugan & Kivett, 1994).

Looking at personal emotional support in light of the criteria used in the examination of a right to social support, would its absence prevent the individual from exercising other rights and pursuing other values? Yes, if the absence of that personal emotional support resulted in depression and thus prevented him or her from meeting societally accepted standards of individual well-being. What has been found, however, is that the absence of personal support for elderly people can result in loneliness and subsequently in depression, not that it definitely will. Social involvement may or may not be rewarding (S. J. Miller, 1986).

We can easily imagine three elderly homebound women living in the same senior-citizens apartment building as Mrs. Smith. Mrs. Clark enjoys having people around her all day. She talks and listens to a number of neighbors who visit, shop for her, and often share what they cook and bake. Mrs. Jones enjoys the same companionship and assistance, but with only two "close friends." Mrs. Kline accepts assistance from a home care agency but does not enjoy one-on-one socializing with any of her neighbors. She prefers to sit alone watching television, reading, and working crossword puzzles. She waves to neighbors as they pass by her window and is comforted by the knowledge that she can call on any number of them in an emergency, although she never has.

It appears, therefore, that the need for and the definition of personal emotional support are individually determined. Some people need it, some do not; some people need it from many sources, some from just a few. Additionally, the homebound client who is capable of making her or his own decisions has the right to make autonomous choices regarding the types and intensity of the relationships—personal emotional support and otherwise—she or he wishes to develop and maintain. It would be difficult to make a case for personal emotional support as a basic right because for some individuals, it is not a precondition to the enjoyment of other rights and the pursuit of other values since they are willing to sacrifice it in the pursuit of other values, for example, privacy. But that is not the deciding factor. We must remember that the critical component of personal emotional support is "mutual attraction and liking." When we refer to the right to personal emotional support, are we actually trying to make a case for a "right to be liked" with a correlative responsibility for someone "to like" that person? Would it be possible to make a case for an individual's right to autonomously choose having a personal emotional support relationship with whomever she or he wishes?

In the case of Mrs. Smith, it would be difficult if not impossible to defend a right to have her family members and neighbors like her, to enjoy being with her, to value her for her personal qualities, and to have her become a valued part of their lives. If her family and neighbors do not like her, they could again choose to act altruistically and respond to her personal emotional support need by spending an hour a day with her watching television or listening to her talk about her problems. They would be responding to her, however, as a person with a need, not as a person who elicits personal feelings. They can respond to her altruistically even if they do not like her. But they could also choose to fulfill their responsibility to act charitably by responding to someone else in need and not to Mrs. Smith. Or maybe spending time with her exacts too high a personal cost. If that is the case, could it be said that they have the responsibility to find an alternative resource, as they did in the discussion of the right to sustenance? What alternative resource exists for supplying Mrs. Smith with a relationship based on mutual attraction and liking? None.

Professional Emotional Support

If a case cannot be made for the right of an elderly person to a relationship with family and neighbors characterized by mutual attraction, it cannot be made for the relationship with professionals and home care aides. The client cannot and should not expect a staff member to be a friend or take the place of a family member.

This fact that a person does not have a *right* to a personal relationship with staff must also be viewed in the context of the *responsibilities* of professionals and home care aides as formal caregivers. The professionals' interventions are governed by their respective codes of ethics, which warn against the potential harm that can result from allowing dual relationships to develop. They cannot at the same time have a professional and a personal relationship with a client. Among the most important characteristics of the professional/client relationship are unbiased objectivity and the ability to prevent self-interest from interfering with professional decision making. Violating the professional/client boundary by allowing a personal relationship to develop puts optimal client care and, therefore, the client's well-being at risk. Because emphasis on the nature of the professional relationship is an integral component of the professional's education and socialization into the profession, if personal feelings for a client do arise, the professional is expected to examine them critically, discuss the situation with colleagues and with his or her superior when necessary, and resolve the issue in the way that serves the best interest of the client.

This is a more difficult situation for clients and home care aides to come to grips with because the types of services provided by home care aides often replace the "function of kin" (Hennessy, 1989, p. 633): housecleaning, performing personal tasks (e.g., bathing), and "socializing" in the client's home. In everyday life, these functions, especially socializing, are accompanied by mutual attraction, personal sharing, and interdependence. It is understandable, therefore, that because of the intimate nature of some of the services provided by home care aides, a client will misunderstand the relationship being offered and view the socializing as well as other interactions as being personal rather than professional. The misunderstanding is often exacerbated by the home care aide who may have entered this field because of a sincere desire to "help people" but has not received appropriate training regarding the nature and necessity of friendly but objective interventions.

To say that the client does not have a right to a personal emotional relationship with staff does not mean that the need of some elderly people for intervention because of the possibility or reality of loneliness and/or depression can be dismissed. The elderly may have a right to professional emotional support: the empathic, caring, but objective responses given in professional/paraprofessional relationships.

The client's desire to have the skillful, efficient performance of tasks carried out by a person who has genuine concern for her or his well-being as an individual and not as just another client should be recognized and honored. It is very important for all staff to hold the belief that the client not only has the right to the effective and efficient performance of tasks, but that she or he also has the right to "virtuous motives": concern, compassion, sympathy, and the like (Beauchamp, 1991). It is equally important for staff to be able to apply these virtuous motives in the correct context of a professional (caring but objective) relationship and not a personal (family or friendship) relationship.

Earlier we looked at the need for personal emotional support as a basic need and right and decided that it did not qualify because it did not appear to be a minimum reasonable demand upon the rest of society since people do not have the right to someone else's affection. We will use the same needs and rights framework to examine professional emotional support.

If a person needs professional emotional support, she or he needs it because its absence will make her or him unable to meet societally accepted standards of individual well-being; the need for or the absence of professional emotional support ought not to exist. Another way of saying this is "Society values the provision of professional emotional support to vulnerable, elderly individuals." A closer look at this value reveals that it may actually be referring to three values: virtuous motives, professional counseling, and socializing. The first one, virtuous motives, has already been addressed: "Society values the compassionate provision of concrete services."

The second is "Society values the provision of professional counseling to vulnerable elderly individuals who are dealing with issues of loneliness, isolation, loss, and the like." Is this a need for something whose absence ought not to exist, and is this type of professional counseling a precondition for the pursuit of other rights and values? The answer to both is yes, since professional counseling is often needed to maintain or enhance mental health, without which the individual cannot meet societally accepted standards of individual well-being. The individual will not be able to pursue other rights and values if she or he is depressed or lonely.

The third is "Society values the provision of 'socializing' services to homebound elderly individuals." This refers to the friendly interchanges about the events of the day or other topics for the purpose of preventing loneliness or as an additional intervention in support of professional therapeutic counseling. This is usually provided by paraprofessionals who are purposeful and objective in their intentions. Is this a need for something whose absence ought not to exist, and is the receipt of socializing services a precondition for the pursuit of other rights and values? The answer here is yes, the absence ought not to exist if the person chooses to have socializing services. Although the lack of these services could lead to loneliness, depression, or other mental health problems, that is not always the case, and some people will choose privacy over socializing.

We have decided that the homebound elderly have the right to social support services: legitimate concrete service needs and the three components of professional support. Using the right to socializing as an example, we will examine certain features of rights, an understanding of which will be useful in the discussion to follow.

Features of Rights

Some may argue that socializing is not a right because by no stretch of the imagination is it a minimum reasonable demand upon the rest of humanity. That argument would have weight if we were talking about a universal right, a right belonging to all people. We are not, however, referring to healthy, active individuals who bear a great deal of responsibility for their social lives. Rather, we are talking about a particular right, one belonging to a specific category of individuals: those vulnerable homebound elderly people who, not by choice, find themselves without friends or confidants.

One of the problems with the examination and determination of rights is that often we look first for the right in order to determine whether or not a responsibility exists. For example, if society decides that a right to socializing services exists, then the correlative responsibility is accepted. But if society decides that the existence of a right to socializing services does not exist, then neither does the responsibility to provide those services.

It is possible, and some would say much better, for society and its individual members to take another approach and examine first whether or not the provision of socializing services to those who need them is the responsibility of a decent society. If Heschel's observation that the test of a people is how it behaves toward the old is heeded, the answer is yes, and society will make the effort to provide these services through its social service system. In this case, the right exists because a responsibility has been recognized and accepted and a promise has been made to the homebound elderly. Society, through public policy, makes funding available to agencies who then announce (promise) that certain social services are available to those individuals who qualify as clients.

No matter how society explains the existence of any social service right as the basis of a responsibility or as emanating from one, it is important to note that very few rights are absolute, that is, never to be weighed against other rights. For example, respect for persons is an absolute right. Most rights, however, are qualified rights and can be weighed against others when all cannot be honored. For example, the right to make autonomous choices is a qualified right.

DISCUSSION

Providing social support to the elderly in the community is only beginning to receive attention from ethicists. There has been a fair amount of exploration of the ambivalence surrounding the case/care managers' role in relationship to their clients, agencies, and funding sources. Far less has been written about the provision of home care, despite the fact that this is the fastest-growing area of health care. This chapter has attempted to uncover some of the ethical issues inherent in the relationships found in publicly funded home care programs.

Although all parties in relationships have responsibilities to each other, we will focus on only a few relationships: policymakers, agencies, and the homebound elderly; policymakers, agencies, and home care aides; and home care aides and clients. The discussion is phrased in a manner that assumes the acceptance of certain values and responsibilities. However, we recognize that this is assumption and not necessarily fact.

Policymakers, Agencies, and Homebound Elderly

Policymakers and agencies are representatives of society's value to care for its vulnerable homebound elderly. They, therefore, along with the homebound, value the efficient, effective, and caring provision of concrete services, which include professional counseling and socializing. They also value respect for persons, which includes the individual's right to make autonomous decisions, in this case, decisions regarding her or his home care. It is not difficult to see how easily these values can clash.

As was discussed earlier, the type of program selected at the policy- and/or program-development levels—the disability model or the aging model—determines the amount of control the client has over hiring, training, supervising, and firing her or his home care aides. This, in turn, determines the type of relationship that will exist between the client and the home care aide, employer and employee or agency client and agency employee. In the latter, although the client may be consulted, the agency has the final say on the types of services that can be provided, how often, and when. Additionally, because of limited resources, the agency also may not be in the position to honor a client's request to have a home care aide replaced.

"As we approach old age, we face the tasks of learning and doing within a world of negotiated choices" (Berrin, 1995, p. 1) is a gentle reminder of the harsh reality that the right to make autonomous choices is not a universal, absolute one. Autonomy is, rather, a particular, qualified right: particular because it belongs to a specific class of individuals, those who are decisionally capable; qualified because it can be weighed against other rights. For example, Mrs. Smith has the right to make choices based on her own values unless that right conflicts with someone else's right to safety. Additionally, when Mrs. Smith becomes the client of a certain agency, she has what is called the right to client self-determination. This means that, as a client, she will not have the right to anything and everything she wants or even needs. She will, however, have the right to make choices from among the options available to agency clients.

Because limits placed on autonomy can affect the very identity of the individual, policymakers and agencies have the responsibility to critically examine existing and proposed limits to determine their legitimacy, for example, because of limited resources. Once the limits placed on autonomy are found to be legitimate, the policymakers and agencies have the responsibility to assist the homebound elderly in understanding, accepting, and integrating the limitations in a way that preserves self-esteem, potential for growth, and as high a level of independence as possible.

Policymakers, Agencies, and Home Care Aides

Policymakers and agencies may state that they value the effective and caring provision of concrete, counseling, and socializing services to the homebound elderly. The veracity of that statement is dependent, however, upon whether or not they actualize the following values: respect for home care aides who are responsible for the majority of these interventions and the provision of the appropriate training, supervision, and support necessary for them to do their jobs well.

The relationship between the home care aide and the client is complex, having features of both a professional relationship and a personal one. Home care aides are members of the home care team and are therefore responsible for observing, understanding, reporting, and sometimes addressing the physical and emotional needs of the client. This calls for specialized knowledge, skill, and objectivity, all of which are characteristics of a professional. However, the intimate nature of many of the interventions, the natural human response to frailty, vulnerability, and need, and the extended amount of time spent with the client make it difficult to divorce personal feelings from the relationship.

The home care aide is often expected by the agency and the family to act as a substitute when the family can no longer provide the social support needed by one of its members. In this role, it is not unusual for a home care aide to eventually suffer from the same types of stress felt by family members when they asked for help. In addressing the limits of morality in family caregiving, D. Callahan (1991a) stated, "That we are called on to respond to someone else's vulnerability means that, in turn, we become vulnerable" (p. 167). In discussing what spouses owe each other regarding continued care, Jecker (1995) pointed out that "caregiving can fulfill moral duties only when society prevents caregiving from leading to unwise and unbearable demands" (p. 176). It seems appropriate that in addition to valuing the provision of assistance to families in the care of their elderly members, there must also be the value of supporting the home care aide, who is often expected to shoulder the same "unwise and unbearable demands." Policymakers and home care agencies can make this a lived value by accepting the responsibilities to provide the training, supervision, and support needed by home care aides in order for them to negotiate the complexities of their relationships with their clients.

Although attention must be paid to the budget, these responsibilities should not be considered luxuries. In an environment of scarce resources, policymakers and agencies are justified in weighing the provision of one service against the provision of another. They are not, however, justified in weighing the provision of social support services by properly trained and supervised staff against the provision of social support services by poorly trained and supervised staff. The client may have to accept choosing from among a limited number of options when she or he becomes an agency's client, but she or he should never be expected to accept less than prepared and skilled interventions.

Neither should the home care aide be expected to accept poor, inadequate, or incomplete training. Therefore, in addition to having the responsibility to train and supervise home care aides for the benefit of the clients, the agency has the responsibility to train and supervise them for the home care aides' own benefit. There is a high personal cost paid when an individual views herself or himself as not having the necessary knowledge, skills, and understanding to do her or his job well, when she or he feels incompetent to perform certain interventions, or when she or he does not know how to function within the complexities of the relationship between home care aide and client. The value of respect for persons plays as prominent a role here as the value of providing effective, efficient, caring social support.

Home Care Aides and Clients

Respect for persons is also a critical value in the relationship between home care aide and client. There is usually an immediate recognition of the home care aide's responsibility to respect the client's individuality, needs, and values. It is not so readily apparent to everyone that the client has the responsibility to treat the home care aide with respect and dignity. A case can be made for the client's being temporarily rude or unpleasant because of the many losses she or he has suffered, or for her or his being occasionally rude because of the events of particular days. But consistent rudeness or unpleasantness should not be acceptable either to the home care aide or to the agency.

This type of difficulty is usually easier to handle than those that stem from cultural insensitivity, disrespect of persons from dissimilar races and cultures, and/or a demeaning attitude toward those perceived to be of a lower class. Although attitudes cannot be dictated or legislated, policymakers and agencies have the responsibility to demand the respectful treatment of home care aides. Policymakers and agencies should also be able to expect clients and home care aides to share a respect for honesty in their dealings with all involved parties. This includes, but is not limited to, hours worked and wages owed.

CONCLUSION

Whether the provision of social support services is a value, a responsibility, a right, or a combination of these, it appears to be an accepted response to the needs of the vulnerable homebound elderly. The home care aide as well as the relationship between the home care aide and the client are essential components of the successful provision of a great number of these services. The role and the relationship appear to be unique, falling somewhere between the professional and the personal, having characteristics of each.

Unraveling the complexities of both the relationship between the home care aide and the client and the home care aide's role in order to clearly define them is a daunting task. Its success depends upon the understanding of first the policymaker and client relationship, the policymaker and home care aide relationship, the agency and client relationship, and so on, until all possible combinations have been critiqued. Then the interplay of all of these relationships must be examined to fully understand, respect, and integrate into practice the combined array of values and responsibilities. The commitment of society and its professional community to the homebound elderly will be actualized by valuing the role of the home care aide and the individuals who function in that role.

12

Ethical Issues in Family Care

Jennifer Crew Solomon

Families tend to create enduring patterns of reciprocal support between older and younger members. Family social care is provided both by younger family members for older family members and by older people for younger. The focus of social care is providing assistance that increases a person's competence and mastery of the environment, rather than increasing his or her dependence (Hooyman & Kiyak, 1996). From a life-course perspective, social care begins with nurturing and socializing the young for participation in society. At the other end of the life course, social care provides assistance with tasks of daily living and personal care in cases of extreme disability. The specific type of assistance is determined by the family member's functional ability, living arrangements, and the gender of both caregiver and receiver. A discussion of ethical issues related to family social care must take into account different types of assistance, family structure, gender, age, and racial/ethnic characteristics of caregivers and receivers.

Bound up in these family caregiving contexts are ethical values, issues, and dilemmas. Ethical values (e.g., autonomy, beneficence, justice, fidelity) provide a basis for deciding what a person in a particular situation morally ought to do. A number of ethical issues arise when these values are applied to situations involving the provision of social care by family members. For example, what is the level of cognitive development required for a person to function autonomously? Ethical dilemmas are created by conflicts between ethical values. Should an older person be allowed to continue handling his or her own finances (autonomy) in spite of consistent money mismanagement (nonmaleficence)? In other words, should a person be protected from harm that results from his or her own bad decisions?

This chapter begins with a discussion of the wide range of assistance provided by family members to other family members and the characteristics of both caregivers and receivers. This is followed by a presentation and analysis of scenarios that illustrate how ethical considerations for autonomy, privacy, beneficence, justice, fidelity, nonmaleficence, and accountability apply to family social care provided by adult children for parents, older parents for adult children with developmental disabilities, and grandparents for grandchildren.

Ethical principles not only provide a basis for examining particular types of caregiving by family members but are woven into policies and legislation that influence behavior more broadly and impact U.S. society in general. Thus analytical strategies, models, and paradigms are presented as a basis for decision making on issues related to family social care. This includes assessing how well U.S. society addresses the needs of family caregivers and receivers; recommending improvements in policy, practice, and research; and making projections about the future needs and resources of family caregivers and receivers.

A discussion of ethical models illustrates the complexity of implementing decisions based on various ethical values. At the theoretical level, the ethical value of autonomy, for example, may be applied to all persons involved in the family. In practical terms, one family member's decision-making rights often impinge on those of another family member. Jamison (1995) warns that our society has placed increasing emphasis on autonomy to the extent that it becomes "almost pure hedonism" and is not balanced with "qualities of altruism and benevolence" (p. 43). Moreover, the family is also a moral community with certain rights and responsibilities, and therefore, family autonomy should not be ignored (High, 1991). Placing ethical values within the context of an ethical model not only highlights complexity but also provides criteria for deciding between alternative ethical decisions.

ETHICAL VERSUS LEGAL ISSUES IN FAMILY SOCIAL CARE

Family members provide most of the care for other family members of all ages, and their actions illustrate the ethical values of beneficence, nonmaleficence, fidelity, accountability, privacy, and justice. Families, however, do not act in isolation from the larger society and other social institutions. Laws and public policy affect family caregiving. In other words, the ethics of family caring is not confined to members of the family and their views of rights and duties but operates within societal institutions as ethical entities. For example, the ethical issue of justice may be difficult to interpret and act on in a society that is stratified by social class, race, ethnicity, gender, and age.

However, according to Kapp (1991), "In terms of practical impact on the lives of dependent older persons being cared for at home by their families, ethical considerations will tend to predominate over legal ones" (p. 6). Although family members cannot ignore the dependent person's well-being to the point of neglect, family members are not required to provide the actual care themselves. They may hire formal caregivers. Thus Kapp suggests that families in general provide care based on ethical rather than legal considerations.

Moreover, legal intervention has questionable application in areas of everyday decision making related to benevolence and autonomy such as hiding the car keys or locking up the liquor. Issues of privacy and accountability may also be raised with regard to the flow of information. Kapp (1991) points out that "the family members are in a position to monitor mail, telephone calls, television, radio, visitors, and other sources who might provide the client with information" (p. 21) as well as information from physicians and other formal caregivers.

Caregiving in nontraditional relationships (i.e., cohabiting same- or opposite-sex partners) may, however, require more specific legal or public policy attention. For example, including certain cohabiting arrangements in the concept of family would help ensure the application of the same legal and ethical responsibilities now assumed by "traditional families."

TYPES OF FAMILY SOCIAL CARE

The family as a social institution functions as the primary source of physical, social, emotional, and financial support for its members. Provision of various types of care flows back and forth between generations. For married couples, a spouse is the primary source of care. However, adult children care for parents or grandparents; aging parents provide assistance or care to developmentally disabled adult children; siblings help each other with housekeeping and transportation; and grandparents raise grandchildren.

Significant demographic and social changes have affected the size and structure of the family and thus the nature of family social care. Increased life expectancy and earlier childbearing in some generations have resulted in the growth of families spanning four or even five generations. For example, 10% of people over age 65 have a child who is also over 65 (U.S. Senate Special Committee on Aging, 1991). Thus a person may be both child and grandparent with care needs and resources based on both roles and life stages. For example, a 45-year-old grandmother may still turn to her 65-year-old mother for emotional or social support; however, as a grandparent, the same person is expected to be concerned with the welfare of her own children and grandchildren.

Another change in the structure of the family that impacts family caregiving is the existence of fewer age peers within a single generation (i.e., siblings and cousins) and more relationships across generational lines (Bengtson, Rosenthal, & Burton, 1990). Consequently, there are fewer younger family members available to care for older members. In addition, as a result of divorce and remarriage, adult children may find themselves caring for their biological parents, current parents-in-law, and former parents-in-law to whom they are still emotionally attached. These middle-aged adults may also find their young adult children returning home due to divorce, economic need, or drug-abuse problems (E. M. Brody, 1981; Cantor, 1994). Thus this so-called sandwich generation is faced with competing responsibilities to both older and younger generations.

Moreover, cohabitation by both same-sex and non-same-sex partners has increased, and little is known about their ability or willingness to provide various types of assistance. The ability of cohabiting partners to provide care for each other is partly related to formal legal rights and duties that will be debated in the courts. The willingness of partners to provide care is based on informal norms of responsibility that must be individually negotiated and then widely acknowledged. However, both ability and willingness may be dependent on the extent to which cohabiting relationships are viewed as similar or equal to the traditional concept of family.

FAMILY SOCIAL CAREGIVERS

Families provide nearly 80% of the in-home care for older relatives with chronic impairments (U.S. Senate Special Committee on Aging, 1992). The primary forms of assistance to older family members are social, emotional, and financial support, instrumental activities such as meal preparation, shopping, housework, and transportation, personal care (e.g., bathing, dressing, and feeding), and help with accessing social service agencies.

Care is principally provided by a single individual, the primary caregiver, with assistance from one or more others, secondary caregivers. The majority of the primary caregivers for spouses are their wives or husbands (Older Women's League, 1989; Stone, Cafferata, & Sangl, 1987; E. M. Brody, 1981). Most older men are married and thus receive needed care from their wives.

If the older person is not married or the spouse is ill, an adult daughter or daughter-in-law most often assumes the caregiving role, followed by a sister, niece, or granddaughter. This order represents a preference based on the caregiver's relationship with the older person, geographical proximity, and traditional gender roles. Adult children are primary caregivers to older widowed women and older unmarried men and serve as secondary caregivers for married couples.

The type of assistance given is influenced by the older person's functional level, place of residence, and the gender of the caregiver. For example, personal care is most often performed by wives or daughters (Cantor, 1991; Tennstedt, Crawford, & McKinlay, 1993). Over 80% of caregivers to the chronically ill are women. Nearly 29% of primary caregivers are daughters, 23% are wives, and 20% are other relatives or female nonrelatives.

Although siblings are seldom primary caregivers (Cicirelli, Coward, & Dwyer, 1992), they are sources of companionship and provide emotional and instrumental support for other siblings when a spouse or adult child is not available (Cicirelli et al., 1992; Peters, Hoyt, Babchuk, Kaiser, & Ijima, 1987). In particular, childless and unmarried elderly tend to rely on siblings rather than on other relatives for assistance (C. L. Johnson & Catalano, 1981). Older women are more likely than older men to receive help and support from siblings, especially sisters (Gold, 1989; O'Bryant, 1988).

RACE/ETHNICITY AND FAMILY SOCIAL CARE

The preceding discussion highlights general patterns of caregiving. However, there are subcultural differences. For example, multigenerational households are more prevalent among African American, Latino, and Asian families (R. W. Beck & S. H. Beck, 1989; Tennstedt et al., 1993). Social support and various types of assistance are exchanged within these extended-family households (Silverstein & Waite, 1993; Speare & Avery, 1993). Although such households may be formed on the basis of need, research indicates that even when controlling for need, racial/ethnic minorities are more likely to live in extended families. They provide assistance with finances and activities of daily living as well as social support between generations (Silverstein & Waite, 1993; Speare & Avery, 1993). For example, a larger proportion of black grandparents than white grandparents care for grandchildren (U.S. Bureau of the Census, 1991). Horwitz and Reinhard (1995) found that black siblings report more caregiving duties associated with caring for siblings with mental illness than do white siblings.

The traditional value systems of Asian Americans and Hispanics emphasize the importance of family and family obligations. However, implementing these values becomes increasingly difficult in today's mobile society in which jobs require relocation. Thus urbanization and modernization may have weakened patterns of intergenerational exchange (Maldonado, 1975).

Discussions of ethical issues in family caregiving need to be sensitive to differing cultural values and living arrangements. For example, issues of fidelity may be well understood in larger extended-family households, while beneficence may be complicated when more people are affected by decisions associated with providing dependent care.

GENDER AND FAMILY SOCIAL CARE

Women are the caregivers in society. They provide social, emotional, and instrumental care to the young, the old, the ill, and the disabled—sometimes simultaneously to various types of dependents. Men seldom engage in primary personal care and tend to provide personal care and instrumental aspects of care such as cooking and cleaning only when no women are available (N. J. Finley, 1989; Foster & Brizius, 1993; Kaye & Applegate, 1990; B. Miller & Cafasso, 1992). Sons are less likely than daughters to provide care in their own homes for a dependent parent. In general, men tend to focus on financial and concrete assistance (Hooyman & Kiyak, 1996). Many men, however, are primary caregivers (E. M. Brody, 1985; B. Miller & Cafasso, 1992), especially husbands for their wives.

A discussion of the ethics involved in family social care must address this unequal gendered division of caregiving responsibilities. Furthermore, power differentials within patriarchal families may complicate ethical decision making (Hanks & Settles, 1988–1989). For example, perceptions of who has the right to make decisions may influence views of autonomy and justice.

CASE STUDIES

Younger Family Members Caring for Older: Adult Children Caring for Older Parents

The provision of care by younger family members for older members may lead to the discussion of a number of ethical issues as well as produce ethical dilemmas when two or more ethical values clash. The following case study of adult children caring for older parents is useful for elaborating some of the ethical issues and dilemmas associated with this type of family social care.

Case 1: Martha is 75 years old and lives alone in the house where she and her late husband Michael raised their three children—a daughter and two sons. Her financial situation is tenuous, and she suffers from a number of chronic diseases, including arthritis and diabetes. She is, however, able to live independently with the help of her married daughter, who provides assistance with household cleaning, shopping, and transportation, and with financial assistance from her sons. Martha also receives social support from her daughter and grandchildren and regular visits and phone calls from her sons, who live in another state. Although Martha's current situation is fairly stable, family members realize that they will eventually confront caregiving decisions as Martha's health begins to deteriorate.

Ethical Issues	Ethical Dilemmas
Beneficence	Autonomy versus beneficence
Autonomy	
Fidelity	Justice versus fidelity
Accountability	

Family members have supported Martha (fidelity), emphasized her best interests (beneficence and nonmaleficence), and respected Martha's autonomy and privacy by making it possible for her to live independently and remain in the home filled with so many memories that it has become a part of her self. They have provided both the instrumental and financial assistance needed for Martha to continue functioning in her preferred environment (autonomy). Moreover, family members have been truthful about their abilities to help Martha (accountability) by explaining the limits of their financial resources.

Unfortunately, Martha's physical health is worsening, and her medication affects her equilibrium, resulting in dizziness and vulnerability to falling. In addition, her daughter has a full-time job that prevents consistent attention to Martha's care. Martha, nevertheless, expresses the desire to remain in her home and downplays the significance of her changing health and functional status.

Family members want to respect Martha's right to make her own decisions, but question her competence. Their main concern is for her physical well-being, which they view as endangered as a result of her deteriorating health and thus declining ability to take care of herself as well as the increased danger that she may inadvertently harm herself. For example, the dizziness associated with her medication could cause Martha to fall down the stairs in her two-story house.

From her family's perspective, her well-being may be better maintained by overriding Martha's wishes to continue living independently in her home. Thus family members illustrate continued beneficence in terms of concern for her physical well-being. They may also feel that they are maintaining Martha's autonomy through acting in her best interests. This action may, however, be defined as paternalistic and a violation of Martha's autonomy—her right to make decisions involving her health and well-being. Family members believe that Martha's dizziness jeopardizes her well-being. Furthermore, the family may assume that she is unable to recognize the potential hazards caused by her dizziness and believe that they are more aware of Martha's abilities and limitations than she is and thus are more qualified to decide the best living arrangement for her. In other words, family members may think that Martha does not recognize her limitations or see her dizziness as a problem. Therefore, they may view Martha as incapable of living alone not only because of her dizziness but also because she does not recognize her limitations and potential hazards. Martha, however, may understand her limitations very well but be willing to trade the risk of falling for continued privacy in familiar surroundings.

Furthermore, moving Martha to a more physically secure living environment may have negative consequences for her psychological, social, and spiritual well-being. This highlights issues associated with the ethical values of beneficence and autonomy. When broad terms such as well-being or personal welfare are used, people are sometimes forced into dichotomous thinking. For example, an action must be evaluated as either enhancing or diminishing a person's well-being. However, well-being can be broken down into different aspects: physical, psychological, social, legal, economic, and spiritual.

If well-being is multidimensional, then which aspects take precedence when all components cannot be achieved simultaneously? Under what conditions is it right to sacrifice psychological or social well-being for the sake of physical well-being? In other words, is it beneficent to protect a person from physical harm when it means restricting his or her social interaction? At what point does concern for physical safety cross over the line to paternalism?

Issues related to accountability also compound the difficulty of this decision-making process. Physicians may not provide patients with appropriate information about the nature and extent of their problems, the prognosis, or courses of actions. In many cases, this information may be given to family members, but not to the patient himself or herself (Latimer, 1991). This lack of accountability makes it difficult for the patient to act autonomously in his or her own best interest and fosters paternalism. Some physicians view paternalism as appropriate, especially within the physician-patient relationship. Family members, however, need to consider their obligation to be truthful in providing care or assistance to other family members.

Further complicating the dilemma between beneficence and autonomy in discussing paternalism is the fact that older people may interpret paternalism as beneficence. Only recently has there been an emphasis on individuals making their own health care decisions. Therefore, older patients may be less concerned about autonomy and expect physicians to be paternalistic (Knight, 1994). If adult children support this type of paternalism, the older person will not have access to information on which to make his or her own decision. Moreover, for some older people, acting autonomously may mean choosing to let someone else (e.g., the physician or adult children) make decisions for or about them or simply choosing not to choose for themselves.

A second ethical dilemma is that between justice and fidelity with regard to the daughter's current responsibilities and the pressure she may feel or receive from her brothers to increase her caregiving. Martha could remain contentedly in her own home if her daughter provided more continual and extensive care for her. This is a fact that all members of the family recognize. From Martha's perspective, it is clearly the best situation, but what about her daughter's rights?

The same ethical principles that apply to Martha also apply to her daughter. The daughter should also be able to act autonomously, making decisions about her own health and well-being and receiving the full support of other family members. In fact, support from other family members could help both Martha and her daughter maintain autonomy. For example, various family members could provide assistance that maintains Martha in her own home and at the same time relieves some of the responsibility from the daughter.

The ethical issues surrounding Martha's care and well-being must be juxtaposed with those of other family members as well as the family as a whole. It becomes very complicated to sort out ethical priorities. The scarce resources of time, energy, and money become decisive factors in ethical decision making. For instance, if Martha's daughter had the time and energy or her sons the money, Martha could be provided with the care she needs to retain her independence.

The ethical issues and dilemmas in this scenario could be further complicated by such factors as a care receiver with a terminal illness or with Alzheimer's disease or some other dementia affecting the mental functioning of the older person. In the previous example, if Martha had Alzheimer's disease, the issue of maintaining her autonomy may rest on family members acting in her best interest or making a substituted judgment of the kind of decisions Martha would make for herself, but without the benefit of Martha's current opinions on issues.

Moreover, the progression of the illness requires that family members provide increasing levels of assistance for Martha with decreasing levels of competent input from Martha. Thus family members' obligations to maintain her well-being (beneficence) become more and more difficult and may negatively impact their own well-being and autonomy.

Long-standing conflicts within the family, poverty, caregiver illness, competing needs among family members, and other family members requiring assistance add other dimensions to a consideration of the rightness or wrongness of decisions concerning family social care. For example, long-standing conflicts based on behaviors of the older care receiver, such as alcoholism, influence the attitudes of potential caregivers. Research has shown that perceptions of a person's culpability for his or her current disability affect caregiver response (Olsen, 1993). People are not as willing to help if they feel that the person needing help is responsible for the condition, for example, an alcoholic with liver disease.

In the current example, a solution that would preserve everyone's autonomy and produce good for all does not seem possible as long as the family is left to deal with the situation on its own. Solutions to ethical issues and dilemmas may not reside solely at the family level but at the societal level as well. For example, businesses could allow more flexible work schedules and paid leave for family caregivers.

One way of resolving some of the ambiguities in applying ethical values such as beneficence, autonomy, and accountability to this situation is to use a context-based ethics, such as the feminist ethics of care (Gilligan, 1982), which emphasizes relationships and nonhierarchical communication. A feminist ethics of care highlights the influence of existing socioeconomic and political structures of inequality in dictating caregiving responsibilities and, consequently, interpretations of ethical values such as autonomy, beneficence, and accountability. For example, what is Martha's experience of autonomy if she expected her husband to make all the "important" decisions? She may now rely on her sons to make decisions for her and experience their decisions as maintaining her independence.

Parents as Caregivers to Adult Children

A second context for family social care is that of parents with adult children who are developmentally disabled. The definition of developmental disabilities requires that the onset of the disability be prior to age 22 with the expectation that it will continue indefinitely. The conditions (e.g., mental retardation, epilepsy, and autism) impair the person's ability to function normally in society in terms of three or more of the following activities: self-care, language or communication skills, learning, mobility, self-direction, and the capacity for independent living or economic self-sufficiency. Consequently, parents of developmentally disabled children continue to provide care beyond the normative expectations of the parent-child relationship. As these parents age and experience age-related changes in health, caring for the adult child becomes increasingly difficult and may require the assistance of other family members. Moreover, the cumulative nature of the care demands of developmentally disabled or chronically mentally ill adult children often compounds the stresses experienced by aging parents (Kelly & Kropf, 1995; J. Jennings, 1987).

As life expectancy in general has increased, so has life expectancy for individuals with developmental disabilities (DDs). For example, 50 years ago the life expectancy of a person born with Down's syndrome was 12 years. It is currently only slightly less than that of the general population (O'Malley, 1996). Moreover, people with developmental disabilities are now more likely to live at home, in group homes, or in communal settings within the community rather than isolated in large institutions. Many require only minimal supervision or function well enough to live alone (O'Malley, 1996). The following case will serve to illustrate various ethical issues and dilemmas associated with this type of family caregiving.

Case 2: Janet is 45 years old with the testable intelligence of a 2-year-old. She lives with her parents, Mick and Molly, who are 67 and 65, respectively. Mick and Molly have another daughter, Eve, who recently divorced her husband. She lives within an hour's drive. Mick and Molly are currently in good health. Molly has primarily worked inside the home raising Eve and caring for Janet. Mick has recently retired and now has time to assist Molly with Janet's care. However, lately Janet has become physically aggressive toward her mother, who provides most of her personal care, and Mick has suggested moving Janet to the state hospital. Molly refuses to consider this option.

Issues	**Dilemmas**
Beneficence	Justice versus beneficence
Justice	Fidelity versus beneficence
Autonomy	Privacy versus justice
Privacy	Beneficence versus autonomy
Fidelity	Beneficence versus nonmaleficence
Nonmaleficence	
Accountability	

Mick and Molly have always provided Janet with a comfortable, loving environment (fidelity and beneficence). They have tried to protect her from harm (nonmaleficence), which is not always easy when dealing with a 2-year-old mentality in an adult-size body.

Issues of accountability, privacy, and autonomy are difficult to apply to people who are not considered mentally competent. Accountability in this case is not so much a matter of Mick and Molly being truthful with Janet as being trustworthy in their commitment to Janet's well-being. Janet does not have the intellectual ability to understand the basis of her parent's decisions, and thus they are not ethically responsible for sharing that information with her. However, they do have an obligation to continue to do what they have committed themselves to doing in the past—acting in Janet's best interests, which may include seeking assistance when problems occur that are beyond their capabilities.

In general, privacy refers to the right to restrict the dissemination of personal information and the right to associate with those of one's choosing, as well as to choose one's living arrangements and to engage in activities as long as they do not cause harm to others. Do these rights of privacy assume a certain level of intellectual functioning? Even 2-year-old children display choice in preferences for toys and being held by certain persons. What are Janet's choices with regard to living arrangements and activities?

It may be possible to apply the feminist ethics of care to this particular situation. Gilligan (1984) suggested that the ethics of care involves developing the "ability to perceive people in their own terms and to respond to their needs" (p. 164). Thus it might be possible to take into account the level of Janet's abilities and define autonomy as she experiences it at the 2-year-old level. Parents seem to recognize expressions of independence in 2-year-old children. Perhaps similar characteristics can be used to determine Janet's experience, for example, irritability at being ignored. On the other hand, young children do not always know what is best for them, and thus parents must act in the children's best interest.

Another issue to be considered is that of nonmaleficence or protecting a developmentally disabled person from harm—perhaps from harming himself or herself. What measures are appropriate? Should tranquilizers be used, or physical restraints, or locked doors? All of these could be considered strategies that protect the developmentally disabled person from harm, but they could also be viewed as harming the person in some way as well. This leads to a dilemma between nonmaleficence and beneficence in which family members, in trying to protect the care receiver from harm, cannot at the same time fully promote his or her well-being.

Another dilemma inherent within this caregiving situation is that of beneficence versus justice. Based on the concept of beneficence, Mick and Molly are obligated to maintain Janet's current level of well-being or improve it. They should also treat her with respect at all times and not discriminate against her in response to her disability. On the other hand, justice requires that the same ethical principles that apply to Janet also apply to Mick and Molly. Therefore, Mick and Molly have the same right to family resources as does Janet and an obligation to maintain their own well-being. What happens when Molly's well-being is threatened by the presence of Janet in their home? In addition, Mick and Molly have two small grandchildren who could also be endangered by Janet's physical aggression. The dilemma, simply stated, is whether Janet's well-being takes precedence over that of everyone else and how justice can be applied equally to all those who are involved.

For example, does their daughter Eve, who was recently divorced, have a right to expect that her parents will provide her and her children with temporary housing until she can afford her own place? There is an increasing trend of middle-aged and older parents experiencing the return of adult children to their household and to some kind of dependence on the parent. The percentage of unmarried adults age 18 to 24 living at home grew from 43% in 1960 to 55% in 1987 (U.S. Bureau of the Census, 1988). In some instances, these adult children return to their parents' home bringing their own children with them. Thus older adults may become responsible for various types of care to grandchildren as well as their adult children, and perhaps their own parents at the same time. How is it possible to act beneficently toward all concerned, to apply justice, and to respect everyone's autonomy?

A second ethical dilemma is that of beneficence versus fidelity. In general, these two ethical values should reinforce each other. That is, beneficence is shown by the maintenance or enhancement of a person's well-being, and fidelity requires that people be reliable in time of need. However, in this example, Janet's well-being may necessitate removing her from a familiar environment—her home—to a more secure but unfamiliar environment staffed by professionals who are trained to deal with her needs and control her aggression. It could be argued that although her parents are continuing to assist her and not abandoning her (fidelity), from Janet's perspective the move to an institutional setting does not maintain, let alone enhance, her well-being (beneficence). How many 2-year-olds want to be separated from their parents?

An additional issue relates to the ethical value of privacy. Janet's presence in the home, especially since she had become physically abusive toward Molly, infringes on Mick's and Molly's privacy rights—the right to associate with others of their choosing. For example, their daughter Eve and her children may be unable to visit or temporarily live with Mick and Molly for fear that Janet will direct her aggression toward them as well as toward Molly.

Furthermore, the value of privacy—keeping information about the care receiver's condition secret—may also conflict with beneficence. Families of children with developmental disabilities often have small or nonexistent social support systems (O'Malley, 1996) because other family members or friends may not be aware that the parents, for example, need additional help or respite from caregiving duties. In other words, privacy can threaten the caregiver's ability to provide quality care (beneficence). Parents may hesitate to seek assistance because of an unwillingness to share personal and possibly embarrassing information with others.

Additional factors that compound the ethical considerations have been mentioned earlier, such as long-standing family conflicts. Mick and Molly's daughter Eve is a potential source of support; however, she may feel resentment for the amount of care and attention Janet has received from their parents. She may believe that she has not been treated justly by her parents (Siegel & Silverstein, 1994). If her parents recognize this and feel guilty, they may not expect Eve to help with Janet's care.

One solution that could benefit most family members would entail placing

Janet in an institution or group residence; however, ethical considerations would remain relevant. Although institutional staff provide various types of care, residents still require personal monitoring and attention from family members. According to Josh Greenfield (1993), speaking of his son Noah, who resides in a state hospital, "Someone always has to speak up for him. To check his actual living conditions. To provide him with the dollop of love every human being requires" (p. 63). Therefore, ethical values such as beneficence, justice, and fidelity continue to apply to family social care even when the care receiver is institutionalized.

Grandparents Raising Grandchildren

According to the U.S. Bureau of the Census (1991), an estimated 5% of U.S. children under 18 currently live with grandparents, and in at least a third of these households neither parent is present. Many older people who must cope with their own health and financial problems are faced with the additional stress of child care that may exacerbate existing health problems. Several recent studies indicate that grandmothers alone raising grandchildren experience particular difficulty because of their high incidence of poverty and poor health (Minkler, Roe, & Price, 1992; Minkler & Roe, 1993; Solomon & Marx, 1995). In addition, the circumstances under which grandparents take on parenting their grandchildren are often traumatic, such as drug addiction or death of the parents (L. M. Burton, 1992; L. M. Burton & Bengtson, 1985). Therefore, grandparents may need medical, psychological, and legal assistance as they address the needs of their grandchildren (Minkler, 1994; Minkler & Roe, 1996). The following scenario takes into account common features of these surrogate parenting relationships.

Case 3: Virginia is a 60-year-old widow. She heads a household containing her 10- and 15-year-old grandchildren, whom she has raised since the death of her daughter and son-in-law when the youngest child was a baby. Virginia's income is slightly above the poverty line. She suffers from a number of chronic illnesses that sometimes restrict her activities. When this occurs, the role of caregiver may be reversed, with her grandchildren taking care of her. Virginia has a married son who lives 5 miles away, and she relies on him for help with yardwork and repairs around the house.

Ethical Issues
Autonomy
Justice
Beneficence
Privacy
Accountability
Fidelity
Nonmaleficence

Ethical Dilemmas
Justice versus beneficence
Autonomy versus beneficence
Privacy versus beneficence

Virginia has faithfully provided her grandchildren with a loving, caring home (fidelity). She has tried to protect them from harm (nonmaleficence); however, her limited finances result in limited access to health care, and sometimes the children have been left alone without adult supervision while she worked. She feels that it is her duty to care for her two grandchildren—that they have a right to receive her support and care (justice). However, Virginia often downplays her own health problems (justice versus beneficence) to protect her grandchildren. She worries that the children will be removed from her home and placed in foster homes if she becomes unable to provide care (privacy versus beneficence). Is Virginia's inclination to hide her problems (privacy) in the best interests of her grandchildren or her own welfare? This is also an accountability issue. Does Virginia have the right to hide her health problems from her grandchildren?

This type of decision making also reflects the tension between the values of autonomy and beneficence. When Virginia makes choices to ignore her own health problems, she may preserve the existing family living environment for her grandchildren and sustain their current level of well-being; however, lack of attention to her health could lead to future disability that might result in the responsibility for her care falling on the grandchildren. Therefore, what is the time frame in which beneficence is calculated? Ignoring health problems now may be in the children's current best interests, but it may jeopardize their future well-being.

A factor that would further complicate the situation of grandparent raising grandchildren and produce additional ethical dilemmas is assuming care of grandchildren as a result of drug addiction or child abuse by parents. This is also a situation in which the legal rights of the parents may supersede ethical considerations for the children. For example, parents must be judged incompetent to care for their children before their legal rights as parents are terminated. Proving incompetency may be difficult. Thus children may remain in abusive situations that do not promote their well-being (beneficence) because of legal requirements for proving the unfitness of the parents.

Multifamily households with grandmother, daughter or son, and grandchildren (and perhaps great-grandchildren) compound the ethical issues and dilemmas, as reflected in research by L. M. Burton (1992). Whose autonomy and privacy take precedence? Is it possible for beneficence to apply equally? What about protecting some family members from harm by other family members? Accountability may be a problem when drug abuse occurs. How does truth telling and trust play into family relationships when some members are addicted to drugs? Should some family members be forced to leave the place of residence when their actions suggest a lack of accountability?

Families clearly provide various types of social care between generations, and a number of ethical values are evident in these caregiving situations. For example, the ethical value of fidelity seems operative, as illustrated by the sheer number of family members involved in a wide variety of caregiving relationships between generations. Evidence for the values of beneficence, nonmaleficence, and autonomy is also suggested by the fact that most people prefer not to be institutionalized, and thus family members manage to provide care in a home setting for as long as possible. In addition, the dependent older person may be concerned about being a burden on other members of the family, illustrating a concern for justice and respect for others' rights. The ethical values of privacy and accountability may apply to a narrower range of caregiving relationships. For example, privacy is often important for families with developmentally disabled children. Accountability requires truthfulness and trust, but may be dependent on the care receiver's cognitive level.

The ability to implement action based on ethical values is influenced by cultural roles and structures of inequality. For instance, women are especially active in providing needed assistance to both younger and older family members and sometimes to multiple generations at one time. In a society in which women are expected to be caregivers and in which women have less power than men, actions based on ethical values such as fidelity and beneficence may be intertwined with obligation and coercion.

The context of family social care is also influenced by cultural values. In contrast to Caucasian families, which emphasize independent living, African American, Latino, and Asian American families are more likely to share households across generations. These multigenerational households provide an existing and ongoing context for needed assistance to flow back and forth between generations. Regardless of racial or ethnic background, family members care for other family members and in the process encounter decisions that raise questions based on ethical issues and dilemmas.

ANALYTICAL STRATEGIES, MODELS, AND PARADIGMS

Analytical strategies, models, and paradigms can be used to explore and suggest answers for some of these ethical questions as well as provide a basis for decision making. A number of ethical models or paradigms can be applied to situations involving the provision of care by family members. Some models focus on the consequences of the behavior (teleological theory), while others suggest that consequences alone may not determine the rightness or wrongness of an action (deontological theory) (Martin, 1995).

Two contrasting teleological theories are "utilitarianism" and "ethical egoism." Utilitarianism is probably the most prominent teleological theory. There are two types of utilitarianism: act and rule. The basic principle of act utilitarianism is that in any particular situation, a person should behave in such a way as to produce the greatest amount of good over evil, taking into account everyone who might be affected by the action. The morality of an action is related to the specific situation and may not generalize to other similar situations.

Applying act utilitarianism to the example of Mick and Molly, who are caring for their developmentally disabled daughter Janet, would provide a basis for moral decision making. One of the problems in this scenario was that of whose well-being should be considered. According to act utilitarianism, the best interests of the whole family must be taken into account. Concern for any one person (i.e., Janet) should not override the well-being and functioning of the entire family. Therefore, if Janet's continued presence in Mick and Molly's home puts other family members at risk for physical abuse and impinges on Mick and Molly's ability to associate with their daughter Eve and her children, a decision to institutionalize Janet would be ethically justified.

Whereas act utilitarianism applies to action in specific situations, rule utilitarianism specifies that an action is moral when acting in accordance with a particular rule would produce the greatest balance of good over evil, everyone considered. Both forms of utilitarianism take the focus off the individual and take into account others affected by the decision or action. Because rule utilitarianism specifies action based on a generalizable rule, it could be the basis for policy decisions as well as individual action. For example, a federally funded home health care program could support the ethical value of autonomy as reflected in a rule stating that autonomy is best expressed by and within a person's preferred living environment.

In contrast to both act and rule utilitarianism, which emphasize the implications of a person's action for others, ethical egoism bases morality on what promotes a person's own self-interest. This is obviously a very self-centered basis of morality but may nevertheless have important implications for family caregiving. Many decisions that people make concerning themselves have ramifications for other people. For example, lifestyle decisions concerning eating habits, smoking, drinking, and exercise may result in disease and/or disability requiring care provided by others. As previously mentioned, the perception of the care receiver's responsibility for the disability or illness influences his or her access to care. Thus the person who defines his or her own good as eating nutritious meals, exercising regularly, and not smoking cigarettes may receive better care than the person who defines his or her good as drinking excessively or smoking cigarettes.

Furthermore, people who act ethically according to this theory would evaluate the extent to which providing care has a positive impact on their own self-interest and well-being. For example, if Martha, in the first scenario, is generally enjoyable to be around and family members respect her contributions to the family, then it may be in their self-interest to work out a living arrangement that maintains Martha in her own home. Furthermore, family members may decide to share living arrangements with an older family member because they find that the additional income provided by the older person's Social Security check or retirement income substantially enhances their household income.

Kantian deontology is the second broad category of ethical models. This paradigm is based on respect for persons as elaborated in "the Categorical Imperative," which states that a person should "act only on that maxim through which you can at the same time will that it should become a universal law" (Kant,

1964, p. 88) and "act in such a way that you always treat humanity, whether in your own person or in the person of any other, never simply as a means, but always at the same time as an end" (Kant, 1964, p. 96). From these moral bases are derived a number of duties, both "perfect duties" and "imperfect duties." The following are examples of perfect duties for which there are no legitimate exceptions: do not kill innocent persons, keep promises, do not lie. There are perfect duties not only to others but also to oneself. Thus a person should have respect for himself or herself as well as for others. For the family caregiver, this would suggest issues of beneficence and justice. The family caregiver should consider his or her own well-being as well as that of the care receiver and respect the rights of all involved.

For instance, family caregivers, usually women, are often willing to assume caregiving responsibilities in spite of the negative consequences to their own well-being in terms not only of health, but also finances, personal freedom, and privacy (Hooyman & Kiyak, 1996). The concept of caregiver burden is a subject of concern in the research literature. Caregiver burden can be subjective or objective. Subjective burden refers to feelings such as worry, sadness, anger, or resentment experienced by the caregiver (Braithwaite, 1992). Objective burden refers to the physical demands of caregiving and its effect on family relationships, income, and social life.

According to Kant, by taking the degree of caregiver burden into account, it would be ethically reasonable to withdraw from a caregiving relationship when the caregiver's own health or financial well-being were at risk. The obvious consequence of this ethical reasoning is that many caregivers would cease providing care, and people such as Martha and Janet would have to rely either on other family members or institutions for needed assistance. Overwhelming evidence indicates that this seldom happens.

Another model, offered by W. D. Ross (1930), may illustrate why the relinquishing of caregiving responsibilities just mentioned seldom occurs. Ross is a "duty ethicist" who shares Kant's basic orientation but rejects Kant's notion that certain duties are absolute. Ross's approach is particularly appropriate for discussing family social care because he addresses the situation where people are confronted with a conflict of duties. How does a person decide which one takes precedence?

According to Ross, duties are based on relationships, such as that of parent to child, friend to friend, and spouse to spouse. Each of these relationships is the foundation of what Ross calls a "prima facie duty." Prima facie duties are derived from the rights and obligations associated with specific reciprocal role relationships. For example, parents have certain obligations for the care of their children.

Ross, however, notes that people may be faced with a number of duties at one time—a situation commonly experienced by family caregivers, especially members of the well-known "sandwich generation" who may be raising their own children while providing care for older family members. Ross suggests that some duties (i.e., prima facie duties) may be cancelled out by other duties when considered within a particular context. For example, caring for a child who cannot take care of himself or herself takes precedence over caring for an older person who is able to wait on or to provide minimally for himself or herself. A problem with applying Ross's model to caregiving by adult children for older parents, older parents for adult children with developmental disabilities, and grandparents raising grandchildren is that these caregiving roles are outside the norm and have no clear-cut expectations for the provision of care.

The previous models focus on the primacy of duties. However, duties imply rights, and certain ethicists contend that it is rights that provide the foundation of morality, not duties. Duties arise only because people have certain rights. According to John Locke (1960), the most basic rights of people are human rights, such as the rights to life, liberty, and property. All people have rights just by being people. Moreover, these human rights are "inalienable"—they cannot be taken away. A person can decide not to exercise a right or assign someone else to be responsible for acting on his or her behalf (e.g., power of attorney or guardianship), but this does not negate the basic human right to autonomy and having control over decisions that directly affect oneself.

How does a consideration of inalienable rights take into account people with dementia who can no longer make their own decisions or assign decision-making power to others? It might be possible to anticipate the decline in mental abilities and encourage the person to assign decision-making power while he or she is still capable. Autonomy is thus maintained but would necessitate accountability in the form of telling the person the truth about the prognosis of cognitive decline. While this approach may address the ethical values of autonomy and accountability, such a decision may not be very beneficent. Being told of one's eventual cognitive decline may even create a self-fulfilling prophecy that accelerates the loss of mental ability. For example, what should Martha's family tell her about their concern for her forgetfulness?

Besides inalienable human rights, there are also "special moral rights" that are created by relationships or commitments, such as those of children to be cared for by their parents. Do older family members have special moral rights to be cared for by younger family members? Do the special moral rights of children get transferred to grandparents when parents are not capable of caring for the children? A basic issue here is that of fidelity and the obligations created by certain relationships.

A. I. Melden (1981) suggests that there is one ultimate right from which other rights are derived: the right to pursue one's legitimate interests, which are those interests that do not impinge on or violate other people's similar and equal rights (Martin, 1995). Moreover, Melden (1981) suggests that people may need help in pursuing their basic rights, and furthermore, people have a right to this assistance, particularly when it involves the provision of necessities for a decent existence. Melden calls these rights positive rights or "welfare rights." This theory implies that the state as well as families is responsible for the care of other family members. For instance, grandparents raising grandchildren would benefit from policies that gave them access to financial assistance (e.g., AFDC or foster parent programs) in raising their grandchildren.

In contrast to the previously discussed models, feminist ethics suggests that moral decision making should not focus narrowly on rights, rules, and abstract notions of justice but rather on the "ethics of care" in concrete situations that take into account the point of view of both the caregiver and care receiver (E. B. Cole & Coultrap-McQuin, 1992). The foregoing discussion of ethics as based on rights and duties reflects a largely male-centered exploration of morality. Men's experience has often involved economic transactions, and thus their ethical theories contain such terms as rights, duties, property, and rules.

Feminist ethics takes into account women's experience and values (Gilligan, 1982). Ethics based on care does not refer to abstract universal rules but requires responding to real people's needs in actual situations. In addition, feminist ethics requires nonhierarchical decision making and emphasizes communication (Walker, 1989). Similarly, Nel Noddings (1984) argues for an "ethic of caring," which includes two elements. The first is a "disposition to care" that entails an openness to the needs of others. The caring relationship is characterized by the caregiver's ability to understand the care receiver's point of view, needs, and expectations. Thus the care receiver experiences autonomy and responds by developing himself or herself.

The second element is the obligation to "care for" by acting in ways that address the care receiver's needs. Manning (1992) describes daily interactions as creating expectations of reciprocal caring based on role relationships. Although "caring for" may require self-sacrifice, she warns that a person should guard against "caring burnout," which could be avoided in a "caring society" in which not only individuals but social institutions recognize and respond to the needs of its citizens for care. Because women are the caregivers at all levels of family social care, a feminist ethics based on caring has particular relevance to the discussion of ethics of family care.

One of the dangers cited concerning the feminist ethics of care is that it may lead to a restrictive view of women. Baier (1985) observes that women's responsibility for the care of others is imposed on them by asymmetrical power relations in society. The emphasis of feminist ethics on caring, empathy, and nurturance has the potential for justifying a limited view of women as caregivers by nature rather than because of the influence of socioeconomic and political structures. Moreover, Mary Dietz (1985) argues that feminist ethics emphasizes "maternal thinking" that narrowly confines care to family relationships rather than the broader context of social responsibility.

Feminists want to emphasize that caring is an important ethical basis for providing assistance. At the same time, feminists caution that an ethics of care does not justify women's continued exploitation as society's caregivers. Thus the notion of care must be combined with the concept of justice to broaden the context of care.

AUTONOMY

Many ethical issues and dilemmas are associated with the value of autonomy. An elaboration of this important concept may broaden the discussion and offer a reference point for action. Autonomy is typically defined as self-determination or self-governance.

Kant and Mill both emphasize the importance of autonomy. Kant (1959) clearly stresses autonomy with his emphasis on humans as self-determining subjects who should always be treated as ends in themselves. Mill (1979) expresses similar notions of autonomy when he speaks of "individuality" and the ability of persons to choose between various options based on reflection and reason and without coercion. However, a person's autonomy may be limited by external factors such as coercion, deception, and lack of information or by internal factors such as mental incompetency, strong emotions, or severe pain. Are there conditions under which a person's autonomy may be justifiably restricted?

The concept of paternalism provides a way to discuss exceptions to the morality of autonomy. Paternalism, according to Gerber (1995), is a major ethical concern for elders and their caregivers. Paternalism is limitation of a person's autonomy that is justified by reference to the needs or welfare of that person. Justification may be based either on the benefit to the individual or on prevention of harm to the individual. Mill (1969), who highly values individual autonomy, argues that while preventing harm to others may sometimes justify interference with autonomy, preventing harm to the individual never does because the individual is always the best judge of his or her own interests. For example, Janet's aggressiveness toward her mother could be a basis for restricting Janet's autonomy (i.e., placing her in an institution), but restraining her to prevent self-harm would not.

This individual that Mill is speaking of, however, is "in the maturity of their faculties.... Those who are still in a state to require being taken care of by others, must be protected against their own actions as well as external injury" (1969, p. 135). This statement seems to open the door for considering the use of paternalism based on the mental abilities of the person and could be applied not only to children who have not developed these abilities but to others with reduced intellectual capacities such as older persons who suffer from certain forms of dementia or the developmentally disabled.

In a similar vein, the following set of "liberty limiting principles" (Feinberg, 1973, p. 33) is used to justify restrictions on autonomy: (1) to prevent harm to others, (2) to prevent a person from offending others, (3) to prevent a person from harming himself or herself, (4) to benefit that person, (5) to prevent the person from acting immorally, and (6) to benefit others. The prevention of harm to others is the most accepted limitation of autonomy. What are the implications in the ethics of caregiving for limiting the autonomy of a person for whom providing care causes harm in the form of stress, depression, and physical illness for the caregiver?

PUBLIC POLICY

In the area of public policy, Kapp (1991) indicates that there should be little external monitoring of family caregiving relationships: "society cannot legislate lovingkindness" (p. 11). However, some families are dysfunctional, and thus elder-abuse and neglect laws seek to prevent harm where ethical considerations for nonmaleficence are inoperative. Public policy addressing elder mistreatment must not simply punish but also address issues of autonomy and support for families.

One public policy approach would be the creation of programs that support family caregiving, for example, training family members to provide certain services for the dependent family member. Financial compensation to family members who provide care would be an added incentive (Kapp, 1991) that might also reduce the financial burden assumed by families in providing care, especially when caregivers are required to quit paid work in order to take care of the older person. For example, public policy changes in criteria for foster care programs would provide an additional income source for grandparents raising grandchildren.

By enhancing family members' ability to care, public policy encourages both beneficence and autonomy. Autonomy in financial management can also be enhanced by legal devices such as ordinary power of attorney and joint bank accounts. In this way, an older person who cannot physically conduct his or her financial business can make decisions and assign a substitute person to go to the bank or write checks. Public policy considerations should focus on enhancing the older person's autonomy while protecting him or her from harm (Kapp, 1991). Grandparents raising grandchildren may also need legal assistance and legal rights in order to acquire medical care for their grandchildren.

FUTURE NEEDS AND RESOURCES OF FAMILY CAREGIVERS

The family will continue to be the primary source of physical, social, emotional, and financial support for its members. Demographic changes such as increased life expectancy, the large baby-boom cohort, and fewer age peers suggest that there will be more older family members to be cared for by fewer younger family members. Although caregiving in aging families brings to mind images of younger members providing care for older members, care tends to flow from older to younger members as well. Older people provide care for each other, their children, and their grandchildren. Siblings also provide care for other siblings who have no spouses or children to rely on.

Moreover, unless gender-role socialization practices change, women will still be considered the primary caregivers to both the young and old. To further complicate both ethical and practical issues surrounding family social care, women are now also more likely to be working outside the home. Consequently, they are likely to need more public as well as private support for their caregiving efforts.

In addition to family forms based on traditional definitions of family, the number of new and diverse family structures such as cohabitation by unmarried heterosexual and homosexual couples and communal living has increased. Little is known about the ability or willingness of these types of families to provide care that may require creating "surrogate families" to replace the traditional family support systems. For example, gays and lesbians who have experienced the loss of family support earlier in life are less likely to rely on family members to assist them in old age. Consequently, they develop strong friendship networks to replace family supports (Friend, 1991; Quam & Whitford, 1992).

In the future, family forums can assist family members in learning the best practices of care. Families of all types will need social policies and programs that are broadly supportive of family members at all stages of the life course, for example, AFDC or foster parent programs that include grandparents; day-care, adult day-care, and respite-care programs; family leave policies that ensure job security; and affordable, accessible health care. Families provide a public good in the form of caring for dependents, both young and old. Political and economic institutions need to acknowledge the essential contribution families make to society and respond with programs designed to support the ethical values involved in the provision of family social care.

13

Ethical Issues in Legal Care

Marshall B. Kapp

Mr. M, a 78-year-old retired corporate executive, walks into his attorney's office. Other than moderate, medically controlled hypertension of many years standing and the beginning pangs of arthritis, he is in good general health, as is his spouse. He realizes, though, that at some juncture in the future his health is likely to deteriorate, perhaps to the point where he will require admission to a skilled nursing facility. Mr. M has come to his attorney for the express purpose of planning for that contingency and specifically for advice about taking advantage of legal devices that will protect his considerable financial assets and income for the benefit of his spouse and adult children while permitting him to exercise an entitlement to Medicaid coverage for his skilled nursing facility care.

Mrs. Y, an 83-year-old widow with a substantial inheritance, enters the attorney's office with her oldest adult son (the one who made this appointment). The son does virtually all of the talking, explaining that Mrs. Y increasingly is experiencing problems in managing her finances and would like to delegate that responsibility to this son. The son requests that the attorney draft for Mrs. Y's signature a durable power of attorney or other legal document to accomplish this delegation.

Mr. K is a 70-year-old man who has been treated for the past several weeks in Holy Smokes Hospital, where he was admitted with a stroke. Prior to this hospitalization, he had lived alone for many years in a single-family house in a rural area 40 miles from the hospital. Although his cognitive status is good, he is physically weak, and his health care team believes that he would have substantial difficulty in doing even minimal activities of daily living if he returned home at this time. Despite the discharge planner's strong warning that his home environment now would be unsafe for him and her recommendation that he should go into a skilled nursing facility for a period of rehabilitation, Mr. K intends to exert his legal right to refuse to follow that professional recommendation and to take his chances at home. He even declines advice that he hire a home health agency to assist him, since he would have to pay a large portion of that expense directly out of pocket.

As these brief, common scenarios illustrate, complex ethical issues frequently arise in the context of attempts to protect and promote the legal rights of older persons. As is true for other aspects of geriatric care, advocating for the rights of the elderly is usually an interdisciplinary and interprofessional endeavor, and the ethical questions implicated are multifaceted. After enumerating some of the kinds of rights affecting older persons for which society has devised various legal protections, this chapter outlines a few of the most salient ethical conflicts and conundrums that confront advocates, health and human services providers, and society during the process of considering, utilizing, and evaluating these legal protections.

ELDER RIGHTS

American society has created a substantial array of legal rights for, or at least potentially applicable to, older persons. These legal rights, emanating from statutes, regulations, and judicial interpretations of constitutional and common-law principles, fall into two categories. Liberties, or negative rights, consist of an individual's shield against unwanted external intervention or interference. For example, the Age Discrimination in Employment Act's prohibition against employers treating employees or potential employees differently (i.e., less favorably) because of their age constitutes a liberty right or freedom for the employees or potential employees. The Nursing Home Quality Reform Act (part of the Omnibus Budget Reconciliation Act of 1987) and its implementing regulations contain entire sections guaranteeing resident rights (e.g., rights to privacy, religious practice, and communication) against unwanted intrusions by nursing facilities.

Conversely, positive rights or claims entitle an individual to demand some affirmative benefit from someone else. The Social Security, Medicare, and Medicaid acts create such entitlements for designated older persons. So, too, do provisions requiring reasonable accommodations—not merely equal opportunity—from employers or businesses serving disabled persons under the Americans with Disabilities Act.

Over the past two decades, the field of elder law has become recognized as an intellectual subdiscipline and a specialty area of legal practice. The implications of this development are profound for older persons, their professional caregivers, and society. Older individuals now are firmly entrenched as distinct legal-services consumers and beneficiaries of the law, as are agencies that serve the elderly. Laws and practices that target the elderly for particular protections or entitlements are tools that both reflect and help to shape heightened social attitudes toward, and respectful treatment of, the nation's older inhabitants. The application of these laws and practices, however, may also raise many thorny ethical questions. It is to an examination of a sampling of these questions that this chapter now turns.

ETHICAL ISSUES AND CONFLICTS FOR ADVOCATES

In their attempts to obtain and/or exercise legal rights, older persons often rely upon the advice and representative services of attorneys and professional nonattorney advocates (e.g., ombudsmen or case managers). The advocate's role acting on behalf of the older person may be fraught with ethical conflicts and ambiguities (Green & Coleman, 1994). Existing ethical standards (American Bar Association, 1981, 1983) have contemplated poorly, if at all, many of the situational contingencies encountered in the service of elderly clients and as a result generally do not provide helpful guidance for resolving ethical quandaries arising in real daily practice.

In the first case presented, for instance, the attorney is asked to assist an older client who could afford his own eventual long-term-care costs to avoid personal responsibility for the costs of his own care by shifting that responsibility to the taxpayers. Although this strategy is permissible under current Medicaid law, it clearly was neither intended nor envisioned by the drafters of that law, and a strong public policy argument may be mounted in favor of outlawing asset transfers conducted for Medicaid eligibility purposes so that public dollars can be used on behalf of the legitimately needy. The attorney here must decide whether it is ethically appropriate, or perhaps even obligatory, to help the client legally manipulate a law that, from a societal perspective, might be characterized as ethically dubious (Crosby & Leff, 1994; Working Group on Divestment, 1994).

The second hypothetical scenario set forth at the beginning of this chapter raises a panoply of ethical concerns for the attorney who has an older person as a client but who is receiving instructions about the client's legal wants and needs from that individual's family member(s). Specific issues to be addressed either directly or tangentially in this difficult but not uncommon type of intergenerational (Collett, 1994; Working Group on Intergenerational Conflicts, 1994) or joint spousal (Pearce, 1994; Working Group on Spousal Conflicts, 1994) situation include but are not limited to (*a*) determining the older client's cognitive and emotional capacity to engage rationally and voluntarily in the sort of decision-making process involved in the legal activity at hand (e.g., making a testamentary or living will, executing a durable power of attorney, selling real property) (Roca, 1994); (*b*) in the case of clients with compromised decisional function, balancing the attorney's responsibility to be a zealous advocate of the client's autonomy or self-determination, on the one hand, with the ethical imperatives of beneficence and nonmaleficence to do good and prevent harm by protecting the best interests of those who are vulnerable and helpless against threats of harm (even harm from themselves), on the other (Margulies, 1994;

Rein, 1994; Tremblay, 1994; Working Group on Client Capacity, 1994); and (c) the extent of confidentiality obligations and how to finesse their observance appropriately (Powell & Link, 1994; Working Group on Client Confidentiality, 1994; Wydra, 1994).

A variety of other kinds of ethical considerations may complicate the work of advocates for the elderly. For example, particularly in legal-services–type advocacy organizations, there may be a strong temptation to use the particular client more as a means than as an end in himself or herself, thereby violating Kant's categorical imperative (Kant, 1938). More specifically, advocates pushing for "social change" (i.e., public policy modifications more consistent with their own personal values and interests) (Sowell, 1995) are acting unethically when they treat individual older clients merely as necessary tools (e.g., to achieve standing in litigation or as appealing photo opportunities in legislative hearings) for achieving that political change, regardless of the actual impact on the client herself or himself (G. P. Lopez, 1996).

ETHICAL ISSUES AND CONFLICTS FOR SERVICE PROVIDERS

Professional and agency providers of health and human services are expected, as part of their fiduciary or trust relationship (Frankel, 1983) with the older persons they serve, to respect and promote their clients' legal rights. In fulfilling this function, ethical dilemmas are bound to materialize. For descriptive purposes, we shall examine the contexts of guardianship and elder abuse and neglect.

Guardianship is a legal relationship, authorized by a state court, between a ward (the person whom a court has declared to be incompetent or incapacitated to make particular decisions) and a guardian (whom the court appoints as the surrogate decision maker for the ward). Terminology regarding this relationship varies somewhat among jurisdictions.

The ethical justification for state (i.e., judicial) imposition of a surrogate decision maker for an incapacitated individual in the realm of both personal and financial decisions is found in the two fundamental and related principles of nonmaleficence ("first, do no harm" to others, or *primum non nocere*) and beneficence, or "doing good." These ethical principles have been transformed into the legal doctrine of *parens patriae* (literally, "father of the land"), the inherent responsibility and authority of a benevolent society to intervene, even over objection, to protect people who cannot protect themselves. Thus, instead of abandoning cognitively and/or emotionally incapacitated individuals to a superficial, meaningless autonomy to make harmful decisions or to neglect their own basic needs, the state may exercise its authority to protect even unwilling disabled individuals from their own follies or deficits.

When guardianship for an older person is contemplated or initiated for benevolent purposes, that is, to help and protect a person who really is at risk because of serious deficits in decision-making ability, the ethical issues for geriatric service providers are difficult enough. When guardianship is employed, as often happens, more to serve the psychological, financial, or risk-management interests of others, such as family members, financial institutions, business associates, and service providers (Schmidt, 1995), the ethical considerations can become yet more complicated.

Any consideration of the appropriate use of guardianship takes place within the context of a tension between our commitment to individual autonomy—the right to be left alone to "do one's own thing" without external interference—on the one hand, and society's commitment to *parens patriae*, built on the principles of beneficence and nonmaleficence, on the other. Dedication to the autonomy principle is quite vigorous in the United States, as reflected by the numerous substantive and procedural due-process safeguards built into state guardianship statutes as intentional obstacles to the imposition of guardianship; in Great Britain, by contrast, a clear beneficence-dominated, medically oriented model vastly eases the process of guardianship imposition (Barnes, 1992).

Despite the elevation of personal autonomy to a preferred place among our ethical principles, a number of critics articulately posit that guardianship is inherently and unavoidably an excessive exercise in professional and familial coercion and intrusion. According to this view, benevolent motives (let alone situations in which guardianship actually is sought to further a third party's agenda) inevitably lead to paternalistic and therefore objectionable behavior (Frolik, 1981).

Even assuming the philosophical legitimacy of guardianship, the current guardianship system in the United States has been criticized widely for its practical weaknesses. As previously noted, one outgrowth of our concentration on the principle of individual autonomy is an extensive set of substantive and procedural due-process requirements that must be fulfilled prior to the imposition of guardianship. Although the vast majority of guardianship petitions are uncontested, their processing still usually involves a significant expenditure of time and money, as well as the fomenting of emotional turmoil and stigma for the proposed ward, family, and care providers. When the petition is contested, the costs are higher yet and the outcome uncertain.

The costs associated with the procurement of a guardianship implicate ethical concerns. When a service provider asks a family to invest the time, money, and emotion to have an aging loved one publicly, officially stigmatized by being declared to be less than a fully autonomous adult person, questions regarding respect and compassion for persons may be raised. Time and finances devoted to the guardianship process by service professionals and agencies invoke considerations about distributive or social justice and the most equitable or fair use of precious resources. For example, might not the money and time that service providers need to invest in obtaining a guardianship order for a patient be more appropriately spent on direct, therapeutic care for that patient or others?

Another concern about guardianship involves the quality of the monitoring process in most jurisdictions. Performance monitoring and evaluation, let alone corrective action, for court-appointed guardians is minimal or nonexistent in most places, negating the ostensible prophylactic function of the guardianship system. Hence the principles of autonomy and nonmaleficence call into question the propriety of a process that arguably produces costs and harms without necessarily achieving the desired benefit of protecting the ward against abuse and neglect.

Specific ethical concerns for geriatric clinicians may revolve around (1) the initiation of guardianship (e.g., At what point should, or must, the clinician become involved in instigating the initiation of a petition, either by the health care institution or by the family?); (2) questioning the guardian (e.g., At what point do a guardian's decisions so diverge from either the ward's own preferences or his or her best interests that the clinician can no longer acquiesce in good conscience?); and (3) the clinician's role in the guardianship proceeding (e.g., When the clinician notes procedural deficiencies that imperil the individual's rights, such as automatic waiver of the proposed ward's presence and/or absence of legal counsel to contest the petition, does the clinician have any moral responsibility to try to protect the person's autonomy rights in the proceeding by at least raising questions on the person's behalf, or is fulfilling the more neutral information and opinion-rendering function sufficient?). Ethical quandaries for the service provider are also embedded in various planned and unplanned alternatives to guardianship for older persons with diminished ability to fend completely for themselves. Through these alternatives, we attempt to respect elders' rights while protecting them from harm.

Advance financial and health care planning by currently capable individuals (through, for example, durable powers of attorney, trusts, and living wills) generally fosters continuing autonomy and helps ensure that when the current exercise of autonomy is no longer feasible, decisions are made and implemented for the individual in the least restrictive or intrusive manner reasonably available. The least-restrictive-alternative (LRA) principle, a well-established tenet of American constitutional law incorporated into the Fourteenth Amendment's due-process protections of liberty, is predicated on the ethical ideas of autonomy, nonmaleficence, and beneficence. A central objective of advance planning is to keep private decisions within the private (i.e., nonjudicial) sphere. Health care and human services professionals have a major role to play in facilitating advance planning.

Service professionals also play a significant role in determining at what point an individual who earlier executed an advance directive has become so decisionally incapacitated that the directive should become operative. Declaring that decision-making power has shifted from one individual to another, even someone else named personally by the delegating individual, is an ethically weighty task.

Although it usually works reasonably as intended, advance financial and health care planning sometimes goes badly awry. The professional geriatric caregiver may become aware, for instance, of an agent named under a now-incapacitated person's durable power of attorney who is misusing or exploiting the person's finances, abusing the person, or grossly neglecting the person's vital needs. In such circumstances, the professional, upon whom the older individual depends for both care and advocacy, confronts ethical quandaries about whether to initiate a guardianship proceeding or otherwise request court involvement. To a large extent, the success of advance-planning mechanisms relies on the good faith and integrity of the participants; if these virtues turn out to be deficient, ethical questions multiply about how to make up for these deficiencies and about the professional caregiver's role in such a situation.

The majority of people who become decisionally incapacitated have failed to take advantage of the advance-planning mechanisms alluded to previously. For this bulk of the cognitively impaired population, alternatives to standard plenary, private guardianship fall into two categories: alternative forms of guardianship and alternatives to guardianship.

Recognition of the least-restrictive-alternative principle has fueled a modern trend toward limited or partial, as opposed to global or plenary, guardianship orders when the proposed ward is able to rationally make certain decisions but not others. Caregivers can promote the ethical principle of autonomy, in situations in which limited guardianship is appropriate, by providing information to the court and involved parties (especially the attorneys) distinguishing as precisely as possible those areas where a minimal level of decisional capacity is lacking from those areas where, with adequate assistance and support, the individual could autonomously—albeit perhaps imperfectly—manage.

For a growing number of older persons whose cognitive and/or emotional impairments would technically qualify them for guardianship, plenary or limited, the most pressing practical problem is the unavailability of family members or close friends who are willing and able to assume guardianship responsibilities. Various forms of guardianship-by-stranger arrangements, in which bureaucratic values may predominate, raise special ethical considerations for cooperating professionals beyond all of the factors present when the guardian is a family member or close friend who knows the ward. In the absence of either a personal or a bureaucratic guardian for an incapacitated person, the service provider usually ends up functioning as a de facto surrogate for the person, a phenomenon presenting members of the caregiving team with the ethical challenge to act consistently with the person's substituted judgment or best interests.

Where a willing family member is present, state family-consent statutes and the informal, long-standing practice of looking to "next of kin" ordinarily substitute for the initiation of guardianship proceedings on behalf of incapacitated older persons. Ethical qualms may arise (potentially leading to invocation of judicial intervention) when the service provider believes that the family is acting contrary to the individual's well-being.

In the elder-abuse and neglect context, legal approaches to the elder-mistreatment phenomenon raise a number of vexing ethical questions for health and human service providers. Many of the most difficult ethical issues emanate from the analogy generally drawn by state legislators and program administrators between elder mistreatment and its counterpart in children, and the consequent development of elder-mistreatment strategies built on the child-abuse and neglect paradigm. A number of critical commentators and health and human service practitioners have raised substantial philosophical and practical doubts about the validity and workability of the elder-child analogy in this context (Quinn, 1985). Unlike children, these critics remind us, adults are legally presumed to be capable of making decisions about their own lifestyles and to be able to seek help if necessary and desired (Gottlich, 1994).

It has been argued that reporting mistreatment and providing protective services (including perhaps even physical relocation) over an adult's objection are affronts to that individual's autonomy. If an older individual prefers to protect an abusive or neglectful family member from punishment or to stay within an abusive or neglectful situation rather than risk involuntary transfer elsewhere (perhaps a nursing facility), then is it ethical for the adult-protective-services system to override that preference?

Furthermore, doesn't violating the duty of confidentiality ordinarily applicable to a professional, fiduciary relationship gravely damage the foundation of trust upon which that relationship was built? In practical terms, the fear of being treated like a child in this respect, with purported protection overwhelming autonomy and expectations of informational privacy, may deter some older people from seeking needed professional care or encourage them to be less than candid in providing information when they do seek it.

Another major conundrum in this area is the insufficiency of resources available for effective, individualized follow-up and intervention after situations of elder mistreatment have been identified, reported, and investigated. The paucity and lack of coordination of resources are often cited as an explanation for the low rate of professional compliance with mandatory reporting laws, let alone professionals opting to report under voluntary statutes. Choice among realistic remedies for mistreated elders rarely encompasses a meaningful continuum of community services in any one location. Instead, the individual's menu of alternatives usually is highly constrained, namely, tolerating the present abusive or neglectful situation versus being subjected to unwanted nursing-home placement.

Under these circumstances, many practitioners and commentators believe that the act of reporting probably would make matters worse instead of better by creating unrealistic expectations and interfering with family situations that are lamentable but preferable to available alternatives. The situation is exacerbated by law-enforcement and court systems that are as underfunded and unprepared for dealing with the elder-mistreatment problem as are the aging-related health and human service systems.

Other difficult philosophical and practical ramifications of elder mistreatment exist, including the need to distinguish neglect from legitimate, perhaps laudable, family decisions to limit aggressive medical interventions near the end of life on the basis of calculations of likely benefit versus burden. We also must clarify the values of the older person and the impact of cultural factors on the characterization of particular patterns of family behavior as acceptable versus abusive. In this vein, for instance, acts of raising one's voice, shouting insults, or striking with the hand may be part of a broad spectrum of conduct and quite acceptable in certain ethnic and religious groups. To what degree should American law and professional behavior be sensitive to and tolerant of such cultural variations?

The issue of self-neglect—that is, an individual's failure to provide for his or her own basic life necessities—as the basis for involuntary intervention in an older person's life is a topic meriting careful scrutiny. Considerations of individual self-determination make it problematic to utilize often competently made lifestyle choices by older persons as the springboard for initiating unwanted government interference, especially when legislation singles out the nondisabled elderly for special intrusive treatment.

Additionally, when detected elder mistreatment sets into operation a formal legal response, what are the implications for involved families? While a dysfunctional label may be attached to many families in which elder mistreatment happens, it is unclear that destroying or irreparably damaging the existing familial structure and relationships best serves the values and the welfare of older persons at risk in the long run, except in extraordinarily bad circumstances.

ETHICAL ISSUES AND CONFLICTS FOR SOCIETY

Ethical issues and conflicts for society arise in at least two different contexts affecting the protection of older persons' legal rights. First, we must consider moral questions about the development of public/social policies that purport to protect and promote elders' rights. Second, a juxtaposition of elders' legal claims against those of other segments of the American population should often engender deep reflection about the social or distributive-justice implications of limited resources being allocated to address infinite demands.

In the first category, those charged with shaping public policy affecting the lives of the elderly could learn much from counterparts in the mental disabilities rights movement. This latter group has in the past decade begun to evaluate its efforts in terms of therapeutic jurisprudence (Wexler, 1990; Wexler & Winick, 1991). Based on the ethical precept of beneficence and the categorical imperative that persons are to be considered as valuable ends in and of themselves, the theory of therapeutic jurisprudence posits that law should act therapeutically as well as procedurally and that to accomplish this result, advocates and lawmakers must converse much more closely with workers in the field and the intended beneficiaries of legal actions.

Under this philosophy, those who influence or make legal policy should consider not only rights, but also such things as economic factors, public safety, and the therapeutic ramifications of proposed rules and their alternatives as relevant normative values influencing the result. This relatively new approach is consistent with the older theory of legal realism, which insists on an evaluation of any part of law in terms of its effects (Llewellyn, 1931).

For example, federal nursing-home law was amended beginning in 1987 to place more emphasis on the right of residents to make their own autonomous choices about their plans of care—certainly a praiseworthy development. However, this well-intentioned legal initiative has engendered a number of unintended and undesirable consequences. For example, for residents who are de facto but not de jure incapable of rationally making their own decisions, the federal law has made nursing-facility providers much more nervous about clearly identifying (especially in the resident's medical record, which will be examined by state surveyors) a third party who possesses definitive, unimpeachable legal authority to make decisions on the resident's behalf. At least according to widespread anecdotal reports, this anxiety is encouraging some nursing facilities to pressure families and other resident sponsors to initiate formal guardianship proceedings concerning residents in order to clarify the legal-authority question.

While potentially benefiting nursing facilities' anxiety level, a proliferation of avoidable guardianships (particularly of the plenary or complete type) seems in many cases to be an unnecessarily restrictive intervention into resident autonomy and an unwise infliction of expense, time commitment, and emotional turmoil on all parties. Given the devastating consequences to a ward's legal adult status of being judicially declared incompetent, such guardianships are likely to accomplish more in providing the nursing facility with psychological and risk-management comfort than in assuring ethical protection for the vulnerable resident.

The Medicaid planning scheme depicted in this chapter's first case scenario illustrates society's public policy dilemma in balancing entitlements for the elderly against legitimate, competing claims of other generations. As already noted, a strong argument may be made against both the wisdom and the fairness of existing law that permits this sort of elder financial hocus-pocus at the expense of others (Kapp, 1997).

CONCLUSION

Protecting the legal rights of older adults raises a variety of challenging ethical questions for advocates, service providers, and society. This chapter has attempted to illustrate how there is much more to a thoughtful inquiry about legal rights for older persons than merely announcing those rights in the abstract and proclaiming our undying support.

14

Ethical Issues in a High-Tech Society

Gari Lesnoff-Caravaglia

Contemporary deliberations regarding the effects of technology upon society have their roots in debates that originated as far back as seven centuries ago. It is important to recognize that long before the dramatic changes precipitated by the Industrial Revolution could be firmly implanted on a large scale, such changes had to be foreshadowed by a slowly evolving reorientation of human wishes, habits, ideas, and goals.

Viewing the growth of technology as springing from a network of relationships tied to a host of other cultural factors leads to a better understanding of the present applications of technology, the areas of technological growth and expansion currently being fostered, and present attitudes with respect to present and future possible uses of technology, as well as the ways in which technology has altered not only the exterior but also the interior worlds of human experiencing. Such a broad view also allows for an evaluation of the level of acceptance or rejection of technology, along with the range of fears that technological expansion has engendered.

Within the contemporary context, the unprecedented rapid growth of technology has given a new cast to such development. Furthermore, technology is being increasingly coupled with yet another unprecedented historical event, that of a burgeoning older population. The presence of large numbers of persons aged 65 or older in the nation is leading to changes as novel and dramatic as those experienced during the First Industrial Revolution. Such population changes, experienced for the first time with no historical models to draw upon, are necessitating wide-scale alterations within society that only a uniting of this demographic phenomenon with technology can hope to meet. Such changes were only just beginning to be felt at the end of the nineteenth century, were made manifest during the twentieth century, and will blaze forth in the twenty-first century, creating what can be easily regarded as the Second Industrial Revolution.

The aging of the nation has meant that as larger portions of the population have diminished capacities for coping with the activities of daily life, there has been a concomitant decrease in the labor force of persons capable or willing to assist with such tasks. The absence of support groups in the home such as children, spouse, or relatives due to distance, divorce, death, or their own advanced old age has also meant that reliance upon people as an appropriate resource is no longer a real alternative. The provision of such services must come from a new source—technology. If sufficient numbers of people are not available to perform requisite tasks, then machines must take their place.

Every phase of human existence, from the provision of necessities to sustain life to modes of recreation and to participation in the world of work, requires alteration. New techniques that will keep more people healthy and active and longer lived can also be harnessed to the workplace to make the work environment more hospitable to the older worker. Technology from this perspective will serve as a liberating force for the aged population.

FEARS OF TECHNOLOGY

The impersonal quality and the anonymity frequently associated with technological development also carry with them the fear that the society itself will be swallowed up by the "machine." Any form of civilization based upon technology that might minimize the role of the individual also gives rise to the fear that particular persons or groups of individuals might be regarded as extraneous to the mainstream of society and thus expendable. This fear may be particularly experienced by older persons, for whom the quality of life is closely linked to social participation and particular significance as individuals. The diminishment of roles for older persons, both in the world of work and within the family itself, has also fostered a perception of the world as a place accessible only to those who are not only more physically able, but who are also more in consonance with the contemporary culture, that is, the age of technology.

An additional fear is that the presence of machines will dictate the number and nature of human lifestyles. For example, if an individual is a particular age, weight, or sex, then it might become appropriate that such individuals adopt specific lifestyles dictated by the availability of particular machines. The aged thus would be expected to avail themselves of particular machines and to adapt their lives accordingly. Loss of mobility, for example, might mean not ever going outdoors again because a television screen can transmit environmental information to the homebound individual. Not to accept such a substitution might mean being regarded as someone who is "acting out" or aberrant in behavior, uncooperative, mentally ill, or even possibly suicidal. The range of choice may become seriously circumscribed. What was intended as freedom may result in fettering human personal decision.

To say "no" to the machine may require the kind of inner strength and moral conviction that few are capable of mustering. Will the weaker, then, become harnessed to the machine, or will the machine eventually become the basis for determining what is normal in old age? To grow old alongside one's machines may be the expected model.

We face increasingly the problematic situation of when to say "no" to the machine, particularly when the machine may mean the extension of life, or the prolongation of death, or possibly a little of each. We are unprepared as to how to deal with such dilemmas. We appear to be more ready to resolve such dilemmas, however, when they concern the elderly.

The primary question remains: Must everyone accept the machine? What if to select the machine at one's bedside or chair or in one's living room means having your home adopt the look of a laboratory or a garage, or the mechanical accoutrements of outer space? Such unaccustomed alterations may not be aesthetically pleasing to the older individual and may be unacceptable. If the use of the machine carries any implication of gross disability or being "something special" or "different," it may be rejected by older individuals. Not only the appearance of the apparatus, but how it is introduced to the older population must take such sensitivities into account. To define one's future self and life in terms of a machine as one's constant companion may not be compatible with one's self-image or identity. A crutch, a wheelchair, or a bed may have gradually been accepted as part of one's identity in illness and old age. Perhaps the machine, if it promises freedom, will be more easily accepted than we might predict. Its introduction, nonetheless, must be treated with some circumspection.

Herein lies the importance of utilizing older persons as an advisory body to assess the possible objections to some forms of technology and how they might be rendered more easily acceptable or useful. Older scientists and laypersons can easily provide a perspective often missing from decision-making bodies. The utilization of such groups will mean an initial screening by people who would view such apparatuses from the perspective of potential users.

The fear of the "takeover" by technology is nonetheless very real. Because of their independent source of power and their semiautomatic operation even in their cruder forms, machines have seemed to have a reality and an independent existence apart from the user. The most durable conquests of the machine, however, lay not in the instruments themselves, but in the modes of life made possible via the machine and in the machine (Mumford, 1963). The refrigerator and the automobile are but two common examples of machines that have altered existence in an irremediable way. Few would willingly return to the days of the icebox or travel by foot.

Mechanical devices have also served as pedagogues and teachers to us all. Their presence has taught us new ways of moving forward and adapting our space to create new forms of liberation. No part of the environment, no social conventions, could be taken for granted once the machine had shown how far order and system and intelligence might prevail over the raw nature of things.

The clue to modern technology was the displacement of the organic and the living by the artificial and mechanical. In the past, the irrational and demonic aspects of life had invaded spheres where they did not belong. It was a step forward to discover that bacteria, not evil brownies, were responsible for curdling milk and that an air-cooled motor was more effective than a witch's broomstick for rapid long-distance transportation (Mumford, 1963).

Fears of technology, however, can be practically dispelled if we recognize that the machine has developed as a parallel or complement to the kind of society that has evolved. As part of such total development, the machine shares with society a common past, present and future. The machine thus has no role apart from that which society chooses to give it. The difference between the First and Second Industrial Revolutions may lie, however, in the intense rapidity with which various contemporary technologies are introduced and applied. Nonetheless, the technical triumphs of the machine cannot be separated from the general human achievements of a particular era.

No matter how completely technology relies upon the objective procedure of the sciences, it does not form an independent system, like the universe. We cannot ignore the psychological as well as the practical origins of the machine. Technology exists as an element in human culture, and it promises well or ill to the same degree that the social groups that exploit it promise well or ill.

THE BRAVE "OLD" WORLD

The world has taken another step in a unique evolutionary process. We have become accustomed to the notion of the physical world linked to an evolutionary process, but we have yet to come to grips with the fact that the material construct of the world—the world created by human ingenuity—has also developed and grown in a manner that strongly suggests an evolutionary progression (Lesnoff-Caravaglia, 1988).

For example, if we do not possess arms long enough to reach a desired object, we develop artificial means for either reaching an item or having that object brought directly to us. Should we wish to speak to an individual who is miles away, we no longer have to devise special drums or whistles to attract attention, to make smoke signals, or even to write. If we wish to witness an activity that is occurring some miles distant, we do not have to move physically, but can have the incident portrayed for us over a screen. When we wish to move to a location that is some miles distant, we do not worry about personal physical endurance or plan on how much food to dry and store in preparation for a trip.

In this particular evolutionary process, we augment our capability to perform certain actions without physical changes to our person. We do not grow longer, sharper teeth or claws; instead we invent tools or methods for processing materials. The telephone has become our new voice and ears; the television our new eyes; the automobile and airplane our feet; the computer our messenger. For sustenance we have developed, unfortunately, "fast food."

We have long considered in some trepidation and fascination the concept of the year 2000. It once appeared as a far-distant point on our horizon. In much the same fashion, we have conjectured about changes in demography and the increasing presence of persons aged 65 or older in our midst. Unexpectedly, as well, without plan or preparation we face two parallel but slowly converging trends that are without precedent in human history: (1) an increasingly older population throughout the world and (2) an accelerated development of technology.

This is the first time in human history that so many persons have lived long enough to reach the ages of 65 and beyond. This is the first time in human history that technology has intruded so definitively into personal individual life space extending to the world of work, recreation, family life, health care, and religion. How we live our lives with machines at our sides is a multidimensional ethical issue of enormous magnitude.

Today it is possible to consider intervention and prevention strategies in caring for older persons that were inconceivable as recently as 10 years ago. This capability, in turn, has fomented debates in the areas of ethics, economics, and health care that have troubled the very fabric of our society. Such issues, as they impinge upon health care, personal autonomy, and decision making, play a significant role in determining the level of independence and freedom accorded older individuals. They also raise the spectre of the amount and kind of dependence the presence of technology fosters and give rise to the question: Will such accelerated advances in technology eventually lead to superplaypens for the elderly in the form of automated homes? Although automated homes may be regulated by older persons, they may create an electronic lifestyle that permits social interaction of a very particular kind. Such restricted social interaction could obviate the need for the physical presence of other human beings.

On the other hand, the increase in numbers of older persons and persons with disabilities could present problems that only the presence of large amounts of new technology can resolve. Future life may be conducted in an atmosphere of limited human interaction, with technology providing life support, communication, and entertainment from an encapsulated environment. The life of the astronaut may be duplicated for those of extreme age who present with serious disabilities.

With advancing age, the issue of dependency becomes very real. There is a slow erosion of the locus of control in the lives of persons as they live into the eighth and ninth decades of life. Such an altered locus of control will continue markedly in the future unless technological interventions are instituted.

Advanced technology and a world increasingly populated by older persons appear as two very dissimilar and unrelated events. They are, however, being increasingly viewed from a single perspective. It is the potential of technology to meet the needs of the larger numbers of older and disabled persons that provides the link. Due to the force of circumstance, both events are being regarded as parallel occurrences that can mutually nurture one another's growth and positive development. In fact, much of the technology currently available, including that which can be transferred from military to civilian use, is technology that is applicable to the needs and interests of the older population. The situation of many older persons resembles that of the astronauts in space, and the resemblance may increase in the near future. Older persons, much like astronauts, frequently exist in a restricted environment that is beset by problems related to activities of daily living, physical activity, and recreation.

Furthermore, the crisis in health care personnel has led to an even closer scrutiny of the potential uses of technology in long-term-care settings. If there are insufficient numbers of persons available to perform services, machines (robots) must do the work. For example, with the reduction in adequate numbers of personnel, clerical work often performed by nurses can be more efficiently accomplished by computers, allowing nurses more time for individualized nursing care.

Another example is in the lifting and moving of patients. This can be more easily and safely accomplished through appropriate devices, thus reducing the number of staff required, as well as lessening the severity of back problems sustained by health care personnel. The debate with respect to "high touch versus high tech" has virtually vanished from the scene because it is now patently clear that it is possible to have high touch aided by the presence of high tech.

The challenge is to find ways to mutually enhance the development of technology and to seek out appropriate applications to offset the restrictions and disabilities of old age. Technological advances can significantly affect the quality of life for older persons as they continue to live longer lives and lives that may well include some elements of disability. Lifestyles of caregivers, such as family members, can be appreciably ameliorated through the introduction of technologies in the home environment. The ability to remain in control of one's life even in very advanced old age allows for individual dignity and self-esteem. Both elements are significant factors in the maintenance of physical and psychological well-being.

As the population continues to age, the numbers of persons who are octogenarians, nonagenarians, centenarians, and centedecinarians continues to grow. What is also significant about this population is that in large numbers, as they grow older, they also become more frail and more dependent on other resources for the maintenance of life. It is the linkage between such increasing dependency and advanced technology that prompts the new evolutionary progression.

States of dependency are made up of a variety of factors. They include experiencing multiple chronic symptoms; a limitation on personal options; dependency on the physical environment that was once taken for granted; and dependency on persons drawn from the family unit or public agencies. To grow old and to be well has not been a common human experience. Increases in life expectancy mean that persons can live long lives without experiencing many limitations. Once they begin to experience some restrictions, dependency becomes a source of deep and abiding frustration.

SHRINKING OF THE WORLD

Older individuals tend to use less and less of what can be termed the total environment. This gradual restriction often begins when the person leaves the world of work at retirement. A second point at which there is a reduced level of participation in the outside world occurs when the individual experiences the onset of a chronic illness. Further restrictions are put into play as the individual ages and sensory deficits, such as vision or hearing losses, become more intensified. Such physical alterations can at times be sufficiently severe to constitute a need to alter individual lifestyle. A frequent change is to limit outside activities, with a concomitant increased usage of the home environment.

Home environments are utilized at a much higher rate by older persons due to physical constraints, economic difficulties, and even psychological conditions such as fear. The location of the residence of the persons plays an important role in the perception of safety within the environment and the view of the outside environment as being essentially hostile. Such a restriction to the home environment leads to what can be termed a "basic-needs orientation." Requirements for the carrying out of activities of daily living (ADLs) take on increasing importance as the limitations due to senescent changes and disabilities due to disease continue to escalate.

Independence in this shrinking environment continues to be eroded, and there is the necessary enlistment of outside resources. The entrance of other family members, health care personnel, social service agencies, and a host of other assistive groups into the individual's private life means the lessening of decision-making power by the older person. As the individual gradually loses control of his or her personal life due to illness, immobility, or sensory loss, the control of that life is assumed by outside agencies. Such a decrease in control is usually followed by further constrictions of the individual world.

Even when the person continues to reside at home, there is a progressive diminished utilization of all of the home space and features. Such diminished utilization can begin with the individual's not using the basement, attic, garden, or garage. Outdoor activity is reduced and eventually ceases. Particular rooms of the home are no longer utilized, such as the living room, dining room, or spare bedrooms. Should the person have difficulty using stairs, the bedroom may be moved to a first-floor room and use made of a first-floor bath when it exists. Some home modifications may be necessary to achieve such a move. The individual may remain on the second floor if such accommodations to a first level are not possible.

Restrictions of the life space eventually center on "the areas of survival." These areas are the kitchen, the bathroom, and the bedroom. The circle of experience also perceptibly narrows, and control slowly, but inexorably, moves away from the individual. As the person continues to age and become more dependent, even possibly bedfast, the locus of control becomes more decidedly assumed by outside agencies. The final area of control, the most personal, is taken over by someone else at the bedside.

The types of activities that usually suffer some restriction generally fall into the categories of instrumental activities of daily living (IADLs) or activities of daily living (ADLs). Although many of these activities are considered routine, their performance reflects upon individual functional capabilities. Problems in the performance of such activities are frequently the basis for a determination as to whether or not the person can live independently and whether institutionalization needs to be considered.

One intervention that can help offset some problems is the development of augmentative technologies that permit persons to perform many of the actions they had been used to carrying out in their own homes. Decreasing abilities to use particular appliances, to utilize the entire living space, or to provide for the accommodation of sensory losses, reduced mobility, and the reduction in physical strength can all be counteracted by modifications of existing homes or the construction of homes that are prosthetic in nature. The conventional home may be a lethal environment for the elderly. Just as environments for special populations, such as children, take into account their special needs, environments for older persons require a careful assessment to determine their suitability.

Furthermore, the functional capability of the individual allows for decision making in terms of how life will be scheduled and structured. Deciding how to spend one's day, or what the daily menu will be, is often regarded as routine and a matter of course. When such decisions must be made in concert with other individuals, or when decisions regarding such issues are determined solely by others, the locus of control has effectively moved away from the individual. When such control includes areas such as dressing, feeding and toileting, the loss of control becomes almost complete.

The situation becomes one that can possibly be best described as Maslow in reverse. In Maslow's pyramid (1968), persons satisfy lower basic needs and move up to the top or pinnacle of the pyramid to reach a personal sense of achievement in intellectual or spiritual arenas. Older persons have spent their lives in striving to reach the top of the pyramid, and many achieve this task successfully. Now that they are at the top of the pyramid and are aged, they must move downwards, backwards, if you will, and this is a negative progression that is not happily attempted. To move down from the pyramid's top means preoccupation with biological and psychological functioning. Furthermore, since such basic needs had once been mastered, there may be anger and frustration at having to attend so exclusively to meeting these needs again, particularly when one's tolerance and ability to cope are waning. This move also constitutes a radical change in self-image, and those intellectual, spiritual, or professional achievements that form part of self-identity pale against the reality of negotiating a steep flight of stairs or opening a food container. For older persons, intellectual, professional, spiritual, aesthetic, and avocational growth seems to have been dismissed, disregarded, or diminished in meaning.

Physical movement also is restricted as the environment shrinks. Contrary to the dictates of human health requirements, older persons become more sedentary and engage in less exercise. Part of this reduced physical activity results from reduced participation in the environment because of physical or environmental barriers. Environmental barriers can include the structure of the home, its layout, and the presence of stairs. Storage spaces and appliances may be difficult to access or use, thus cutting back on the person's activity. Shrinkage of the environment due to the nature of the environment itself means that there is a lack of fit between the person and the environment. Such a lack of consonance means that the person is less stimulated by the environment and finds it to be more of a frustration. Increasingly, drawing away from the environment and curtailing their ability to manipulate the environment to their own best advantage results in persons losing control of their lives and, eventually, of themselves. Both physical and mental deterioration may result, and it is at this juncture that a loss of interest in life may manifest itself. Coupled with such negative views of the self are the feelings of impotence and uselessness. Suicidal ideation becomes a possibility.

The social climate in which many older persons experience aging is often bereft of caring friends and family members. Support groups may not be available due to several factors, including three principal ones: death, distance, and divorce.

The longer a person lives, the greater is the likelihood of the experience of the death of a loved one. Such death experiences may be multiple, and the person begins to feel like "the last leaf" and to question the purpose of continued existence. Due to the shrinking of the world, fewer persons are available to fill the gaps left by the dead.

Not only do the elderly suffer from the presence of death, but they are also plagued by distance. They themselves may have moved a number of times during their lifetimes and not have developed lasting friendships. Relatives, due to the mobility of society, may be scattered across the globe. Despite the advertisements of telephone companies, long-distance calling is not an effective substitute. Relationships are maintained only through persistent and ongoing contact, and distance attenuates many once-close relationships.

Divorce effectively divides older persons from potential support groups. Women who are divorced in old age have difficulty in finding new partners. Men are more likely to rebuild personal lives with new partners due to the greater presence of older women and society's sanction of older men's marrying women of much younger ages. A man can have two or three families throughout life, whereas many women are limited to one. The longer life expectancy afforded women continues to exacerbate this problem.

With the presence of multiple families, the obligation to care for an older person becomes more problematic. Divorced parents frequently are estranged from children or have a series of children, both of their own and of their succeeding partners, such that responsibility for the older parent is often muddied. There is much confusion as to with whom the moral responsibility for an aging parent lies. Should it be the daughter who has never lived in the mother's home? A step-granddaughter? The deceased husband's natural daughter who resided with them while attending high school? When children are available, they are faced with responsibilities for several sets of older relatives. These may include one's own parents, parents-in-law, aging aunts and uncles, and older siblings.

Older individuals may also be called upon to repeat their nurturant roles in old age. A not-unusual scenario is that of a woman of 82 who is caring for her son who is 63 and a mother who is 101. The restrictive world in which the older woman lives due to physical health problems and an ineffective environment make the provision of such care even more problematic.

TECHNOLOGY AND AGING

Technological innovations and applications must be appropriate, affordable, and accessible. The aesthetic component of design must not be dismissed lightly. The appropriateness of technology designed for the use of older persons needs to be of such a nature as to bridge the gap between age and control. The ultimate goal should be to restore control or help ensure that control of personal life will be left as much as possible to older persons.

Older persons, through a series of technologies, can be in control of automated homes. New innovations in home development and construction can lead to utilization of existing technologies such as the telephone and television to provide control of appliances, security and safety, home maintenance, and entertainment. The increase in independence that the presence of technologies can make will lead to increased self-esteem and general well-being. Such positive results have an effect on both physical and psychological health.

It is also important to bear in mind that the elderly are not the handicapped. Their concerns and problems may stem from similar dysfunctions, but the problems of the elderly are precipitated and experienced in old age and are often brought on by the process of normal aging. It is also important to note that we do not have sufficient anthropometric data on the elderly. We do not know enough about reaching capabilities or the strength potential of older persons. Functional body measurements are needed that define not only what the elderly are, but what they can do in terms of body movements, ambulation, arm and leg reaches, and task performance—the kinds of data needed by engineers who deal with the design of housing, health and chronic-care facilities, transport vehicles, appliances and equipment, and prostheses. Most of the studies done in these areas have been based on males in their mid-20s, leaving a serious research gap. Much of the application of technology also assumes its utilization by younger clients and must be modified to suit the needs and capabilities of older persons. This is particularly true of the development of wheelchairs.

In order to provide for a continuity of experience for older persons, surveys or assessments of homes should be an ongoing activity. Such inventories or assessments can evaluate what is presently available to the individual, as well as what can be added to the environment to ensure greater independence. There needs to be a degree of choice permitted the older person in the inclusion or dismissal of particular technologies. As changes are required to adequately accommodate the needs of older persons, home arrangements and the additions of technologies need to be a steady feature of the provision of care. Since accidents figure so prominently in the health care of older persons, safety is an important aspect of all home assessments.

The danger of infantilizing the older individual can be counteracted by including the older person in the survey process and asking what types of interventions might be necessary. Educating older persons to potential hazards and the need for modifying the environment is an important aspect of the provision of care. Increasingly, older persons have experience with a wide range of technologies because more of the population aged 70 or older has lived through the experience of rapid technological change in areas such as transportation (horse to airplane), food processing and purchasing, telephone, television, and hair dryers.

Providers of services to the elderly can also utilize many of these housekeeping technologies, with the added bonus of having those chores that are boring, repetitious, demeaning, or fatiguing performed through mechanical means. The presence of technological devices can significantly add to the interpersonal exchanges between caregiver and client due to less time being given to routine activities. The cost of such home health care would be markedly reduced due to reduced labor costs.

EDUCATION AND ATTITUDES

In order to introduce a wide array of technologies, the attitudes not only of older persons, but of caregivers, researchers, industry, and the general public must be taken into account. Do these groups agree as to what types of technologies are appropriate? Is the negative attitude toward all things old, including people, a deterrent? An educational program to counter such negative views and attitudes needs to be instituted at a variety of levels. In particular, marketing individuals and industry must be led to see this new and growing market as one to explore. The aging bias that is seen in research must be offset by a recognition that new advances in technologies that can be used with the elderly are often of such universal design that they can be widely employed by a whole host of groups.

Furthermore, as we continue to experience larger and larger numbers of older persons in the population and begin to more adequately meet their needs, the realization grows that the elderly have been too globally perceived and that demarcations as to age groups are exceedingly important if this group is to be served adequately. Unfortunately, we continue to use a number of euphemisms to describe the older population, and researchers have used terms that in some cases have virtually esoteric meanings. Such terms include senior citizens, golden agers, young old, old old, oldest old, the long-living, the frail elderly, the well elderly, or simple designations like "the risky" and "the frisky." Other designations include the slow-go, the no-go, and the go-go. Such labeling, by and large negative, has hampered our ability to deal with the older population both conceptually and scientifically.

A return to terms supplied by the dictionary would aid considerably in reducing the confusion provided by such terminology. Septuagenarians are persons in their 70s; octogenarians are in their 80s; nonagenarians are in their 90s; while centenarians have reached 100. There is probably a need for the development of neologisms to cover the increasing numbers of persons over the age of 100, with a designation of centedecinarians for persons in the age range 110–119 and centeventenarians for persons 120–129. A further advantage to the use of such nomenclature is that these terms have a Latin base and allow for international comprehension of the terms used to describe particular age groups.

LOSSES IN OLD AGE

The range of losses experienced by older persons cannot be equated with losses experienced at any other time in an individual's personal history. Many of these losses are of a permanent nature and strike at the very heart of personal identity: work role, social role, loss of sensory acuity (who is prepared to grow old and blind?), the death of nearly everyone one has known, and an alteration in the relationship between the self and the environment. When physical, economic, and familial changes are the norm, individuals begin to question their personal identity. Neighborhood changes are often viewed as a form of death. Once initiated, many of these changes are irreversible.

Further, social roles undergo change without the person's being able to intercede in such alteration. They are caught in the flow of time. In role repetition, for example, the aged mother frequently experiences the return of her adult children to the nest, and she repeats her nurturing role (as may be the case with the return to the mother's home of an ill and aging son by the daughter-in-law, or the return to the home of an adult daughter whose husband has divorced her and left her for a younger woman). In role equivalence, both mother and son may be in the same nursing home and are both regarded by society at large as "old." Generational differences are snuffed out (aging families engage in discussions of the merits of different nursing homes in much the same way they once discussed the advantages of particular schools or colleges), and family visits may be carried out by moving from floor to floor of the same nursing home. In role reversal, the mother is frequently the recipient of care by children who may in fact become her "guardians." Such role alteration is fraught with resentment and discomfort on both sides. People are not prepared to be long-living either economically (the recent barrage of sales of the jewels of famous aging women provides a good contemporary example) or psychologically. Never in the history of humankind has this opportunity for such long life presented itself to so many as a common projection of self.

Another interesting factor that has important implications for the acceptance and use of technologies is the fact that the older population is made up principally of females. Females in our culture are given little exposure to things mechanical or technical. One exception is the older female population of the former Soviet Union. Following World War II, with the male population practically decimated, Russian women had to take on all forms of labor. The herculean effort undertaken by the women is today commemorated by a national Russian holiday. This also is why nursing-home residents (principally women) in Russia are accorded the status of war veterans.

HEALTH CARE

The fit or lack of fit between the person and the environment has a determining effect upon when aging occurs and how the process is made manifest. The environment as the locus for aging provides a significant point of interaction that largely influences why particular changes are experienced with advancing age. Environments that do not adequately match the needs and interests of the elderly often serve to accelerate the aging process, resulting in premature aging. Prosthetic environments that are malleable to the needs and interests of the elderly can be regarded as augmentative in that they serve to extend the capacities of aging persons and are geared toward promoting continued maximal functions.

Traditional home, institutional, and work environments can maximize or restrict optimal functioning in the elderly. The incorporation of both high and low technologies in such key settings can offset the decrements of age. Their employment, however, is fraught with ethical dilemmas. Such interventions can be person oriented or environment oriented. Person-oriented changes include such adaptations as false teeth, cosmetic surgery, and organ transplants. Environment-oriented changes have taken on a wide variety of constructs derived from computer technology. Electronic cottages that permit people to continue to conduct a variety of occupational roles while remaining in the home setting are but one example.

In much the same way that the experience of a life long lived is altering the needs and wishes of the elderly, their own increasing sophistication and knowledge of their own health status and the health care system convince them that most traditional health care settings are inappropriate. As the educational level, political acumen, and economic status of the elderly continue to rise, the demand for health care within the home setting or the community will also rise.

Not only does technology provide the freedom for the making of personal decisions, but it also frees caregivers from routine activities and allows for more time to be spent in meaningful personal interactions. The use of robots, for example, in health care settings can increase the quality of care and the level of job satisfaction—two principal concerns of health care providers and their employees. Robots can be developed to assist in the activities of daily living, as well as for the provision of respite to caregivers. Reminding technologies can be developed set to the speed of understood speech and can utilize the caregiver's voice or that of a family member (Engelhardt, 1989). Examples of ways in which robotics can be used in health care settings include the following:

Transfer of patients (lifting)

Housekeeping

Ambulation

Physical therapy

Depuddler (cleaning of human and pet wastes)

Surveillance

Physician assistance

Nursing assistance

Patient assistance

Fetch and carry

Cognitive rehabilitation

The successful utilization of such technologies rests largely on attitudes of caregivers, patients, and family members.

The robotic systems that will serve the needs of the most severely disabled individuals will be those that have a high degree of machine intelligence. The need for sensitive and delicate touch will be mandatory in a robotic aid intended to help lift or transfer a paralyzed patient whose body or garments must be handled with a confident but gentle touch.

Automated Guided Vehicle Systems technology is already performing materials-handling tasks in industry. This same technology can be utilized in an institutional health care environment to transport meals, drinks, and personal items to patients. Such a mobile robotic device could also move from patient to patient, collect vital-signs data, and, with two-way communication, provide a link with the centralized nursing station. Robots can perform tasks that health care providers find boring, repetitive, degrading, or dangerous. Robotic technologies hold the possibility for playing a role in both patient therapy and therapist training. A system that can deliver range-of-motion exercises for muscle maintenance, if properly designed, can also serve as a teaching tool for student therapists because it could be programmed to mimic certain disabilities.

There are currently a number of technologies that have broad applicability and not only serve in a rehabilitative capacity, but provide freedom for a broad range of activities. Examples of technologies with such liberating features include eyeglasses, hearing aids, pacemakers, talking books, and Kurzweil reading machines. Furthermore, devices such as eyeglasses have no side effects and open up a broad arena of activities for the user in the vocational as well as avocational spheres of life. Devices for the elderly must find such a broad market base in order to ensure their development, utilization, and acceptability as ordinary features of life.

Equally important are those features of daily life that can promote and encourage the taking on of responsibilities by patients. One such possibility lies in the development of reminding technologies. In developing reminding technologies, it is important to place sufficient emphasis upon the reaction of the older person to the technology. Such concern must focus upon how the information is delivered, that is, whether the speed is appropriate, and whether the rate at which the information is given is meaningful. Whether such information is accepted to the point of provoking action or a response may be related to the gender or language of the speaker.

It is even conceivable that robots can be designed that can make the environment so sensitive that it can provide respite care. Sensitive monitoring instruments can serve to offset accidents and to develop an environment that focuses upon interventions and prevention rather than simply custodial or policing care.

TECHNOLOGY AND LONG-TERM CARE

The health of the caregivers and the health of the care receiver must be jointly considered. What benefits the caregiver can result in less staff turnover. For example, the technology that can be employed for patient lifting and moving may not be immediately perceived as having such a beneficial effect, but the reciprocal nature of the provision and the receipt of care is too often lost. The incorporation of technology into long-term-care settings thus plays a dual role that enhances the environment from both the perspective of the patient and the care provider.

The relationship between technology and aging underscores the importance of functional ability for maintaining the independence of the elderly, along with maximizing their options and improving their quality of life. The growth of the aging population is likely to increase the demand for long-term care and the need for increased assistance, principally for those age 80 or older who face a combination of incapacitating and largely unavoidable infirmities.

Technology has been the major factor in the growth of the older population and its increased longevity. Technology can now respond by providing both knowledge and ways to apply that knowledge in the long-term-care setting. It is clear that a major challenge into the twenty-first century will be the maintenance of the health and functional ability of the older population, particularly as the proportion in the oldest age groups continues to rise.

SEX AND AGING

The elderly of the future will have considerably more time to devote to interpersonal relationships, and there will, no doubt, be an increasing interest in personal appearance. Cosmetic surgery offers opportunities to maintain a personal image based on personal preference. After the age of 80, it appears that in terms of health care individuals seem to reach a plateau, and there are no serious disabilities for at least another decade. Since the elderly will have followed healthier lifestyles, their physical condition will be superior to that of the older population of today. Older persons today exhibit what can be termed as "premature aging," brought on by stress, improper diet, unhealthful living conditions and habits, and unsound work patterns. An amelioration of the total environment will not only prolong life, but will add immeasurably to the maintaining of youthfulness. In some cultures long-living men who have led healthful lifestyles are found to possess viable sperm at the age of 100. Women in such environments menstruate until the age of 60 or later (Lesnoff-Caravaglia & Klys, 1987). With the more recent advances in conception and the added possibilities of "rent a womb," there is now the possibility for women to give birth and nurture children at ages much older than had been thought possible.

The sex life of the future may be characterized as being "age independent" and not tied by function to any particular period of chronological age. The enjoyment of family and intimacy may take on entirely new configurations. Romance until death will be the norm. Death, when it comes, may be a brief moment brought on by the wearing out of a machine.

FUTURE PROSPECTS

How can we realize our ultimate goal: self-activating, self-respecting, independent human beings who have lived long and productive lives and who seek self-actualization in ways not too far removed from life as they have known it? How can we ensure continuity and avoid discontinuity to prevent illness, premature aging, desperation, and suicide? That is the challenge facing the "brave old world."

Much freedom can be afforded older persons through technology. Some answers have been suggested through the NASA space-exploration program and the transfer of some of the sophisticated technologies to civilian needs. The challenge that faces us requires that in developing technology for the elderly, it is important to bear in mind the following: How can we return control to the individual to ensure greater well-being for the individual and caregivers? How can we face realistically the alterations in demography and in the work force? How can we provide health care that augments the capabilities of the aged individual? Finally, how can we create a humane and caring environment to accommodate an aging world?

It is important to remember that the introduction and acceptance of new technologies is a human problem of long standing. For example, a newspaper editorial in 1834 said of a medical instrument: "That it will ever come into general use, notwithstanding its value, is extremely doubtful because its beneficial application requires much time and gives a good bit of trouble, both to the patient and the practitioner because its hue and character are foreign and opposed to all our habits and associations. There is something even ludicrous in the picture of a gray physician proudly listening through a long tube applied to the patient's thorax" (Anonymous, 1834). That *London Times* editorial was criticizing the introduction of the stethoscope.

SUMMARY

Acceleration in technological advances, coupled with increases in the aging population, has led to an unavoidable convergence of these two major societal trends. What the blend can look like is largely dependent upon attitudes toward the elderly and the appropriate utilization of technologies in areas such as home health care, education, work/retirement schemes, and adaptive lifestyles. As the population continues to age, it is likely that increasing numbers of those aged 85 or older will face incapacitating and largely unavoidable infirmities. The relationship between technology and aging underscores the importance of functional ability in maintaining the independence of the elderly, maximizing their options, and improving their quality of life. Technology has been the major factor in increasing life expectancy; technology can further respond by providing additional knowledge and avenues to enhance the quality of life in advanced old age.

The aging of the population raises critical concerns for employment, the retirement system, transportation, health care, recreation, and housing. The increases in the numbers of persons aged 65 or older have occurred because of technological advances that have resulted in better control of infections and chronic diseases and improved standards of living. New technologies under development today suggest continued change in longevity and functional capacity. It is clear that the aging of the population will fundamentally change the future economic and social fabric of the world.

Most current projections regarding the impact of an aging population, however, assume an elderly population with characteristics similar to those of persons living in the present day, such as withdrawal from the work force, declining health, increased needs for hospitalization and nursing care, and other characteristics that suggest a highly dependent 65-or-older age group. Improved health care, increased understanding of the physiology of aging, and continued advances in technology may well alter the characteristics of the elderly of the future. In addition, applications of computers, robotics, telecommunications, and other technical innovations in the home and workplace may provide new opportunities for increasing independence, productivity, and quality of life for the elderly.

When the contemporary world is looked upon from a historical perspective, it is clear that there has been an evolutionary progression. Planes have become the wings dreamed of by Daedalus, and we do walk on water, albeit on the decks of ships. We have explored the moon and found that it is not made of green cheese, and we have discovered that it is not brownies who curdle milk, but bacteria.

As we move forward, we develop new mysteries in the world of the computer, robotics, and a host of other systems with equally complex features. Once a technology is invented, it usually advances to be perfected again and again. The process of aging is equally irrevocable; populations will continue to age in vast numbers. Both these unprecedented events have shown enormous evolvement in the contemporary age. As Nikita Khrushchev, the premier of the former Soviet Union, was quoted as saying, "We have moved in one generation from the outhouse to outer space."

15

Ethical Issues in Research on Aging

Beth A. Virnig, Robert O. Morgan, and Carolee A. DeVito

PRINCIPLES OF RESEARCH ETHICS

This chapter examines ethical issues associated with geriatric research. The research discussed in this chapter generally falls under the umbrella of clinical research. This includes research about medical care, as well as psychiatric and psychosocial aspects of health and health care. Few of the issues described are unique to geriatrics. Rather, most topics discussed are common to clinical research in general. The chapter briefly reviews some of the historical development of contemporary research ethics and touches on current controversies and themes that are common in research ethics today.

Commonly cited principles of contemporary U.S. research ethics are voluntarism, nonmaleficence, beneficence, utility, and justice. These principles are remarkably similar to the ethical principles of health care, reflecting the close ties between health care ethics and research ethics.

The first principle, *voluntarism*, is a modification of the autonomy principle. All research subjects must voluntarily consent to participation in research. Lack of voluntary consent can occur in a variety of ways. The most extreme is explicitly forcing subjects to participate completely against their will. The most notable example of forcing subjects to participate totally against their will is Nazi research conducted during World War II. Most other violations of the principle involve not informing subjects that they are research subjects, not informing them that they can refuse to participate, or not providing sufficient information so that they can make an informed decision whether to participate or not. An example of a study that did not inform subjects that they were participating in research is the Jewish Chronic-Disease Hospital Study of elderly patients, including some who were demented, who were injected with cancer cells to examine whether cancer was contagious. Subjects were not informed that they were participating in a research study (Faden & Beauchamp, 1986, pp. 161–162). Other examples are the radiation experiments conducted in the 1950s and 1960s that were recently reviewed by the President's Advisory Committee on Human Radiation Experiments (U.S. Advisory Committee on Human Radiation Experiments, 1996).

While egregious violations of the principle of voluntarism are relatively rare under current regulation and oversight, the principle of voluntarism still faces occasional obstacles. The most common examples are associated with not providing subjects full information to understand risks and benefits of participation. Without proper understanding of the study, people may consent to a study they would refuse to participate in under circumstances of more information. Other violations of voluntarism include providing payments or other incentives to subjects that are large enough to be coercive, and linking participation in research to other services such as routine clinical care. A classic example of providing incentives to encourage participation is the Willowbrook Hepatitis Study. That study was designed to test the efficacy of a new hepatitis vaccine. The study was conducted on retarded children living in a state-run home. The protocol included deliberately infecting children and adults with the virus, and participation in the research was made a requirement for admission to the home (Faden & Beauchamp, 1986, pp. 163–164).

The second principle, *nonmaleficence*, holds that subjects should not be harmed or knowingly subjected to harm through participation in research. This principle does not deny that most clinical research involving drugs or procedures has some level of risk involved. The principle does hold that the risk involved should not be significantly greater than what the subject would face during the normal course of clinical care unless the subject understands these different risks and knowingly consents to face them. The standard allows for different risks as long as the risks of the new drug are not significantly worse than those of the old drug without any difference in potential benefit. For example, most cancer chemotherapies involve some side effects. The standard for a new chemotherapy would be that there is no reason to believe that subjects face greater risks than they would if they received "standard therapy" or that, despite greater risks, there are greater probabilities that the new therapy will be effective.

Third is *beneficence*. Whenever possible, people should be better off having participated in research than if they had not. Later, in discussions of randomization, this issue will be discussed in more detail with regard to the issue of conditions under which subjects can legitimately be assigned to different treatments in a research study.

Fourth is *utility*. This principle holds that conducting the research should result in some broad societal benefit. If the research does not have any promise of helping people through the development of new treatments or adding to the scientific knowledge base, then any risks, however minor (including something as benign as inconvenience), cannot be justified. While utility is a central component of research ethics, it comes into play after the first three principles are satisfied. That is, research cannot be justified on the grounds of utility alone if it allows subjects to be harmed or does not involve voluntary consent. In the past, much harm to research subjects has been justified by utility alone (e.g., it was used by Nazi researchers as a defense during their war-crimes trials). The current ordering of ethical principles recognizes the importance and also the limitations of utility.

Finally, there is *justice*. Discussions of this principle have shifted slightly since the first codes of research ethics were developed. Originally, the purpose was to guarantee that the risks of research be evenly distributed across population groups. This principle was in response to a history of conducting potentially harmful research on marginalized groups such as the elderly, the handicapped, the poor, minorities, and prisoners for the benefit of others (Beecher, 1966). Recently, however, the emphasis on justice has shifted to guaranteeing that the benefits of research are evenly distributed across population groups (Rothenberg, 1996). This shift reflects recent changes in public perception of participation in research from being inherently risky to being more beneficial than harmful.

The first modern code of research ethics is the Nuremberg code. It was included in the judgment in *United States v. Karl Brandt* at the Nuremberg trial of the horrifying conduct of Nazi researchers (*United States vs. Karl Brandt*, 1948) and represents the values violated by Nazi researchers during World War II. Similarly, the Helsinki Code (18th World Medical Assembly, 1964) and the Belmont Report of 1978 (U.S. National Commission for the Protection of Human Subjects of Biomedical and Behavioral Research, 1978) represent translations of research abuses into specific values and explicit rules (Jonsen & Toulmin, 1988). All three reports emphasize the same underlying values of autonomy, nonmaleficience, benificence, utilitarianism, and justice.

While the research codes serve many purposes, one obvious purpose was to establish explicit criteria to determine what is ethical conduct and thereby guarantee that future subjects would not be subjected to abuse in the name of science. In addition to clarifying codes, institutional review boards (IRBs) were developed as human-subjects-research ethics committees and are regulated by the Office for Protection from Research Risks (OPRR) of the National Institutes of Health and the Food and Drug Administration (FDA). Institutions and organizations (including universities, hospitals, and drug manufacturers) voluntarily complying or obligated to comply with federal guidelines must establish an IRB that follows the rules outlined in the Belmont Report. In brief, before any research using human subjects in any form (including examination of cells, review of medical records, and direct patient contact) can begin, the IRB must approve the study and its detailed protocol. From this, the IRB will determine whether the subjects need to sign a consent form, and, if necessary, approve the content of the written consent form. The IRB is charged with examining the research to ensure that subjects are fully informed of its risks and benefits so they can make their own (autonomous) voluntary decisions about participation. The purpose of developing these codes and instituting IRBs was to create clear rules that could be applied to a wide range of human-subjects research. This combination ensures that researchers will be actively monitored and, if necessary, forced to comply with the rules. Without such oversight, it was feared that outrageous abuses of human subjects would continue.

RESEARCH DESIGN

Discussions of clinical research design cover two broad types of studies that involve direct contact with subjects: observational studies and interventional studies. In interventional research, something about the way the subject is treated is determined by research design. For example, an interventional study comparing the effect of chemotherapy to chemotherapy plus radiation would assign subjects to one of the two treatments. In contrast, in observational research, patients are watched in various ways, but nothing about the way the patient is treated is affected by participation. In an observational study comparing the effect of chemotherapy to chemotherapy and radiation, researchers would note which treatment each patient was prescribed by his or her doctor, but would not attempt to change the decision in any way.

Interventional Research

Interventional research uses three main types of design: randomized clinical trials or randomized control trials; open-label studies; and group randomized studies. The primary ethical issues with interventional studies are the following:

- Voluntarism
- Nonmaleficence
- Justice
- Privacy

Understanding how each type of study is conducted and what it aims to do makes attempts to balance these issues more understandable.

Randomized control trials assign individual subjects by chance (i.e., flipping a coin or computer-generated random assignment) to one of two or more groups. The groups are each assigned a different protocol of some "treatment" being studied. Use of the term "treatment" in a research context can be somewhat misleading. By definition, the purpose of research is not to directly benefit individual subjects, but rather to further science. However, because "treatment" is a well-understood general term that broadly applies to medical care, it will be used in this discussion. Treatment can include being given different drugs or doses of drugs, being offered different tests, or otherwise being treated differently. The purpose of randomization is to make sure that the groups are similar on factors other than the treatment being studied. With randomization, differences between the two groups can be attributed to the treatment rather than to other factors. If important differences between the two groups other than treatment remain, there will always be a question of whether any differences in effects (outcomes) were due to the treatment or to the other differences.

Ethically, for a trial to use random assignment, there must not be compelling evidence that one treatment is better than the other(s). If such evidence existed, denying some people a treatment known to be beneficial would violate the principle of nonmaleficence (doing no harm). For example, routine screening for cervical cancer through Papanicolaou (Pap) testing is well established and has proven benefit (U.S. Preventive Services Task Force, 1996). For this reason, a study that randomizes women to having a Pap test or not having one would be considered unethical. However, screening for prostate cancer using the prostate-specific-antigen (PSA) blood test has not been proven to be beneficial (Guide to Clinical Preventive Services) and, for that reason, could still be tested using randomized trials. The requirement of compelling evidence does not mean that a particular researcher may not believe (or suspect) that one treatment is superior. Rather, the compelling-evidence requirement means that there is no consensus in the scientific community about the relative merits of the two treatments. A particular physician who has strong beliefs about the relative merits of the treatments may not want his or her patients to enter the trial, but the trial itself would still be considered ethical.

Often new treatments are compared to whatever treatment is standard medical practice for the condition of interest. This standard treatment is also called "usual care." In many randomized trials (but not group randomized trials), it is best if the researchers assessing subject response to the intervention (e.g., deciding whether the patients improved) and even the patients themselves do not know which treatment they received. The process of keeping the exact treatment received by a particular subject hidden until the end of the study is called "blinding." In a "double-blind" study, neither the researchers who are in direct contact with the subjects nor the subjects know which treatment they received (however, some member of the research staff always has access to treatment information for emergencies). Single-blind studies, which are less common, keep either the researcher or the subject from knowing treatment status but not both. Blinding is thought to prevent unintentional bias in assessing or reporting function that might be associated with researchers or subjects having different expectations for the performance of different treatments. Studies that use blinding are required to have a mechanism in place for informing doctors which treatment the patient received in case of emergency. This is called "breaking the blind." For conditions where the treatments vary in form (e.g., one is an injection, the other a pill), a placebo might be used. A placebo looks like the treatment but is not thought to have any active impact on the condition being studied. Placebos are sometimes called "sugar pills." Placebo versus treatment studies can only ethically be used in situations where there is no established treatment for a particular condition. That is, if there is an established treatment (even if there is evidence suggesting that it does not work), then a placebo control will not be allowed.

Subjects are also protected from potential risks of participating in clinical trials by requirements that clinical trials continually keep subjects informed of new information that might change the subject's willingness to participate in the trial. This includes monitoring subjects for adverse events and informing subjects of any findings that would be related to informed consent. That is, if information becomes available after subjects consent that might make them reconsider participation, they must be given that information even if it means that most subjects withdraw from the study. To fail to provide subjects with all information available is in violation of the principle of informed consent.

Many clinical trials also have decision criteria established before the start of the study that outline a procedure for ending the study early if large-enough differences between treatment groups are found. For example, the Physicians' Health Study was a broad study that included a randomized, double-blind study of the effect of daily aspirin use on the incidence of myocardial infarction (heart attack) and on cardiovascular mortality. The study enrolled more than 22,000 subjects and was designed to last eight years. After five years, the aspirin study was terminated after observing a highly statistically significant ($p < .00001$) and practically important (44%) reduction in myocardial infarction associated with aspirin use (Steering Committee of the Physician's Health Study Research Group, 1989). The study ended despite the existence of remaining questions about the possible benefits of aspirin for particular subgroups (e.g., men under age 50) or for other outcomes (e.g., hemorrhagic stroke). In other words, once the large reduction in myocardial infarction associated with aspirin use was identified, it would be unethical to deny some subjects the benefit of aspirin despite the existence of other questions of scientific interest.

For there to be voluntary, informed consent for participation in any clinical study, subjects must be informed of treatment options beyond participation in the study. Rarely are there conditions for which participation in research is the only option initially available. This does not mean that subjects will not choose to participate in the trial; rather, they must fully understand their choices.

While many of the examples reported in the media as well as those discussed in this chapter involve serious conditions where death is a potential outcome, it is important to keep in mind that interventions covered under the umbrella of interventional research do not need to be limited to extreme conditions. For example, Kasper, Mulley, and Wennberg (1992) conducted randomized studies on whether providing unbiased information to patients and their families helped them make informed treatment decisions. While probably not directly affecting survival, this study underscores the point that all aspects of health and health care are potential topics for interventional research.

Some clinical studies are not meant to treat patients with a particular condition; rather, they are designed to establish the safety of a particular treatment (i.e., show that it does not harm people to take it). These studies provide the first test of a drug's or device's effectiveness—that the drug can be taken safely. There is nothing unethical about conducting these safety studies. However, it is important that subjects who are asked to participate in such studies, which are not aimed at providing some treatment, clearly understand that the intent of the study is not to directly or indirectly treat their condition. Further, potential subjects must be clearly and fully informed of the potential risks associated with participation in the study.

In contrast to blinded, randomized trials, *open-label studies* are typically nonrandomized studies in which all subjects receive the same treatment and everyone—the subjects and researchers—knows it. Open-label studies are often used to monitor the effectiveness of a drug in "routine clinical practice." That is, investigators adjust the dose of the drug as the subject's condition requires rather than according to some preestablished protocol. Open-label studies are also a way for subjects to continue using an experimental drug after clinical trials have been completed, but before the FDA approval process is complete.

In contrast to randomized clinical trials and open-label studies, in which individual subjects are enrolled, the *group randomized study* enrolls entire groups into a protocol. These studies are effective ways of assessing the impact of program or policy changes that affect an entire institution or intact group (T. D. Cook & Campbell, 1979). Examples of group-level research include examining the impact of staff education on patient care; monitoring the effect of programs aimed at reducing psychotropic drug use on how frequently nursing-home residents fall; and examining the impact of new staffing or charting procedures on office efficiency. Studies of this sort are widely thought to be the best way to evaluate efforts to improve institutional care for the elderly. From a researcher's perspective, group randomized studies are usually thought of as relatively unproblematic studies in terms of ethical concerns; however, they probably deserve a second look. The following example illustrates the importance of considering ethical issues associated with group randomized studies.

A study involving 20 nursing homes was undertaken to evaluate the effectiveness of structural changes to the institutions (e.g., safe areas and concealed exits) to prevent wandering and fall-related injuries by dementia patients. Evaluation included review of patients' medical records, a survey of patients whose cognitive functioning was sufficiently intact, and the maintenance of incident logs. Patients and their families were asked to consent to medical-record review and interviews. The son of one patient objected to participation and stated that he did not want his mother's physical environment changed. He insisted that she not be affected by the study in any way—including the modifications to the physical environment of the nursing home. The son was offered the opportunity to move his mother to another institution. He refused, contending that it would be a very disturbing move for his mother, and that this was not an appropriate solution to the problem of her participation. The nursing home and the researchers faced a dilemma. They believed the changes to be beneficial to all residents of the home, wished to participate in the study at an institutional level, and were comfortable with not including the woman in evaluation. However, they were also concerned about the woman and her well-being (Orgren, 1995).

By definition, group randomized studies affect all members of a group. It would be virtually impossible to conduct many group randomized studies if every member of every group were required to consent to the intervention. This is a particular problem in settings such as hospitals and clinics, where it can be impossible to identify in advance all people who will use the setting during the study period. The result, however, is that the only option for persons strongly opposed to participating in such a study is to leave the group.

Subjects are allowed to decide whether to participate in data collection. The interventions are usually considered to be benign and to pose little if any risk. Occasionally, however, situations arise in which a patient or family member is outraged at this practice. In the preceding example, the staff were concerned because their goal was to improve the nursing-home environment for all patients who wandered. They did not feel that it was in the woman's best interest to leave the home where she had lived for so many years, yet it was difficult to cancel a potentially beneficial program because of the objection of one patient.

This case illustrates several difficulties that can arise in group randomized studies. In studies of individuals, people can refuse to participate for any reason and do not need to articulate their reason or have it based on any real or perceived harm. Group randomized studies would be almost entirely shut down by a standard requiring all persons potentially affected by an intervention to consent before research could commence. Group randomized studies are an important method for assessing whether programs designed to improve care for the elderly are effective, but resolving ethical components while allowing studies to continue will not be easy. The ultimate solutions are not clear and remain open for discussion.

Observational Research

Observational studies, as the name suggests, involve watching people without doing anything that will affect their clinical care. Depending on how long they last, and whether they collect information at one period in time or over a series of days, months, or years, observational studies are categorized as cross-sectional (one point in time) or longitudinal (over time).

Although observational research is research based, there are generally fewer ethical issues associated with it than with intervention. However, several issues remain, in particular, voluntarism and privacy. Observational studies use many of the same measures as interventional studies: interviews (telephone, in-person, and mailed), reviews of medical records, and physical examinations. As with interventional studies, researchers must obtain informed consent for all research involving direct contact with subjects. Consent must be voluntary, and subjects must understand that they will not be adversely affected by decisions to not participate. If the observational research is conducted in a clinical setting, they must clearly understand that participation in the study is not meant to constitute treatment of any sort.

IRBs generally permit researchers to review preexisting records (e.g., hospital medical records) without informed consent (that is, the subjects do not have to consent for their record to be reviewed) if the IRB is confident that the information collected contains no individually identifying information and does not pose a threat to any subject whose record might be reviewed. An additional source of data for some observational studies is administrative data obtained from agencies that collect the information for routine record keeping and billing. Data of this sort include Medicare billing (claims) files maintained by the Health Care Financing Administration (HCFA) and vital-statistics information (births, deaths) collected by state health departments. These data are released to researchers who can guarantee confidentiality and who have research questions that the data can appropriately help answer. These requests, too, must be approved by an IRB. Studies using administrative data often provide good information about the experiences of a larger population than can feasibly be studied using other methods.

RESEARCH POPULATION AND SETTING

Ethical issues also arise from the population being studied and the setting in which the study is being conducted. Certain settings may have a greater likelihood of raising concerns about coercion or the ability of subjects to provide informed consent. Coercion issues arise when there is the possibility that the setting in which the research will take place will make subjects reluctant to refuse participation in research. In part, these concerns stem from the Nazi era when defendants at the Nuremberg trial insisted that they asked Jewish prisoners if they wanted to participate and only included in research protocols those who agreed. The Nazis cited World War II–era research conducted on conscientious objectors as equally coercive. Likewise, prisoners often have seen participation in research as a way to demonstrate their "good behavior" that might lead to early release. Due to fear that the potential of early release is coercive and prevents informed consent, there have been calls for banning research on prisoners. Less obvious examples of coercive situations include patients who are asked to participate in their physician's personal research, and virtually any research where potential subjects may worry that their health care or living situation will be affected by their decision to participate. Many of these coercion issues have been alleviated by including in written consent forms a statement that other care will not be affected by decisions to participate.

Fear of coercion leads easily to subjects' concerns about privacy. A great deal of potentially confidential information is collected in the process of conducting a research study. This includes the names of participants, responses to interview questions, information from medical records, and results of laboratory tests. All of these could be potentially embarrassing or damaging if inappropriately released. Yet suggesting that no confidential information may be collected would shut down most human-subjects research. Likewise, forbidding researchers from having a mechanism to link a particular response to a particular subject would make all longitudinal (conducted over time) research impossible and make publishing of other results very difficult (because many journals request comparisons of the population eligible to participate with the population who actually participated). As a result, several protections have been put in place. First, federal regulations (the Public Health Services Act) protect data collected for federally funded research from being subpoenaed for legal purposes with very few exceptions. The most notable exception is that persons who have a positive HIV test conducted for research purposes where the test can be linked to identifying information are not immune from public health reporting laws.

IRBs and most funders now make researchers justify collecting identifying information and, if necessary, require that identifying information be kept separate from the other data collected. When the study no longer needs access to identifying information (e.g., after the follow-up period has ended), identifiers must be destroyed, but the data may be kept. While identifiers are attached to data, the data must be securely stored where no one outside of the study can access them. Third, when research results are published or shared, no individual or individuals may be identified or identifiable (by a combination of characteristics that might be unique) in any way. For example, the HCFA does not allow publishing information on groups of fewer than seven individuals. Finally, subjects must be informed whether data will be kept confidential and must be clearly notified prior to data collection if there are any exceptions (e.g., for many studies of investigational drugs, the FDA and the company that produces the drug will need the ability to access original data).

Questions of Competency

Beyond issues of the information that must be available to potential subjects to obtain a valid informed consent are issues of determining who is capable of providing an informed consent. Although most elderly are not demented and suffer no cognitive impairment (Ostfeld, 1980), the frequency of dementia and other cognitive impairments is substantially higher in elderly populations than in younger populations. Thus any policy about ability for elderly persons to provide consent needs to keep both in mind.

Many researchers complain that in general, IRBs seem more concerned with obtaining the proper consent document (Lynn, Johnson, & Levine, 1994) than with determining who is competent to consent or monitoring the quality of the consent. Researchers often view this obsession with procedural formalities as a barrier to research (Campion, 1985). In an attempt to make consent forms comprehensive, some researchers develop forms that are essentially incomprehensible (Lawton, 1980). They argue that strong emphasis on written documents is of concern because it misses the purpose of ensuring voluntarism and instead is preoccupied with legal niceties. Often IRBs exhibit little interest in examining or regulating the consent process as it actually takes place (Rothman, 1991). Interestingly, while the IRB process may seem to overemphasize legal aspects of research, it is likely that actual monitoring of the consent process—including comprehension, quality of understanding, and confirming voluntarism—would be more difficult for researchers, not less.

Determining Consent for Adults with Questionable Competency

While few claim that competent adults should be denied the opportunity to consent or refuse to participate in research, there is less agreement about how to handle consent for adults whose competency is questionable or absent. There is currently no standard way of determining competency for research subjects. Most research protocols either rely on observers to determine competency or use a standard instrument that tests memory and cognition (e.g., the Mini-Mental State Exam; Folstein, Folstein, & McHugh, 1975). Observers can be unreliable and subject to their own biases, and a single measurement of mental status may not differentiate between transient and long-standing problems.

Whether to allow someone to consent or refuse to participate is a difficult and important ethical component in the conduct of human-subjects research. As noted earlier in this chapter, voluntarism is one of the most important principles of contemporary U.S. research ethics. Barring people who can provide a valid consent from this process is a clear violation of the principle. Equally, however, allowing someone to consent who lacks sufficient competency violates the principle of voluntarism. Thus attempting to conduct research on populations that include subjects with questionable competency requires a careful balancing of these concerns.

The group of "borderline competent" individuals is large and diverse. It contains persons with a wide range of functional abilities, from older adults with occasional problems with memory and reasoning to borderline retarded adults or those with temporary losses or lapses in competency due to medication, extreme stress, or illness. Competency for older adults can change over relatively short periods of time in response to acute changes, including grief and unfamiliar situations. These changes are frequently not permanent, despite how serious they may seem at a particular point in time. Likewise, some people are very adept at masking substantial problems. In other words, competency questions can run in both directions—over- and underestimating a person's abilities. Failure to acknowledge these sometimes dramatic shifts can cause substantial problems. However, with such subjects, caution is clearly warranted even once the competency problem has apparently cleared.

With borderline groups, the problem of consent is clear: failing to allow a competent person to consent limits his or her autonomy and violates the principle of voluntarism, yet allowing an incompetent patient to consent does not promote autonomy, does not further the patient's best interests, and might lead to harm. Options for obtaining consent for "borderline" populations must take into account both the risks of failing to allow adults to exercise their autonomy and the risks of allowing incompetent adults to make decisions. For these reasons, the best option for obtaining consent is one that allows the subject to maintain a role in decision making. Dual-consent protocols require two persons to consent to participation in research. The subject and either a surrogate or physician must consent. Under this model, the subject is given some control over the decision to participate in research, but he or she can only participate if his or her decision is supported and approved by another decision maker. This solution protects each person's right to decide whether he or she wishes to participate in research while also providing extra protection to ensure that vulnerable people are not placed at undue risk.

Problems of competency are inherent in research in elderly populations. Ethics codes and ethics committees alike emphasize the importance of voluntarism as a sign of respect. Protecting and promoting this value for special populations and in special circumstances is sometimes difficult and always must be handled with care. The options describe ways of handling consent for subjects with impaired or questionable competency and ways of promoting voluntarism while also allowing participation in research. Achieving this balance is essential for the ethical conduct of human-subjects research.

Determining Consent for Incompetent Adults

Consent for research for incompetent adults is usually handled in one of three ways: proxy consent, advance directives, and complete prohibition. Between a view that there should be no surrogate consent (complete prohibition) and the opposite view that surrogate consent is always acceptable, the appropriate middle ground is unclear. Robert Cooke (1994, p. 205) states the dilemma of surrogate consent quite clearly:

If normal healthy adults cannot be drafted for research to help others without their consent, should it be possible to give third-party proxy for research on more vulnerable people—the ill, handicapped or disordered? . . . Unless the anticipated knowledge might reasonably benefit the individual subject, any risk that is greater than minimal as defined for [the] nonvulnerable is unacceptable. There is no greater moral obligation for a mentally infirm subject toward others of his disease class, present or future, than for any other person in society. . . . Since it is accepted that normal persons should not be enrolled in nontherapeutic research with more than minimal risk unless they can give informed and meaningful consent, it is doubly unreasonable that the mentally infirm should be so enrolled.

Advance directives for research (ADRs) were suggested as a means of allowing incompetent persons to consent to research that would protect the autonomy of those unable to consent for themselves (Dubler, 1985; American College of Physicians, 1989; Sachs, 1994). In theory, ADRs are an ideal solution: while competent, a person can specify whether he or she wishes to participate in research at some future time when he or she is no longer able to consent. In practice, the difficulties are likely to be much the same as with advance directives for medical care (ADs): most people do not have them, and, when present, the documents rarely contain enough detail to clearly direct decision making. Based on experience from clinical ADs, it can be expected that in the absence of strong, extreme views, ADRs will provide only a broad statement of the subject's view of research (generally likes or dislikes it) and name surrogates who will be responsible for interpreting how this broad direction translates into a decision for the specific circumstances at hand.

From patients naming surrogates through ADRs comes support for use of surrogate decision makers for research (High, 1992). In practice, this option is the usual method for obtaining consent for people who do not have an advance directive and has been in use much longer than advance directives. As with medical care, it is hypothesized that surrogates make decisions using one of two models: substituted judgment and best interest. Substituted judgment asks the surrogate to make the decision he or she thinks the subject would have made had he or she been competent. Best interest asks the surrogate to make the decision that would serve the subject's best interests. In practice, the basis for most decisions is entirely unknown because surrogates are not required to articulate the reasons for their decisions, and except in extreme cases, surrogates' decisions are not questioned (High, 1994a). Information from research (High, 1994b) suggests that they probably use a combination of the two models.

The hard-line approach of "no one can consent for anyone else" appears, on the surface, to protect autonomy, but, in fact, this stance is more likely to limit autonomy than does surrogate consent. The ultimate effect of adopting this hard line is to assume that no incompetent potential subject would want to participate. Autonomy is limited because the patients are forbidden from making decisions about participation both directly (by their condition) and indirectly (because their families are prohibited from deciding for them). Not allowing a decision to be made is making a decision. The only difference is that in one case (complete prohibition) the decision is made by total strangers, and in the other it is made by those who presumably know the subjects best.

The hard-line approach also makes certain types of research impossible: "If we can only perform senile dementia research using demented patients, but should not allow them to participate because they are incompetent, then we are left in a quandary. We cannot ethically conduct senile dementia research using demented subjects because they are incompetent; but we cannot technically perform it using competent subjects because they are not demented" (Ratzan, 1980, p. 36). Thus an extreme view does not avoid making assumptions about subjects' preferences and also limits scientific knowledge that may benefit the patient or, at least, other members of the patient's group.

The ideal solution is for every elderly person to have an ADR and a named surrogate (Dubler, 1985). Unfortunately, this probably will not happen in the foreseeable future (Sachs, 1994). For those people without ADRs, proxy consent is the best option (High, 1992). It preserves autonomy to the greatest extent possible and only allows research in those situations where those closest to the subjects feel that it is appropriate.

CHANGING VIEWS OF RESEARCH

As research progresses and the beneficial results of research protocols become known, the view of research as essential and beneficial activity is becoming more common. Perhaps one of the best examples of the benefit that research can provide for elderly nursing-home patients is associated with studies of physical-restraint use (Miles & Myers, 1994). Physical restraints were, and in some situations still are, commonly used in nursing homes. Their use was based on the best of intentions: preventing falls, limiting injuries to patients prone to wandering, controlling aggressive patients, and maintaining appropriate posture (Miles & Myers, 1994). After a few tragic problems, research was undertaken to quantify the alleged benefits of physical-restraint use. The research showed that restraints were actually associated with increased injuries, agitation, physical deconditioning, and death. Research demonstrated that devices once accepted as good medical care were harmful to vulnerable people and were used inappropriately more often than they were used appropriately. Other research studies designed to assess whether there were harmful effects associated with reduction in restraint use showed no increased risk of falls.

Before the early 1980s, the value of physical restraints was virtually unquestioned; they were common practice. By the end of the decade, the evidence against restraint use was so compelling that the federal government passed legislation aimed at severely limiting their use as part of the 1987 Omnibus Budget Reconciliation Act (OBRA). The clear lesson associated with this experience is that without the unbiased eye of research, harmful but well-intentioned care might have been allowed to continue.

The growing recognition of uncertainty in medical decision making has also contributed to growing confusion about clinical research. Research is simultaneously being described as a right and unethical. Comments like "ethicists and institutional review boards must sincerely consider whether disdained and vulnerable people are being substituted for experimental animals" (A. Novick, 1991, p. 126) are still common, but perhaps less justified. However, for many conditions for which treatment alternatives are lacking (e.g., AIDS), research trials are increasingly seen as a scarce resource that must be allocated fairly. Participation in research is now being viewed as a right that should be fairly distributed across all sectors of society rather than as an altruistic act or, perhaps, a societal obligation. While formerly, members of minority groups, the handicapped, prisoners, and other disenfranchised groups used justice-based arguments to support their claims that they should not be asked to be research subjects (the basis for the value of voluntarism), these same groups are now using justice-based arguments to support claims that they should not be denied the right to participate. Carol Levine (1988) sums up this tension nicely: "The shortage of proven therapeutic alternatives . . . and the belief that the trials are in and of themselves beneficial have led to the claim that people have a right to be research subjects. This is the exact opposite of the tradition starting with Nuremberg—that people have a right NOT to be research subjects" (p. 172).

Yet this transition is by no means complete. The following example illustrates the harsh and often contradictory light under which research protocols are currently examined: Work in prevention of falls in the elderly led to the observation that recent hospitalizations were a major risk factor for subsequent serious falls (Department of Health and Rehabilitative Services, 1990). This was entirely consistent with research showing that prolonged periods of bed rest (often experienced by hospitalized elderly) result in physical deconditioning that is, in turn, a major risk factor for falls (e.g., Sattin, Rodriguez, DeVito, Lambert-Humber, & Stevens, 1991; Simonsick et al., 1993). Physical therapists informed us that although they believe that physical rehabilitation can effectively remedy this problem, Medicare does not currently reimburse for rehabilitation after hospitalizations unless there is a specific motor deficit. While Medicare's policy contradicts much conventional wisdom, the policy is justified because general rehabilitation has not been scientifically proven to benefit the elderly. In truth, the benefit of rehabilitation immediately after hospitalization has never been directly studied. Our group at the University of Miami sought to fill the gap and obtain necessary data to change Medicare's policy. To do this, we proposed a randomized trial to examine the effect of physical rehabilitation after hospitalization for elderly people.

According to our study protocol, elderly persons who consent and whose physician approves would be randomized to usual care (whatever posthospital services their physician orders) or rehabilitation. Our study was criticized by one reviewer because randomization to the control group would unfairly deny someone a treatment believed to be beneficial, and that is unethical. A different reviewer criticized the study because randomization to the rehabilitation program (the intervention) might place subjects at unjustifiable risk, and that is unethical. We were totally unsure how to respond to our critics. The two critiques are a perfect example of the inconsistent way in which ethical evaluation of medical research is viewed. While both reviewers agreed that it was unethical to randomize subjects, one believed that harm was associated with being in the control group, while the other felt that the harm was being in the treatment group. Our experience illustrates the difficulty that can be faced when requirements for proving the efficacy of accepted therapy are reviewed by people who think that such evaluations of accepted therapies are unnecessary and by people who mistrust human-subjects research in general. Researchers are caught between these conflicting views and often find it difficult to conduct studies aimed at verifying things that are accepted but never proven.

CONCLUSION

Ethical issues in research continue to be important and evolving areas of interest. As scientific methodology and areas of research change and, occasionally, become more technologically advanced, the corresponding ethical issues that receive the most emphasis also shift. New therapies and new applications of old therapies are being held to increasingly stringent standards before they are approved for offering on the commercial market or reimbursement by third-party payers for health care. With these standards controlling access to new technology, more and more patients are seeing participation in clinical trials as a real treatment option.

An aging population and growing recognition that the elderly have different health care needs from younger populations and, occasionally, unique problems have resulted in calls for more research on the elderly. Yet these are also the people who experienced much of research's scandalous history. For the elderly, given the history they have observed, mistrust of research is not just understandable, it is rational. The medical community, and researchers in particular, must work together to build the trust of the elderly in research and help them see that appropriately conducted research is a benefit to all.

16

Ethical Issues in Long-Term Care

Laurence B. McCullough, Nancy L. Wilson, Jill A. Rhymes, and Thomas A. Teasdale

SCOPE OF ETHICAL ISSUES ADDRESSED IN THIS CHAPTER

Mrs. G, a 79-year-old widowed, white woman, has been admitted to the short-stay unit of a comprehensive geriatric health care center after discharge from the hospital for hip replacement. She has been discharged to the short-stay unit as part of a contract arrangement between the hospital and the geriatric health care center. Her care plan includes postsurgical follow-up, physical therapy, and planning for the future. Her medical problems include mild heart failure and moderate visual impairment, secondary to macular degeneration. She also has moderate right-side hearing loss. Her poor eyesight contributed to the fall that resulted in her broken hip. This fall occurred at home, where Mrs. G lives alone. She has lived in this home for 50 years and alone in this home since her husband died 10 years ago. She has three children, her oldest, a son, and two daughters, all of whom are married with children of their own. She is closest to her youngest child, who is 49 and has three teenage children of her own. Both she and her husband are working and have started a savings plan to send their three children to college.

Dr. S, the medical director of the short-stay unit, sees Mrs. G each day, and on the third day of her admission, after she has gotten oriented and settled into the new routine after her hospital stay, Dr. S asks her about what she is planning to do when she has completed rehabilitation and is ready to leave the short-stay unit. Mrs. G says that she has begun to look into nursing-home placement and only that morning had asked the unit social worker to get her information on facilities in the area.

Later that day Dr. S notices Mrs. G's daughter coming out of her mother's room, appearing very upset. Dr. S inquires if there is any way that he can be of assistance. Mrs. G's daughter says that she has just learned from her mother that she plans to move to a nursing home when she is ready to be discharged from the short-stay unit. Mrs. G's daughter tells Dr. S—and makes it clear that she intends to tell the unit social worker the same thing—that this is a terrible plan and that she will not hear of her mother going to a nursing home because "it would kill my mother."

It is not hard to see, in this brief case description, the seeds of interpersonal and intrapsychic stress that are beginning to occur and, unless they are addressed prospectively in an effective fashion, about to get worse. Dr. S and the unit social worker, as well as Mrs. G, her daughter, her other children, and their families, are in a position to do something about these potential problems. The decisions that they are about to make could make things worse or better. This chapter is about such cases and the difficult decisions that they prompt in the lives of elders, their family members, and health care professionals every day. Put more precisely, this chapter is about the ethical issues that arise when elders and their family members make long-term-care decisions.

Long-term care has been described as "a set of health, personal care and social services delivered over a sustained period of time to persons who have lost or never acquired some degree of functional capacity" (R. A. Kane & R. L. Kane, 1987, p. 4). This chapter concerns long-term-care decision making by elders, family members, and gerontologists and geriatricians who assist them in the decision-making process. We will address long-term-care decision making at what can usefully be termed the "micro" level of individuals, of everyday life. Obviously, macrolevel considerations of public policy and of institutional practice and policy affect the micro level of decision making about long-term care.

Long-term-care decision making involves millions of elders, family members, and professionals every year in the United States and other countries. In any national or cultural setting, long-term-care decision making has the following characteristics, which must be addressed by ethical analysis and in practice: (*a*) where an elder with long-term care needs should live, for example, whether the elder should continue to live in his or her home or apartment or move to congregate housing or even a nursing home; (*b*) what sort of care the elder needs and ought therefore to have, for example, stimulation that a day-care program might provide or nutrition from a meals-on-wheels program; and (*c*) who ought to provide either the location of long-term care or long-term-care services. Long-term care thus involves a wide spectrum of institutional sites and services, as well as domestic sites and personal services provided by family members and other "informal" caregivers.

Consider, for example, the decision made by Mrs. G to move to a nursing home. Mrs. G will then face decisions about whether to sell her home, what possessions she should bring with her to the nursing home, whether she will seek a single or double room, what activities of the nursing home she will embrace, with whom among her fellow residents she will strike up new relationships, and so on. Her daughter, we saw, prefers that her mother not move to a nursing home. As it turns out, she tells Dr. S and the unit social worker that she is very concerned that her mother not go back home and live alone. Perhaps her mother could move in with her and her family, she tells the unit social worker later that same day. She, her husband, her children, and her mother will then confront many decisions about such matters as which room her mother will occupy, finances, where pets will go, family work schedules, living space, and meal contents and schedules. The decision-making process can be further complicated by the elder's actual or perceived diminished ability, or even inability, to make decisions as a result of physical or mental changes that have been occurring. The elder may thus in some cases not be able to participate meaningfully in the decision-making process. Decision makers also grapple with conflicting interests, uneven distribution of caregiving burdens, especially by gender, uncertain senses of spousal and filial obligations and their limits, lack of clarity about roles and power, and emotional conflicts between and within decision makers. The people involved in the process can change over time. Decision makers may also hold and act on sharply different definitions of the elder's problem and needs and of their own capacities and willingness to meet those needs.

Long-term-care decision making thus frequently becomes a considerably, though not hopelessly, complex process because it involves a series of medical, social, and personal decisions, made incrementally over time by multiple decision makers, rather than a single, well-defined, time-bound decision made, as in acute care, by the dyad of physician and patient. The conceptual and ethical dimensions of microlevel long-term-care decision making have begun to attract the attention and investigation of scholars in gerontology, geriatrics, and bioethics (McCullough & Wilson, 1995).

Long-term-care decisions are, at their heart, ethical decisions. They involve ethical values such as preserving good relationships within one's family, showing respect and gratitude toward one's parents, and protecting elders who are vulnerable from unnecessary harm and injury. These decisions also involve important ethical principles such as beneficence and respect for autonomy. Any adequate account of the ethical dimensions of long-term-care decision making needs to take account of these values and principles. Doing so is the primary purpose of this chapter.

To this end we provide in this chapter a preventive-ethics approach to long-term-care decision making. We begin with a review of developments in bioethics that set the stage for the emphasis on preventive ethics. We then briefly review current policies and legislation in the United States that set the context for and act as constraints on long-term-care decision making. We next provide a brief comparative examination of policies in other countries to underscore the lack of a coherent approach to long-term care in the United States. We then provide an ethical analysis of acute-care versus long-term-care decision making. We go on to identify the implications of this ethical analysis for practice. On the basis of the preceding sections, we set out a stepwise, practical preventive-ethics approach to long-term-care decision making. This process incorporates the values and principles mentioned previously and shows how they can be effectively addressed in geriatric and gerontologic practice. We close with a consideration of the policy implications of this approach to long-term-care decision making.

DEVELOPMENTS IN RECENT BIOETHICS: THE VIRTUES OF PREVENTIVE ETHICS

The dominant approach to ethical issues in the literature of bioethics on the practice of the health care professions remains reactive in nature, just as most of health care in general does. This approach involves developing responses to ethical issues, problems, or crises after they have already occurred. This reactive approach to the ethics of the health care professions has resulted in attention to dramatic issues with which gerontologists and geriatricians have become familiar. These issues include discontinuing critical-care management of patients with advanced dementia who cannot express their preferences and did not do so before becoming gravely ill, discontinuing nutrition and hydration for dying patients, and physician-assisted suicide. The reactive approach to bioethics, including the ethics of professional practice in medicine, nursing, and social work, provides the clinician with tools for addressing and attempting to resolve these very difficult, often wrenching issues.

This reactive approach to clinical ethics does indeed engage the attention and energies of students, practitioners, and the public at large. This is because addressing and attempting to resolve "four-alarm" issues and "dilemmas" requires intellectual work that is interesting and absorbing, even exciting. These features of the reactive approach to clinical ethics help to explain why it has come to dominate the literature and pedagogy of ethics and aging, as well as every other topic in clinical ethics and, more generally, bioethics.

The reactive approach suffers from the striking defect that it does not take account of the possibilities of preventing ethical issues, conflicts, and dilemmas from arising in the first place by taking a prospective and anticipatory, rather than reactive, approach. The reactive approach to clinical ethics may resolve the "problem," defined as a discrete, limited decision in the acute-care setting, but it does not attend preventing problems and preventing the sequelae of decisions about problems in the lives of the individuals affected by them.

Gerontologists and geriatricians who work with elders and families making long-term-care decisions know these sequelae all too well. They include the wife who works herself into illness and a hospital admission taking care of her frail husband; the daughter exhausted by yet one more phone call in the wee hours of the morning from kindly neighbors where her father lives, who have yet again collected her father from the middle of the neighborhood street into which he had wandered; and the social worker who feels manipulated by adult children who attempt to enlist him or her in an effort to take over decision making from their frail mother, just as Mrs. G's daughter might be about to do.

These considerations and others have prompted us to take a preventive-ethics approach (Chervenak & McCullough, 1991; Forrow, Arnold, & Parker, 1993) to ethics and aging in general and to ethical issues in long-term-care decision making in particular (McCullough, Wilson, Rhymes, & Teasdale, 1995). Long-term-care decision making, just like other complex human activities, has the potential for ethical conflict and stressful sequelae built into it. Our own experience in putting preventive ethics into practice has taught us that it would be far better for all concerned if professionals engaged in this decision-making process worked to prevent such conflict from occurring in the first place. A preventive-ethics approach to long-term-care decision making also should make the ethical conflicts that nonetheless do occur more amenable to effective and less stressful management.

In this chapter, we therefore present a preventive-ethics approach to long-term-care decision making. Adopting such an approach in gerontologic and geriatric practice means that the complexity of long-term-care decision making need not so routinely stress, sometimes unreasonably, those who undertake it: elders, family members, and professionals. They can manage that complexity prospectively, with a view toward preventing ethical conflicts that arise almost as a natural function of the complexity of long-term-care decision making. Thus our main focus in this chapter is on a preventive-ethics approach to managing the ambiguities and complexities of long-term-care decision making. We intend in this chapter to equip the professional working with elders and family members to integrate the conceptual tools of ethics into a practical approach designed to prevent ethical conflict in long-term-care decision making. This is a tall order, just as preventive approaches to health care generally are. In this sense, the content of this chapter poses ethical challenges to the geriatric and gerontologic professional to take up the practice concepts that we will present in what follows.

CURRENT LONG-TERM-CARE POLICY AND LEGISLATION IN THE UNITED STATES

In long-term care, as in other aspects of U.S. health care delivery, "form follows funding" (R. L. Kane & R. A. Kane, 1990, p. 416). Because U.S. long-term-care policy and financing are decentralized, categorical, and limited (Benjamin, 1992), there is no long-term-care system but a fragmented array of different programs and many gaps in what is needed, especially outside of institutions. The following facts regarding long-term-care financing are key to comprehending what we must frankly admit is a nonsystem of care (N. L. Wilson, 1995): (1) Major differences and divisions exist between the financing of acute and long-term care for the elderly. These differences create sometimes powerful constraints on access to long-term-care services. (2) Individuals and families pay for a significant portion of long-term care. This means that the burden of caregiving becomes an ethically significant issue in long-term-care decision making. (3) Federal and state funding, provided through multiple program categories, results in fragmentation of benefits for the separate but interrelated medical, social, and income needs of older people. The result is that long-term-care decision making is a demanding and often stressful process. (4) Public financing of long-term care has been heavily biased toward payment for institutional long-term care and medical needs and not for formal home and community care. In our view, public policy expects, exploits, and reinforces family caregiving at home as a matter of obligation, almost without limits. Setting ethically justified limits on family caregiving thus becomes one of the central ethical concerns in long-term-care decision making. Long-term care should not be based on the "value" of endless self-sacrifice.

LONG-TERM-CARE POLICY IN OTHER COUNTRIES

Other industrialized nations have been addressing the issue of rising demand for comprehensive long-term care for many years longer than the United States. There are both similarities and differences in the organization and financing of long-term care in such countries (Schieber, Pollier, & Greenwald, 1991). The differences reflect different values concerning the government's role in providing long-term-care support as well as whether long-term care is viewed from the perspective of being a risk for an individual or a risk for a family. For example, in both Switzerland and Germany, as in the United States, long-term-care services are generally funded by private resources. In those cases where an older person has inadequate income, there are means-tested programs of financing comparable to Medicaid. However, in these countries, the financial status of the older person as well as close family members is considered in determining their eligibility for a financial subsidy. In other countries, as in the United States, there are different definitions of services that can be grouped under the concept of long-term care. For example, the distinction of medical versus social care exists in many countries. In countries such as Great Britain, there are chronic-care hospitals financed through a national insurance program. However, more traditional social services are not centrally financed, and, therefore, community services vary greatly according to local and regional financing. Many patterns of support therefore exist for long-term care in other countries.

One sometimes hears the view that other countries have more adequately responded than the United States to health care needs, including long-term care, through their systems both of financing and of organization. In actuality, because long-term-care coverage is not generally a part of national health insurance, there is only limited noninstitutional long-term care within many countries and considerable lack of coordination between the medical services funded through national health insurance and the more traditional social services. Only in some of the Canadian provinces and Denmark has there been adequate and systematic coordination of long-term-care services across health and social service programs. Consequently, elders and family members confront many of the same micro dilemmas facing persons in the United States (Doty, 1988, 1990), that is, where an elder will live and what services he or she will receive and from whom at whose expense.

ACUTE VERSUS LONG-TERM CARE IN THE BIOETHICS LITERATURE

We defined long-term care at the beginning of this chapter. On this definition, as well as others in the literature that the reader may prefer, long-term care differs significantly from acute care. We will first consider the bioethics literature on acute care and then show how the ethical dimensions of long-term care differ significantly and therefore call for a distinctive preventive-ethics approach.

Ethical Dimensions of Acute-Care Decision Making

Brian Hofland has pointed out that acute care, as a rule, involves well-defined problems as well as well-defined alternatives for managing them. Long-term care, by contrast, exhibits greater ambiguity. Problems are less well defined, and alternatives are therefore more resistant to clear definition (Hofland, 1990). Acute care tends to involve problems that are clear-cut. For example, the patient has gangrene caused by poor vascularization secondary to poorly controlled diabetes or significant occlusion of two coronary arteries with risk of life-threatening or crippling ischemia. In more clinical terms, the patient with an acute problem has or is thought to have an anatomical or physiological abnormality. Pathophysiology falls within the province of the health care professions, medicine in particular. Thus a built-in feature of acute care is that the health care professional, rather than the patient, possesses the intellectual basis for naming the patient's problem.

This dependence on health care professionals to name our problems when we are patients in acute-care settings is one of the sources of the power of health care professionals over patients. This aspect of the healer's power—the ability to make decisions by applying biomedical concepts to clinical situations—is usually not shared with the patient (H. Brody, 1992). The health care professional also exercises power, now in the form of an ability to carry out one's decisions, in an institutional context in which resources for the diagnosis and management of acute-care problems are organized and made available for health care professionals—physicians, in particular—to use in the care of patients. Health care professionals, not patients, control access to these resources, creating yet another dimension of the physician's power to make and carry out decisions in the acute-care setting.

The health care professional also exercises power within a hierarchical structure in which, for example, the physician writes orders that other professionals or technologists then carry out. Physicians recommend management strategies to patients. It is no longer the case, however, that physicians or any other health care professionals issue "orders" to patients, with which compliance is to be "prompt and implicit," as was expected in nineteenth-century American medical ethics (American Medical Association, 1847).

One important implication of the health care professional's role in the acute-care setting, especially in the hospital setting, is that patients experience dependence on their professional caregivers—physicians, nurses, and allied health professionals. This kind of dependence results in a loss of power by the patient, both to make and to carry out medical decisions. The informed-consent process can be understood as a response to enhance the patient's autonomy and therefore presumably the patient's power (McCullough & Wear, 1985). The purpose of the informed-consent process in this respect is for the patient to understand and authorize the physician's use of power on the patient's behalf.

In summary, in the acute-care setting, the health care professional, the physician in particular, possesses the power to name the patient's problem. The physician thus plays the role of chief ontologist, undertaking diagnostic workups to place the patient's reality into the correct pathophysiological category. The patient cannot perform this role, because the patient lacks the relevant scientific knowledge and clinical skills. Increasingly, third-party payers and managers, in addition to the informed-consent process, function as significant counterweights to the physician's power.

The patient's pathophysiology and the response of physicians and health care professionals and institutions to it have significant implications for the patient in other spheres of his or her life and for others in the patient's life. However, these are treated as implications, not matters of central concern, of acute care for third parties to the physician-patient relationship. The interests of the patient are therefore separable from those of family members in the acute-care settings (Arras, 1995).

Ethical Dimensions of Long-Term-Care Decision Making

Long-term care differs sharply from acute care in at least three respects: (*a*) competing realities rather than clearly defined problems; (*b*) less professional control of resources; and (*c*) family interests as intimately intertwined with and not easily separate from those of the elder. We turn now to an ethical analysis of each of these three conceptual components of long-term-care decision making.

Competing Realities

First, in long-term-care decision making the elder may not be a patient at all; quite the contrary. He or she is usually living in some community setting, getting along more or less well enough with his or her life. The physical, mental, or social changes that occur may not be acknowledged by the elder or, if acknowledged, may not be seen as problems or as serious problems—that is, warranting intervention and change—by the elder. Yet family members or the physician may judge these changes to be problems, and indeed, serious problems. In short, there is no chief ontologist in long-term-care decision making. For example, Mrs. G may not think that she is able to live outside a nursing home because her needs can only be met there, while her daughter may have quite a different view.

Consider the following circumstance: an older person living alone who does not have a strong interest in preparing meals just for one may nonetheless regard herself as quite capable of taking care of herself, yet her case manager may notice that this woman's nutritional status seems to be deteriorating. The case manager is expected to notice such changes and respond to them as potential threats to the elder's well-being. This woman may resist such solicitous intervention because she does not agree with the case manager's description of her condition or with the case manager's clinical ethical judgment that this condition poses a potential risk and therefore ought to be addressed. Competing realities constitute a defining feature of long-term-care decision making and a major source of ethical conflict within that process, a taxonomy of which is provided by Terrie Wetle (1995).

The realities of long-term care, as this case example illustrates, have both a factual and an evaluative dimension. The fact that this woman is or might be malnourished or at risk for malnourishment can be in dispute between her and her case manager. What each of them thinks about the importance or urgency of such factual matters can also be in dispute. By training and professional judgment, formed in beneficence-based (McCullough & Chervenak, 1994) regard for the well-being of a client, the case manager justifiably reaches the evaluation that risk of malnourishment is a harm to this woman and should be prevented. Such judgments possess the power to create dependencies like those created in acute care by the power to name the patient's problem. Yet, based on the sort of analysis that Bart Collopy (1995) has offered, the woman's decisions about how she lives may be an expression of her own concept of safety. Moreover, adequate nourishment, in George Agich's language (1993, 1995), involves the interstitial exercise of autonomy, the cumulative effect of which may be a nodal decision, for example, whether to stay in one's own home or move to a more structured setting in which nourishment is assured. Factual and ethical complexities can and do combine differently in professional and lay judgment, resulting in sometimes differing "mapping" of values relevant to the long-term-care decision-making process (McCullough, Wilson, Teasdale, Kolpakchi, & Skelly, 1993).

Thus the competing realities of long-term-care decision making embrace both factual and ethical elements, raising two questions:

1. Is there an authoritative factual description of the elder's situation?
2. What ought the elder, family members, and professionals to think of that situation, or how, reasonably, should they evaluate the elder's situation?

To the extent that matters of health are at stake, the professional's descriptions in response to the first question possess considerable intellectual authority. An individual with clinical symptoms of malnourishment has the burden of proof to show that she was not, in fact, malnourished. However, there exists no smooth, much less automatic, transition from intellectually authoritative clinical descriptions in response to the first question to controlling answers to the second question.

The second question calls for an evaluative judgment about agreed-upon facts; agreement on facts will not by itself routinely produce an agreed-upon evaluative judgment. Long-term-care decision makers form their evaluative judgments on the basis of different perspectives on the elder's interests. Professionals tend to take a perspective external to that of the elder, that is, a beneficence-based judgment about what would be good for any individual at risk for malnourishment. The elder, exercising autonomy, takes her own, personal perspective on these matters. This perspective can be usefully informed—but ought not to be controlled—by the professional's perspective (McCullough et al., 1993).

Family members also have a perspective on the elder's interests. In long-term-care decision making, as John Arras (1995) has argued, family members are not third parties to the decision-making process, especially family members who have been or might become caregivers. Family members are bound to the elder in complex moral relationships, whether as spouses (Jecker, 1995), children (Brakman, 1995), in-laws and stepchildren, or other kinship relationships. Family members bound to the elder by ties of moral obligation—which ought to be equal with respect to gender but in practice may not be—are thus the elder's moral intimates. Their perspective is at once external—they see things from a perspective other than that of the elder—and intimate to the extent that they know the elder well, spouses especially, and have access to the elder's internal perspective on the elder's interests. As Arras (1995) has pointed out, conflict of interest is not a terribly useful conceptualization of this complex moral relationship. Nonetheless, there is surely the potential for confusion in family members' perceptions of the elder's interests.

In the language of philosophical ethics, long-term-care decisions involve a kind of moral realism: situations are defined at their core not only from factually informed perspectives but also by the nexus of moral obligations that define the identity of elders and family members and shape the history of their relationships. The case worker in our case example reaches her judgment of her client's needs partly because she has beneficence-based obligations to protect her clients from unnecessary harm. The client has no such obligations and so reaches a different account of her reality. Moral realism flourished in the eighteenth century in Great Britain and took the view that "is" did indeed imply "ought" when the "is" described a social role that embraced and put into practice a nexus of obligations (Price, 1948). Long out of favor in twentieth-century Anglo-American philosophy, moral realism has recently enjoyed something of a renaissance in which moral realities are thought to "supervene" factual realities (R. W. Miller, 1992). The older version of moral realism is the more appropriate conceptualization of long-term-care decision making: moral realities help to constitute—not supervene or somehow add something to—the situations that trigger long-term-care decision making.

In acute-care decision making, we saw that there is often a chief ontologist whose descriptions of the patient's condition posses intellectual authority and whose moral judgments about how that condition ought to be managed possess considerable authority and power, in an imbalance of power with the patient. In long-term-care decision making, both factual and moral elements can be and are contested from the start. No one has conceptual authority or power to resolve them in the way that a physician has the conceptual power to make diagnoses of disease. The problem of contested reality must therefore be addressed in a preventive-ethics approach to long-term-care decision making.

Control of Resources

Second, the resources that might be marshalled in response to a situation that is agreed to be a problem are not under the sole control of the health care professional. This reflects the nonsystem aspect of long-term care, and health care generally, in the United States, as described earlier. Most of the resources in time, matériel, and money consumed in long-term care in the United States are owned by the so-called informal caregivers, the elder's moral intimates: spouses, children, other kinfolk, stepchildren, in-laws, neighbors, and friends. These individuals do not live in hierarchical relationships to the elder, nor the elder to them. As Nancy Jecker (1995) and Sarah Brakman (1995) have argued, the relationships between elders and family members involve tangled, often inchoate, and negotiable webs of obligations and their limits. Moreover, the informal caregivers do not stand in hierarchical relationships to professionals or to institutions that arrange or deliver formal long-term-care services. In short, the professional cannot issue orders to family members and other informal caregivers, nor they to each other. Power to make and carry out decisions is much more nearly equal among elders, family members, and professionals in long-term-care decision making.

Decisions about the use of resources thus lack the drama that often accompanies such decisions in the acute-care setting, for example, whether to admit a gravely ill patient with a poor prognosis to an already-overcrowded critical-care unit. Power is more diffuse and the exercise of autonomy by elders and family members more subtle and quotidian. In Agich's (1995) terms, once nodal decisions—the large, "either/or" decisions—have been made, for example, to stay at home and accept meals-on-wheels to help prevent malnourishment, many matters of interstitial or everyday decision making move to the fore. Harry R. Moody, adopting the theory of communicative ethics, has argued that requests, compromise, and negotiation are the tools of decision making in long-term care (Moody, 1992). Agich's (1995) analysis helps us see why: interstitial decision making among moral intimates, especially when the burden of care is unequal between genders, involves the subtle skills of negotiation rather than the blunt exercise of power to resolve nodal questions.

Martha Holstein and Thomas Cole (1995) and Nancy Wilson (1995) have shown that powerful historical and policy forces affect the nature and availability of resources for long-term-care decision making. History and policy making define, and indeed create and control access to, long-term-care resources. That most such care is provided by family and community members is no accident. Historical stigmas of poverty are associated with nursing homes, and the lack of publicly funded alternatives de facto exploits the obligations of spouses, children, kinfolk, and friends. This exploitation may increase with changes in Medicaid and Medicare, transforming them from entitlements to government "contributions." In order to control payment for use of formal services and therefore access to them, professionals have been empowered to play the role of gatekeepers. Case managers play this role explicitly, as do others, especially physicians. R. A. Kane (1995) and Wetle (1995) have documented that case managers are increasingly aware of the ethical conflicts generated by their role as gatekeepers.

Public policy constraints, especially regarding payment for formal services, thus do not operate in the background of long-term-care decision making; they often define the very parameters of what is realistically available to elders with long-term-care needs and to their network of informal support. Managing the effect of resource constraints on both nodal and interstitial autonomy of elders and family members and on the constant negotiation and renegotiation of limited obligations to provide care is an essential element of preventive ethics in long-term-care decision making.

The Importance of the Psychosocial

Third, the psychosocial spheres of the elder's life cannot be ignored in long-term-care decision making, because this process shapes the elder's and family members' psychosocial reality. This is because the elder's problem, while it may involve mental or physical change, just as often involves social change. Indeed, the latter can sometimes loom far larger than the former, for example, with change from home to an institutional setting. In our judgment, loss of self-sufficiency counts more as a social phenomenon in the life of the elder and his or her moral intimates than as a medical one. Relocating to receive care or accepting assistance with daily tasks may have a profound effect on an elder's self-identity and opportunity to perform cherished social roles. Acute care pertains mainly to health matters, long-term care to health and to housing, income, self-care, community, family, and personal matters, as illustrated by the case of Mrs. G with which this chapter began.

In other words, long-term-care decisions are prompted by changes that can pose a direct threat to the elder's and therefore to family members', especially the spouse's (N. L. Wilson, 1995), self-identity, as expressed in where one lives and near whom one lives and in one's habits, that is, the values that together give coherence and meaning to a human life. In philosophical accounts, self-identity is appropriately addressed in terms of the necessary conditions for the unity of personal identity over time. Such philosophical analysis focuses on whether continuity of physical or mental identity over time is required for self-identity as its necessary condition. These austere philosophical investigations enjoy the luxury of ignoring the material, sufficient conditions for mundane self-identity and are animated by Enlightenment ideals of the unity of persons.

Mundane, quotidian self-identity in its material sense—one's habits, one's neighborhood, one's friendships—involves long-standing patterns of behavior, expectations, and relationships, including moral obligations as a spouse, parent, or child. Self-identity in its material sense is best understood as a coping strategy with the conditions of human existence at the end of the most violent and rending century in the recorded history of our species. Elders have lived through the worst, most bloody parts of that century, their children through the better, more peaceful part of it. Self-identity in its material sense aims at social, moral, and aesthetic coherence of who one is and hopes still to be in a sometimes hostile and confusing world. In the language of Irwin Lieb (1991), we can say that self-identity seeks to weave the self-as-past together with the self-as-future well enough, that is, in an effort to avoid destructive tension between the two.

Long-term-care decision making sometimes confronts the possibility of such tension. Recent qualitative study of elders' values in long-term-care decision making indicates that preservation of self-identity is an important consideration (McCullough et al., 1995). Respondents in this study expressed their values in this category in straightforward, concrete terms, for example, staying in one's own home, not leaving one's neighborhood of many years, and the like. Long-term-care decisions often threaten the value an elder may place on self-identity, because changes that may be made may radically alter material conditions of that identity. An elder will struggle to remain herself when she moves from home to nursing home, as Mrs. G is contemplating doing.

The decision-making process has more at stake than simply a living setting or care arrangement, because the latter are structured by history, policy, professionals, and institutions in ways sometimes incompatible with maintaining or adapting individual identity. Living independently is a struggle in a nursing home, and living securely can be a struggle living alone in a high-crime area. Thus the ethical dimensions of long-term-care decisions include the following consideration: whether the elder and family members ought to be willing to embrace long-term-care alternatives is partly a function of whether they ought to be willing to embrace the psychosocial realities entailed by those alternatives.

R. A. Kane (1995) and Wetle (1995) have identified and examined value-based conflicts in long-term-care decision making, the awareness of care managers of these conflicts, and the possibilities of effectively addressing these conflicts in practice. The challenge to the health care professional who seeks to manage the psychosocial dimensions of long-term-care decision making effectively is to practice nondirective counseling about value-laden decisions. The ethos of nondirective counseling has been developed to prevent professionals from imposing their own values on clients and patients, a positive development in the ethics of health care professionals. A dangerous implication of nondirective counseling is to conclude that the professional has no role to play whenever value-laden, normative matters—questions about what ought to be done—are at stake. These normative questions, the health care professional may wrongly conclude, are matters for patients and clients to decide on their own, with no assistance from the health care professional. This view of nondirective counseling could amount to a kind of abandonment, especially in the context of long-term care, where elders and family members may not have acknowledged that their problems involve competing realities, interests, obligations, justified constraints on their own resources, and the negotiation of their own self-identity. Nondirective counseling, a key element of preventive-ethics strategies, can identify these issues in the constructive and open-ended way called for by long-term-care decision making.

Summary of the Ethical Dimensions of Long-Term-Care Decision Making

In summary, long-term-care decision making involves competing realities, including competing evaluative interpretations of realities. There will often be disagreement among long-term-care decision makers about whether the mental or physical or social changes that reduce self-sufficiency in activities of daily living have occurred and, when they have occurred, whether they should count as problems. There is no chief ontologist who can claim the intellectual authority to control the outcome of such disagreement, even when the elder is a patient with long-term-care needs awaiting discharge from the hospital. The power to name the problem is thus contested, not settled as it is in the acute-care setting. Second, the power to command resources in response to a long-term-care problem, once it is agreed to be such, is widely diffused among the elder, informal and formal caregivers, and institutions. Because of the important role that they play, informal caregivers function both as major long-term-care resources and as important decision makers with the elder and the physician. It therefore follows that the obligations of family members and their legitimate interests and the obligations of elders to family members are essential to deciding whether family members ought to serve as such a resource. Third, long-term care is inherently biopsychosocial in nature. Such care involves medical as well as social and personal realities that need to be brought together in some coherent way. Indeed, long-term-care decision making, with its competing realities, essentially temporal character, and shifting cast of participants, may best exemplify the biopsychosocial model in health care and social services (Engel, 1980).

IMPLICATIONS FOR PRACTICE

The preceding ethical analysis underscores ambiguity and its management as central ethical themes of long-term-care decision making, in sharp contrast to acute-care decision making. Long-term-care decisions introduce ambiguity by contradiction or the threat of contradiction among the values, hopes, and identities in the moral lives of elders and those who care for them. These ambiguities shape housing and financial decisions, as well as decisions about what care is needed and who can, will, or ought to provide that care. Long-term-care problems and decisions do not come easily into a sharp and steady focus. They are blurred because they are shifting, uncertain, and contested. Any ethical approach to long-term-care decision making must therefore make ambiguity the fundamental category and response to ambiguity the appropriate strategy (Arras, 1984).

Built-in ambiguity cannot be resolved or solved. The language of resolution of conflict that figures so prominently in the bioethics literature, a result of the nearly single-minded focus on acute-care decision making, is therefore inadequate to the ethics of long-term-care decision making. Instead, the language of management of ambiguity and of its potential to generate conflicting obligations and, therefore, preventive ethics move to the fore.

"Manage" comes from an Italian root that pertains to the training of horses—the analogue of the ambiguity, conflict, or problem to be managed and prevented. Every equestrian knows that even the most docile and well-trained horse can turn ornery without warning. The rider does not control a horse, as if the rider were in charge. The rider attends to the horse's signals and responds to them, directing the horse, coaxing, on the alert for the unexpected. The relationship between horse and rider is one of ongoing negotiation with an eye to preventing the worst outcomes and trying to do the best that one can together. So, too, for long-term-care decision making. There are reliable ways for "horse" and "rider" to reach accommodation. Our preventive-ethics approach to long-term-care decisions will have to show the way for elders, family members, and professionals to reach accommodation.

Long-term-care decision making therefore does not lend itself to the theoretical resolution of establishing a priori, that is, without reference to experience, a fixed hierarchy of ethical principles and then applying that hierarchy to cases. Moreover, decision making under conditions of ambiguity is best understood as a fragile process, open to both success and failure, and thus open as well to the need for reactivating the decision-making process when failure occurs. The most appropriate responses of the professional assisting elders and families with long-term-care decision making are to be aware of the ambiguities of long-term-care decision making and to take a preventive-ethics posture toward conflicting obligations and ambiguity. We will describe our preventive-ethics approach to long-term-care decision making in the next section. In our judgment, any adequate preventive-ethics approach to long-term-care decision making needs to address the following conceptual and ethical issues:

First, there exist powerful system constraints at the macro level of policy that are shaped by a long and implacable history, as described earlier. These policies, in turn, shape the long-term-care decision-making process. Second, there are also constraints operating at the micro level of the decision-making process. As we saw earlier in our brief review of American long-term-care policy, these include such factors as a shifting cast of decision makers, decision making as a hurried process depending on the urgency of the elder's need or the family's limits, and failure sometimes to appreciate that a decision needs to be made. Third, these two factors combine with the powerful element of gender bias, leading to the provision of long-term care as a way of life for some women (N. L. Wilson, 1995). Fourth, constraints that can also affect the professional's role include competing realities, time, uncertainty about who is the primary client, the preferences of elders and family members, and multiple roles and "agencies" played by the professional, including especially the role of gatekeeper for payment for formal services. The medical bias of long-term-care policy described earlier influences practice, with a tendency to discount the psychosocial dimensions of long-term care. Fifth, all of the constraints on long-term-care decision making can impair the exercise of autonomy, both nodal and interstitial. However, even implacable constraints on nodal autonomy do not entail such constraints on interstitial autonomy; there is a great deal of independence between the two kinds of autonomy. This represents a significant opportunity to enhance autonomy both of elder and family, an opportunity that can be lost by following a misleading, acute-care–type focus on the nodal issues or decisions as the whole of the story. Sixth, there are competing realities, which should be understood as a complex mix of both factual and moral matters. The latter include the following: (*a*) a concern for safety that seems to override and thus eliminate all other considerations or values, reflecting and potentially reinforced by the dominance of beneficence-based judgments of professionals; and (*b*) treating safety not as an independent value but on a continuum with the autonomy-based value of independence. Seventh, in contrast to the acute-care model, family members may be full participants in both caregiving and decision making and have legitimate, even if conflicting, interests of their own. They should not be considered third parties disabled by conflicts of interest. Eighth, the obligations of spouses and adult children—indeed, of any long-term caregiver—are limited. This is a key ethical consideration in long-term-care decision making because it is not selfish or mean spirited for family members to want to avoid unreasonable caregiving burdens. Family members often find themselves caught between endless self-sacrifice and selfishness as the only two options they can perceive for themselves. There exists a middle ground that a preventive-ethics approach to long-term-care decision making opens for their consideration, namely, legitimate self-interests. These include obligations to one's spouse and children and close friends, and perhaps to one's employer, as well as those activities from which one draws deep and abiding satisfaction and fulfillment. No ethical theory requires that these be routinely sacrificed in one's moral life. Ninth, it follows that elders have ethical obligations to family members and other caregivers to respect their legitimate interests. Tenth, the complex nexus of obligations and interests joining the parties to long-term-care decision making cannot be settled a priori, that is, in theory. This complexity and its moral ambiguities must be negotiated for each case and may result in a trial of a long-term-care arrangement as the outcome. Eleventh, long-term-care decision making is a fragile and potentially unstable process and therefore subject to periodic breakdowns and the consequent need to restart the decision-making process. Twelfth, the professional can play the crucial role of initiating, in a nondirective fashion, consideration of the ethical dimensions of long-term-care decision making from the start of this process, a practice implication of all of the preceding factors. To do otherwise unwittingly, but nevertheless negligently, creates the conditions for preventable conflict and all its stressful and preventable sequelae.

A PRACTICAL, STEPWISE PREVENTIVE-ETHICS APPROACH TO LONG-TERM-CARE DECISION MAKING

Preventive ethics eschews theoretical, a priori resolution of the ambiguous and complex process of long-term-care decision making (Chervenak & McCullough, 1991). Preventive ethics takes a prospective approach to ethical conflict in the decision-making process. The preceding analysis of the ethical dimensions of long-term-care decision making and their implications for practice makes it possible to describe a preventive-ethics approach to long-term-care decision making. This preventive-ethics approach individualizes decision making, thus creating a powerful antidote to the "cookie-cutter" care plans that R. A. Kane (1995) has appropriately criticized.

We have also designed our preventive-ethics approach to check the potential trumping power of beneficence-based professional judgment, especially about safety of the elder, and of family-member preferences by emphasizing respect for the legitimate interests, limited obligations, and autonomy of both elders and family members. Any particular long-term-care arrangement that results from this decision-making process will therefore in principle be open to review and renegotiation.

By the time the professional becomes involved in the process, some long-term-care decisions, nodal as well as interstitial, already have been made, seriously considered, or firmly rejected. Professional involvement in the long-term-care decision-making process can sometimes unintentionally disrupt or even break relationships and "careers" of caring. Using the following preventive-ethics approach, the professional can, in a nondirective fashion, bring some structure and order to both nodal and interstitial long-term-care decisions. While the elements of this preventive-ethics approach are listed in a particular order, the process itself may not always be linear. There are parallels between this preventive-ethics approach to long-term-care decision making and communicative ethics, the details of which are beyond the scope of this chapter.

1. Identify the stakeholders in the decision. Who should be included in the process?
2. Seek an agreed-upon factual account of the elder's condition, especially significant or irreversible changes in capacity for self-care.
   a. Identify the biopsychosocial needs and care requirements of the elder.
   b. Identify whether family members are physically and cognitively able to meet these requirements.
3. Identify formal long-term-care services that are realistically available to meet the elder's needs, given financial, geographic, and policy constraints. Identify the benefits and risks of each alternative to prevent making the assumption that an alternative (especially the nursing home) is risk free.
4. Invite the elder and family members, on the basis of their evaluations, to identify all reasonable alternatives.
   a. Invite discussion of reasonable, justified limits of familial obligations to provide care to the elder.
   b. Invite recognition of gender bias in the family's distribution of caregiving burden and expectations of who can and ought to provide long-term care.
   c. Elicit the elder's views about the obligation to prevent unreasonable caregiving burdens on family members, especially female family members.
5. Elicit the values of the elder and family members and on this basis elicit their evaluations of the elder's condition and realistic alternatives for its management.
   a. Remind the elder and family members that there is usually more than one alternative consistent with each's values.
   b. Encourage the elder and family members to identify and take account of each other's limited obligations to protect and promote the interests of others as an important basis for evaluating realistic alternatives.
   c. Invite careful and thoughtful discussion of the implications of realistic alternatives for self-identity of the elder and family members, especially for relationships that they want to protect and promote.
6. If the professional has recommendations, either from among these alternatives or for one that has been set aside, the professional should offer these recommendations. When possible, recommendations should be based primarily on what appears to be in the elder's and family members' interests, rather than on agency or institutional interests.
7. Encourage agreement on an alternative, recognizing that it may not be permanent.
   a. Remind the elder and family members that the long-term-care arrangement selected may not work.
   b. Encourage the elder and family members to establish a process for review of the arrangement and, if possible, the criteria for its stopping, continuation, or revision.

This preventive-ethics approach to long-term-care decision making takes seriously the time constraints that often affect the decision-making process. As a result of such time constraints, some decisions may already have been made. The health care professional, however, should not regard such decisions as irrevocable, and the elder and family members should therefore be asked if they want to review or reconsider the decision already made. In addition, they should be made aware that even when nodal decisions of long-term care have been made, many everyday or interstitial decisions remain to be made and that these decisions can be made in a way that can indeed take account of the elder's and family members' interests, especially the elder's. That some nodal decisions have been made for the elder does not require that subsequent everyday decisions be made for him or her.

Elders with diminished decision-making capacity should not, on the basis of such information alone, be judged unable to participate in the long-term-care decision-making process. Instead, the multistep decision-making process described here should be attempted for elders with diminished decision-making capacity as a way to determine if they can in fact make their own decisions. We propose this approach to impaired decision-making capacity because the kinds of skills called for in this process are not necessarily well measured by existing, validated mental-status–assessment instruments. If the elder or family member shows himself or herself irreversibly unable to participate in this decision-making process, then that process should be initiated with others acting as a proxy for the elder or family member. The proxy should be asked in step 5 to focus primarily on the elder's values and preferences, as best as these can be known. There will be some distance between the actual autonomy of the elder or family member and any surrogate, but this distance is not totally insurmountable. Conscientious proxy decision making should be the goal, not perfect proxy decision making; holding all proxy decision making to the standard of substituted judgment is simply impossible. There should be appropriate use of a best-interest standard as well.

We find Arras's (1995) reservations about a "low-key, oblique approach" to long-term-care decision making persuasive. Thus the preventive-ethics approach we have described takes an open approach to long-term-care decision making. This approach should, like any clinical intervention, be offered to elders and family members and their consent elicited to undertake the process.

Because the decision for nursing-home placement is so wrenching, as it is about to be in the case of Mrs. G, we consider it here in more, brief detail. The multistep long-term-care decision-making process applies especially to the interstitial, everyday decisions that remain. These decisions provide an important but often neglected opportunity to maximize respect for the elder's autonomy in this domain of decision making. As Agich (1995) has pointed out, the elder's autonomy is very much at stake in the day-to-day decisions in nursing-home life because autonomy finds meaningful and important expression in such decisions.

As Lidz, Fischer, and Arnold (1992) have documented, the nursing home as a "total institution" has corrosive effects on the elder's autonomy. In this setting, the gerontologist's or geriatrician's role is appropriately to advocate for the elder's autonomy in interstitial decisions. The day-to-day issues in the life of nursing-home residents have been discussed in a volume edited by R. A. Kane and Caplan (1990). The health care professional needs to be attentive to and protect such mundane exercises of autonomy as phone privileges, roommate selection, and opportunity for spiritual and religious growth. The health care professional should take advantage of the nursing-home staff's day-to-day knowledge of the elder to identify what is important to the elder, especially elders with severe dementing disorders and diseases. As Agich (1993) has argued, there can still remain in the midst of dementia ethically significant expressions of autonomy, for example, going to a stairwell, not to "elope," but for peace and quiet.

There are implications of our preventive-ethics approach to long-term-care decision making for long-term care per se. This is a very large topic, and so we can touch on it here only briefly. The health care professional should work with nursing-home administrators to create an environment in which the nursing home is not so systemically corrosive of the elder's autonomy. Lidz et al. (1992) call into question nursing-home policies that excessively favor considerations other than autonomy. For example, the health care professional can point out that too much regard for bodily safety can lead to use of restraints that undermine autonomy, making the elder worse off and, in a larger sense of safety, perhaps less safe (Collopy, 1995). Lidz et al. (1992) suggest that patients with different cognitive abilities should not be routinely mixed together, inasmuch as this can erode the abilities of those with the least cognitive loss. In these and other small but incrementally valuable ways, the health care professional can take a preventive-ethics approach to enhancing the autonomy of the elder living in a nursing home by obliging the nursing home to review its policies and practices with a view toward identifying their impact on the autonomy of the home's residents.

IMPLICATIONS OF PREVENTIVE ETHICS FOR LONG-TERM-CARE POLICY AND PLANNING

The preventive-ethics approach to long-term-care decision making that we have proposed here has important implications, still fully to be identified and explored, for public policy and for institutional practice and planning. Public policy and institutional practice and policies can sometimes function synergistically as a source of unnecessary and ethically suspect impediments to preventive ethics. For example, many hospitals have attempted to shorten length of stay for Medicare beneficiaries in response to the economic incentives in the Prospective Payment System used by the Health Care Financing Administration. As a consequence, the discharge-planning process may be hurried and the patient may still be so ill that he or she cannot participate adequately in the decision-making process. The autonomy of the elder can easily be undermined by family members who take advantage of these institutional and policy constraints and simply make a decision for the elder. When they do so, they should be challenged and forced to bear the burden of proof of the ethical justification for the exercise of such considerable power. In short, rethinking the conceptual and ethical dimensions of microlevel long-term-care decision making will, as it progresses, create a policy and practice agenda of reform of macrolevel long-term-care decision making. The core of this agenda is ethical: protecting values such as the importance of one's self-identity and limited familial obligations of caregiving and such ethical principles as respect for autonomy from adverse effects of poorly thought-out policies and practices.

Long-term-care decision making by elders, family members, and professionals calls for nuanced, flexible responses because the changes that prompt long-term-care decisions dislodge elders and family from the nexus of relationships, achievements, sacrifices, and other factors from and in which human beings sustain their identities and worlds of meaning. A spouse dies or a child reaches the limits of caregiving obligations, and support networks unravel. Previously accommodated levels of dependence can no longer be accommodated. The elder confronts a world in which self-identity must be adapted to increased levels of dependence. The adult child confronts a world in which endless sacrifice may shape or shatter his or her self-identity. An elder hospitalized with pneumonia experiences worsening of her congestive heart failure and mental-status changes. The discharge planner suggests to the patient's daughter that her mother will need a significant level of support and supervision if she is to return to her ranch in the hill country, hours away from the city where her daughter lives and works. The issues go beyond where and how to live. The issues become the challenge to this woman and her daughter to forge a caregiving relationship that will shape the self-identity of both.

In short, long-term-care decisions reach into the nooks and crannies of the moral lives of elders and their families because self-identity is an essential dimension of our moral lives. The moral life, as philosophers since Socrates have taught, comprises our obligations to others because acknowledging and fulfilling obligations shape each individual's identity. Forging and, through negotiation, reforging caregiver obligations and care-receiver obligations shape and reshape self-identity and therefore one's moral life. Long-term-care decision making thus roils with complexity, ambiguity, conflict, and stress, just as the moral life generally roils with complexity, ambiguity, conflict, and stress.

Complexity, ambiguity, conflict, and stress are, to put it simply, the normal conditions of the moral life. These features of our moral lives cannot be "solved," that is, eliminated. They are, instead, to be managed—we cope with and adapt to them as best we can by shaping a self-identity in which one still can recognize oneself and intimate others. Thus elders and family members often dedicate themselves to the hard and often needlessly stressful work of long-term-care decision making. Gerontologists and geriatricians can help to make this hard and stressful work less stressful and less exhausting than it often is. Toward this important goal of humane care for the elderly, we have set out our preventive-ethics approach to long-term-care decision making.

17

Ethical Issues in Decision Making: A Balanced Interest Perspective

Tanya Fusco Johnson

In the preceding chapters, the contributions have addressed several important issues and dilemmas in ethics and aging. The seven concepts of autonomy, privacy, beneficence, justice, nonmaleficence, fidelity, and accountability have been discussed with varying emphases. In the process of exploring these aspects, the contributors have noted other important parameters. These include personal ethics, the ethics of relationship, ethics and politics, ethics and power, and ethics in a multicultural and multidisciplinary context. In this chapter, the seven ethical concepts will be examined along with these parameters to show how a "balanced interest" perspective could be applied in each instance. The chapter will close with a brief discussion of my application of Habermas's "communicative ethics" (1990, 1993, 1996), which presents the balanced-interest perspective in decision making.

While it would perhaps make things clearer if I were to adopt a particular ethics ideology or point to propositions or protocols that have guided my thinking, I cannot be that specific. There is so much merit in all of these "camps" that it would be limiting not to encompass all, or at least allow for their application. However, the reader must not lose sight of the fact that as a sociologist, my thinking is oriented toward interaction and reciprocal relations. My education in theology has also encouraged a multidisciplinary view. Finally, it is very much the case that my political orientation with a small *p* is democratic. What follows is informed by these beliefs and biases.

Before we proceed, it is important to define what is meant by a "balanced" interest. The discussion of the five elements that follow will illustrate this notion. The term "balance" implies a steadiness or equilibrium. It suggests that things are stable or on an even plane. However, this is not what is meant here. Its usage here transcends leveling. Balanced interest supposes that all have an equal hand in making decisions. There is sufficient exchange, joint interaction, and sharing of rights and responsibilities so that balance is not making the best of a bad situation, is not achieved at others' expense, and is not a plan just to preserve the status quo. Rather, it is the outcome of a dynamic process in which decisions are crafted in the interchange of ideas.

KEY PARAMETERS IN THE BALANCED PERSPECTIVE

The Ethics Concepts

While some of the contributors to this handbook would disagree, in my view it is better to see the seven concepts in a balanced perspective rather than as a hierarchy. If they are viewed in this way, there is a blending or an integration rather than competition. This in no way does away with the tension between right and responsibility and the positional distance between autonomy and accountability. As we have seen in the contributors' discussions of the issues and dilemmas that emerge when we apply these concepts to aging, there are differences and confrontations with each other, daring the other to show cause for his or her arguments. However, in the balanced perspective, this tension can only be resolved when we see that these concepts are all of a piece. This is like our description of the puzzle in chapter 1. People are not afraid to find opposition because the assumption is that one person's point of view is just as important as another; one professional's point of view is just as valued as another's. The goal, then, is not to conquer but to accommodate.

The parties and the concepts they address are tied together. After all, they most likely share the same goal. It is the means that differ. Fidelity implies accountability. It assumes that beneficence is achieved through fidelity. If we were to be unfaithful, we could do harm that would violate nonmaleficence. Fidelity also implies justice or fair play. It helps preserve privacy and autonomy.

Jennifer Solomon in chapter 12 in the case of Martha shows the interface among the concepts. Family members have supported her autonomy, have promoted privacy, beneficence, and nonmaleficence, and have attempted to be accountable to her, including the fact that there were limits to their financial resources, which calls into question the concept of justice. In chapter 9, Holstein and McCurdy describe "dignity" as going beyond autonomy to include "a crowded moral universe of others" in which there is the need for the older adult to be accountable along with the expectation that others will be equally accountable. The emphasis of one ethical concept over another, or one's rights over their duties, or the interplay of the rights of one juxtaposed against the duties of another in each of these seven contexts will cause an asymmetry in the articulation of concerns. If autonomy supersedes beneficence, the outcome will be win-lose. The older adult may get his or her way, but is likely to experience unnecessary adverse consequences at the hands of others. In like manner, the relative, the paraprofessional, or the professional who centers on his or her rights with regard to justice may violate the autonomy of the older adult. The right to decide what is best for the older adult is part of the scenario. As stated in chapter 1, the older adult is seen in community and, as a contributor, must provide as much as possible as well as receive autonomy, privacy, beneficence, justice, nonmaleficence, fidelity, and accountability. The balanced-interest perspective encourages all parties—older adults, families, informal caregivers, paraprofessionals, and professionals—to be neither indulgent, on the one hand, nor to simply make sacrifices, on the other. Rather, they are expected to develop agreements and honor the interest of others while at the same time ardently advocating for their own. The ultimate goal is a win-win outcome. We will show how this might be achieved in the decision-making process at the conclusion of this chapter when we apply communicative ethics to it.

Personal Ethics

Ethical issues must necessarily start with individual interpretations of the world. This may be done apart from the concepts, propositions, protocols, and decision-making groups who may be party to these issues. If we do not start from the individual's point of view, whether the individual is the client or patient, the professional, the paraprofessional, a family member, or another care provider, we may overlook this essential ingredient in decision making as demands for closure and crisis-based decisions smother individual differences. As Crawford says in chapter 3, we "invent life differently." It is because of this fact that conflicts of interests occur. Nevertheless, if all parties are expected to have input, they must be asked their opinions. Of course, there is a whole range of responses. Some individuals have carefully worked-out opinions, while others have no opinions at all. An autocratic system is certainly easier. It is also likely to be the most efficient method for closure. The problem, however, is that this type of leadership is not the most effective if there is to be reciprocity. What each person involved in the issue or dilemma says impacts on the resolution of ethical concerns as well as success in execution. Back and Pearlman in chapter 5 discuss the issues that arise when patients pursue "alternative therapies." Mitzen and Gruber in chapter 11 note problems that occur when there are cultural differences between paraprofessionals and clients, even when they are from the same ethnic group. In his discussion of abuse, Kapp in chapter 13 observes that some individuals may perceive shouting and slapping as behavioral expectations of their ethnic or religious group and therefore not as abuse at all. These are perceptions that, in the end, come from individuals and how they view their "worlds."

Many of us accept the fact that there is not one reality, but several realities. Further, we observe that we are not likely to agree on one right reality. Therefore, we must continually be sensitive to the fact that a personal ethics may be strongly held and may contradict or clash with others. Or, on the other hand, it may be so weakly held or so dominated by others' views that any hope for self-determination is extinguished. In either case, the failure to have a voice (because of either coercion or submission) undermines any attempt to gain compliance. Therefore, the balanced interest perspective calls for us, whether we are older adult, family member, other informal caregiver, paraprofessional, or professional, to see each individual as a special contributor, equally valued for ideas and recommendations and equally responsible for expressing them. Recall the case study in chapter 1 in which

1. the helping professionals are concerned about the health of the disabled older adult if that person remains in the apartment;
2. the older adult does not want to go to a nursing home;
3. the retarded son just wants to be with the parent;
4. the daughter does not want to look after her retarded brother who is currently living with her parent because of the extra burden of care;
5. the neighbors fear that the older adult's clumsiness will set the apartment on fire while she is preparing a meal; and
6. the landlord is getting threatening phone calls from other tenants, but his hands are tied because there are no legal grounds on which to evict the older adult and child.

In this case, after each party's concerns were aired and pursued, the decision was made to have a live-in paraprofessional caregiver for both the parent and the son. Food and lodging were exchanged for care. The local social services agency provided assistance to the paraprofessional for respite care one day a week and for vacations. With this arrangement, everyone's interests were served without anyone winning at another's expense. This is an example of how balanced interest may be applied to an actual situation.

Ethics in Relationships

When ethics operates in the practice setting, it sets us in relationships that must be worked out in a web of competing solutions. One person's ethical solution may become, precisely, another's ethical problem.

Cromwell Crawford in chapter 3 notes that many of the religions focus on relationships. For example, in Confucianism, *jen* has a dual meaning: man and two. The man of *jen* is one who, desiring to develop himself, develops others, and in desiring to sustain himself, sustains others. Ethical decision making presumes that the older adult and others in relationship, including the professional, are equal partners in the plan. This does not mean that they are equal in expertise or experiences. Rather, they have equal rights and responsibilities to work through ethical decisions. Elsewhere, Cortese (1990) states that we can only be conscious of the other's ethics when we are in a relationship (p. 158). Since from this writer's point of view, the client's values are just as important as the professional's, they constitute the first decision-making team (T. F. Johnson, 1995a). Mitzen and Gruber in chapter 11 caution against the paraprofessional becoming too intimate with the client. Their point is well taken, but maybe there is something between social distance and intimacy. A relationship does not presuppose intimacy. Instead, it supposes a level playing field in communication and a commitment to work toward mutual interests. Social distance can be preserved, but there is, nevertheless, subjectivity as the professional seeks to understand the needs of the older adult. Lesnoff-Caravaglia in chapter 14 talks about "high touch" even when "high tech" is used. Dallas High in chapter 7 uses the example of hospice programs to point out how relationships are important in the successful care of the client. For example, he talks about the need for the hospice provider to listen to and learn from the older adult. Such an encounter, therefore, must be "personal." In his fourth guideline, High notes that medical professionals caring for terminally ill patients cannot afford to be impersonal. High emphasizes that the patient is a "social being" and therefore should be integrated into the communication of care rather than isolated. Achenbaum (1985) also finds this deep affinity in intergenerational relations. "Working with the young, and the middle-aged, older Americans can help all of us see the connections between our personal destinies and our collective fate" (p. 112). As Gilligan (1982) notes, relationships are nonhierarchical. In our understanding of balanced interest, they must be nonhierarchical. The older adult's success is our success when we are in relationship, whether as a family member, a friend, or a professional. The same is true for failure. If the older adult fails, we too fail. We cannot separate ourselves from one another. Paul Blanton makes this case graphically, but eloquently: "An old man—bedfast and alone, lying in his own feces and urine, dying of a malignancy is you. This awareness is fundamental—not whether he is eligible for Medicaid, not if he is mean and deserves his misfortune, not if he has the mental capacity to make sound decisions . . . His need for help, first of all is our need" (1989, p. 31).

As Heintz notes in chapter 8, families may be in conflict, and when this is present, the ethical issues are much more complex. However, avoiding this situation in no way alters the fact that a relationship does exist and must be addressed. There is a commitment to be involved. Back and Pearlman in chapter 5 describe how this works in the "deliberative" approach. McCullough and Wilson (1995) talk about the "nondirective" approach that demands communication. This balanced interest perspective in relationships can be seen in the following case:

1. A competent older adult prefers to live in a potentially abusive situation with her spouse because her religion requires her to remain in the relationship in good times and in bad.
2. This view competes with the adult-protective-services social worker's effort to provide for her safety and the knowledge that the worker will be held accountable if any harm comes to her.

3. This view conflicts with the physician's commitment to preserve her health by placing her in a nursing home.
4. This view counters the court's mandate to seek justice when citizens' rights are violated.

These circumstances return us once again to the question "In whose best interest is ethics operating?" and reminds us that all of these persons are first and last in a relationship of some kind and to some degree. Somehow, solutions must be worked out to achieve a balance of all their interests. Because the welfare of both the older adults is important, the balanced perspective would begin by exploring the relationship between the partners and how they could arrive at a shared definition of the situation. If this can be achieved, we would be using the preventive-ethics orientation which McCullough and Wilson present in chapter 16. If there is no consensus, negotiation will include adult protective services, the physician, and the courts. In this case, the husband agreed to participate in an "alternatives to violence" support group two years ago, and, happily, he has not been physically or verbally abusive to his wife since.

Ethics and Politics

In addition to being circumscribed by relationships, ethics cannot be practiced apart from the society in which it is situated. Doing ethics must necessarily be accomplished in and through the political system in which it finds itself. Therefore, ethics and politics are inevitably bedfellows, at times uneasy, at times quite satisfied, but nonetheless very much involved with one another. Politics can exist without ethics, but ethics cannot function without politics and the structures it provides to work through its application. Margaret Rhodes (1991) shows this union in her book *Ethical Dilemmas in Social Work Practice*, in which she develops three themes: (1) ethics is a part of most decisions by social workers; (2) politics is also involved in decisions because of the need to respond to governmental regulations; and (3) case studies show how ethics and politics are linked. In the case noted in the preceding section, we recognize that professionals—the adult-protective-services worker, the physician, and the courts—are expected to follow specifically mandated legislation in their caregiving functions. However, sometimes these laws do take the needs of the competent individual into account. Ethics as a philosophy is unfettered. As we have seen throughout this handbook, it takes a number of forms. However, once it is tied to everyday life, it must develop its modus operandi within the society's governing system in which it finds itself at a particular point in time.

Ethics is not politics and politics is not synonymous with ethics, but the two intersect and sometimes are in agreement. Jürgen Habermas (1996) points out how the two may differ in his discussion of legal autonomy and moral autonomy. Same-sex marriage between older adults, physician-assisted suicide, and equal access to heart transplants may be ethical tenets for some, but in the political arena, legislation may block these goals. On the other hand, being protected from abuse by others and the mandate for informed consent may be consonant with legislative policies, but may run counter to the ethical prescription one has constructed. Vernig, Morgan, and DeVito in chapter 15 discuss these shifts in policy with regard to using vulnerable persons—the handicapped, prisoners, and disenfranchised groups—as guinea pigs in research. Holstein and McCurdy in chapter 9 consider the degree to which the society may be responsible for mental illness through ambivalence toward aging, ignoring some elderly who live in poverty, and a failure to respond to the needs of those who are more vulnerable to illness because the society has not adequately protected some of its older citizens. They close their chapter with a plug for the balanced perspective: "The hardest task then will be to balance the most desirable approach with the one that might be possible with the sociopolitical context."

Ethics and Power

Older adults, especially those who experience some kind of dependence, find themselves in a number of situations of differential power. Lesnoff-Caravaglia in chapter 14 points out that this is a likely consequence of aging. It tends to erode our control. This erosion may come in the form of another's strong, forceful personality, someone having control of the older adult's finances, someone with greater authority because of his or her expertise, or the authority that the law exerts. If any of these types of situations occur, it may be very difficult for older adults to be partners in the plan. Solomon in chapter 12 discusses power differentials in families and their impact on decision making. Marquis and Ide in chapter 6 observe that 75% of treatment decisions are in the hands of physicians and, further, that decisions may not always be based on medical expertise. Instead, they may be the result of the geographical location in which one practices, value systems such as race and gender, beliefs about aging, or the assessment of the patient's ability to pay. According to Knut Logstrup, even though we may not like it, "eventually we will have someone's entire destiny in our hands," (1971, p. 56). This means that each of us is vulnerable to being exploited and being the exploiter, whether he or she is a layperson or a professional. If such occasions occur, we must be prepared for the right to decide, but also the responsibility that ensues when power falls into our hands. Sometimes individuals prefer to have someone else in control. Heintz, for example, talks in chapter 8 about families who defer to professionals because they are seen as "experts" with histories and track records.

It is important to note that age is not the determinant of power. It is more likely personality. There are some older adults who wield incredible power over their professional care providers, even if they are subject to dependent care. Not all adults are lovely and generous. The balanced interest perspective sometimes requires us to navigate through encounters of dominance and hardheadedness of the worst kind. However, in order to work toward the share taking of rights and responsibilities, it is important both to recognize the power of others along with their boundaries and to know that we too have limits, but we also have possibilities to be in control, even if we are bedfast or blind.

In chapter 16 on long-term care, McCullough, Wilson, Rhymes, and Teasdale talk about power shifts that occur as a consequence of short-term and long-term care. In the former, power is clearly prescribed. However, in long-term care, power is more likely to be distributed among older adults, family, paraprofessionals, and professionals because of the greater ambiguity in the care of the older person. In long-term care, there appears to be a better chance for the balanced interest perspective, but this does not imply that there is no chance for this approach in the short range. It appears that our best hope for implementation is advocacy for this point of view.

We cannot end this section on power without mentioning technology. It too has a kind of power that we must surely reckon with. In reading the chapters, I was struck by the rather negative billing the contributors gave it. Dallas High in chapter 7 uses the phrase the "unbridled use of life-sustaining technologies." Marquis and Ide in chapter 6 express considerable concern as they talk about costly technology that appears to have no demonstrable benefits in health care. Cortese in chapter 2 has a similar concern when he raises the question of whether developing new technology is the best use of our money in the face of limited resources. Finally, Suggs in chapter 4 contends that one consequence of high tech has been to blur the distinctions between life and death. However, Lesnoff-Caravaglia in chapter 14 takes a more balanced view and declares that there is good news and bad news about technology and aging. She points out how technology has allowed older adults to live independently at home, to maintain relationships, and to communicate with others. These positives must be mentioned along with the negatives in order to present the whole picture.

ETHICS IN THE MULTICULTURAL, MULTIDISCIPLINARY SETTING

As the contributors to this handbook point out over and over, we live in a multicultural society. Along with aging being a triumph of the twentieth century, we can also claim credit for great strides in human rights and the respect for persons of differing classes, color, cultures, and creed. In addition, we have recognized the value in seeing the individual in context and with a variety of needs, biological, psychological, social and cultural. The holism in clear. We cannot view an emotional problem as detached from the cultural definition and response, from its impact on our physical health and relationships with others. We cannot view a relational problem with others apart from cultural prescriptions, their impact on our personal identity, and the potential health consequences. The culture's characterizing of members of a social stratum affects their self-worth, the relationships they form, and the health care they receive as a consequence of being classified in a certain way in the society. In chapter 9,

Holstein and McCurdy emphasize this biopsychosociocultural linkage in their discussion of causes and prevention of mental health problems.

It is important to think of ethics in aging as multicultural and multidisciplinary. There is no question that medicine has dominated ethics during the last quarter of the twentieth century. Death has been described as an enemy of medicine, and when issues of life and death arise, ethics is not far behind. The presence of a biomedical centering is obvious in this handbook. Many of the contributors use health as an ethos in which to examine issues and dilemmas in ethics. But ethics and medicine are not synonymous, as Marquis and Ide and Heintz make clear, although Crawford points out that Jesus was both a healer and a moral teacher. Marquis and Ide go on to talk about "lifestyle" illness and the importance of recognizing that health problems that emerge from this source are not just medical problems. Holstein and McCurdy point out the problems with "medicalizing" aging. Crawford also urges us not to "medicalize" aging, a concept that Estes and Binney (1991) have developed. McCullough, Wilson, Rhymes, and Teasdale illustrate this difference by noting that self-sufficiency is a social issue among one's moral intimates, not a medical one. Returning to the use of technology, there is still the perception that its use is exclusive to medicine. John Bond and Peter Coleman (1993) view high and low technology only through the eyes of medicine: "Of increasing concern to the gerontologists in the twenty-first century will be ways in which high and low technology can be further developed and utilized to prevent disease, assist health care organizations to deliver health care efficiently, and to foster independence among elderly people who are frail" (p. 342).

Balanced interest requires a broadening of the scope of concern from the medical to the psychological, the social, and the cultural. All of us are much more than our bodies. In fact, the preservation of the body is dependent on our attitude toward ourselves, the support we receive from others, and the cultural policies that guide our responses to ourselves growing older. To address our whole nature, there has been an increase in holistic care. Such services are variously called, but a common name is the multidisciplinary team approach. With the growth of the multidisciplinary approach to care that High, Suggs, Kapp, and McCullough et al., especially, describe, we are likely to see a more equitable alignment in the biopsychosociocultural concerns. There are signs that this is taking place (Holstein, 1995). As psychologists, sociologists, social workers, lawyers, and clergy (along with other keepers of the psyche, the social conduct, and the culture) increase their involvement in the ethical decision-making enterprise, we may expect to integrate these complex multiple needs of the older adult more effectively. The change in our characterization of the older adult as "consumer" rather than "client" is a testimony to the fact that the older adult is becoming a subject rather than an object of care, with a name, feelings, sometimes strong feelings, and the potential to control his or her destiny.

COMMUNICATIVE ETHICS IN DECISION MAKING

"Communicative ethics" is a systematic method for making ethical decisions. This approach to ethical decision making is described by the German social philosopher Jürgen Habermas (1990). In recent years, Habermas has used the phrase "discourse ethics." However, we will use communicative ethics because the word conveys a better sense of this process—how and what we communicate when we must make ethical decisions in a group setting. Communicative ethics reminds us of the importance of the "dialogic approach" and subsequent give-and-take in an effort to be reciprocal and therefore to reach balance. In his review of Habermas's communicative ethics, Thomas McCarthy points out the importance of the speech act: "What Habermas calls 'communicative ethics' is grounded in the 'fundamental norms of rational speech.' Communication that is oriented toward reaching understanding inevitably involves the reciprocal raising and recognition of validity claims. Claims to truth and rightness, if radically challenged, can be redeemed only through argumentative discourse leading to rationally motivated consensus" (1978, p. 325). Harry Moody has advocated for communicative ethics in his book *Ethics in an Aging Society* (1992) and notes its role in achieving consensus: "The value of a communicative ethic is to find commonly agreed upon ways of negotiating differences when we fail to agree in binding principles and rules" (p. 13).

It is important to note that what follows is this author's interpretation of Habermas's communicative ethics or action. It may be that I have misinterpreted Habermas. I do not presume to comprehend his position in the sphere of meta-ethics, ideology, and applied ethics. Indeed, I would not wish the reader to assume that I have adopted Habermas's very complicated views on Aristotle, Rawls, Kant, and Kohlberg. His writing has merely been an inspiration for this author's views of balanced interest.

Although what follows should be understood to be this author's words, except where there is correspondence with the sense of Habermas's view of interaction in society, it is important to note that Habermas has modeled the kinds of behaviors that make a balanced interest perspective a reality. First, his education at Göttingen, Bonn, and Zurich in the fields of philosophy, psychology, history, and German literature demonstrates a multidisciplinary approach (Outhwaite, 1994). Second, in an interview with Torben Hviid Nielsen in Habermas (1993), he notes how his various experiences from social research to being a teacher of sociology and philosophy have led him to change his point of view over time. It is this kind of openness, personal growth in interpretation, and change that makes his thoughts so fertile and that has informed the notion of the balanced perspective that has been outlined here.

A first step in making ethical decisions is to identify the concerns—the issues (questions) and dilemmas (conflicts) that arise when one seeks to define ethical concepts such as autonomy, privacy, beneficence, justice, nonmaleficence, fidelity, and accountability. Ethical practice or "doing ethics" may be divided into three activities: (1) decision making to determine the appropriate ethical behavior; (2) monitoring the behavior that has been outlined in the decision-making phase; and (3) evaluating the success of the resolution prescribed in the first phase. The discussion that follows focuses only on the first stage, decision making to determine what the appropriate ethical conduct should be, based on the identification of ethical concerns. We have divided this approach into two levels. The first level includes the underlying assumptions—the attitudes that those who come to the table must agree upon in order for this decision-making process to be balanced. The second level includes the steps for implementing balanced interest.

Some Underlying Assumptions in Communicative Ethics

Communicative ethics presupposes that one takes the following conditions for participants and communication as their starting points.

Participants

1. Communicative ethics is a social ethic rather than an individual ethic. As such, it only operates in the context of a group.
2. Competent clients are considered a part of the decision-making team and are partners in the plan for the resolution of issues and dilemmas. If clients are incompetent, primary caregivers are expected to be a part of the decision-making team.
3. All parties in communication have equal status in the decision-making process. There are no hierarchical relationships. One's status, whether professional or layperson, neither elevates nor subjugates one in the communication process. Therefore, communicative ethics is based on the democratic process.
4. The clients' or caregivers' ethics may not be the same as those of the professionals, but are just as valid and valued as those of the professionals.
5. All parties in the decision-making process are expected to enter into a "relationship" that means that one is expected (*a*) to be open to others, (*b*) to be respectful, (*c*) to be trusting, (*d*) to be honest, (*e*) to be fair, (*f*) to make every effort to communicate concerns in a common language that others will understand, and (*g*) to have unconditional positive regard for all members of the decision-making team. The relationship creates interdependency. Therefore, communicative ethics assumes that there is no such thing as a "disinterested" party.
6. All parties understand that decisions will be based on consensus; everyone is in agreement about the process for arriving at a decision.

Communication

1. Communicative ethics requires participants to be political in the sense that they have the desire to create a policy or plan of care. Being political involves advocacy, persuasion, debate, and negotiation.
2. Communication is necessary because there are unresolved issues and/or dilemmas.

3. All parties must make every effort to enter into the process of communication with the utmost seriousness, being truthful in the information one shares and committed to finding ways to understand one another's point of view.
4. Communication is both about advocacy and also appreciating and even affirming views that may be alien to one's own.
5. In the communication process, there is no right answer; the answer is contingent on how the group defines the situation. In this regard, ethical decision making is relative, not absolute. A group composed of other parties may arrive at different outcomes because their values, beliefs, and protocols may be different. Communicative ethics does not presume to set a situation against absolute ethical standards. These standards are brought to the table by the participants and may need to be adjusted to the particular case.
6. Communicative ethics is merely a method to work toward a balance in points of view, giving all an equal right to their points of view. Therefore, the communication process itself guarantees democratic standards, but it is not imbued with any absolute principles on what is right or wrong action.
7. The communication process ends when there is consensus, with everyone agreeing with the plan of action, which is merely a proposal for the resolution of issues and dilemmas, not the resolution. Resolution refers to what takes place in the enactment of the decision and goes beyond the decision-making phase to application.
8. Once the proposal for the resolution is determined, there is no guarantee that it is final. The plan for resolution depends on events in the life of the clients that are always in flux and subject to change. There may be a need to adjust and alter the plan over time if circumstances change.

Implementing Communicative Ethics

There are three steps in the formula for resolving ethical issues and dilemmas: information, deliberation, and negotiation. It is important to keep these phases separate. The goal of the information phase is to exchange positions on the issues and dilemmas. In the deliberation phase, members debate differences. Finally, the purpose of negotiation is to bargain with one another until consensus is reached.

Before the information phase begins, the group should select a facilitator from among its members. The only persons who should not take on this role are the clients, a primary caregiver, or other family member because of their understandably direct involvement in the situation. Facilitators are expected to guide discussion, ensure fairness and open discussion, encourage members to express their opinions, articulate disagreements, and move the group toward negotiation for consensus.

Information

1. Each person shares his or her concerns, stating what he or she believes to be the issues and dilemmas from his or her point of view.

2. Each person presents what he or she knows to be the truth of the situation in a "common language" free of jargon and other language that is discipline specific.
3. Listeners allow the speaker to have the floor without interruption and may only ask for clarification when the speaker is finished. Listeners should identify points of congruence as well as differences in preparation for the deliberation phase.

Deliberation

1. Each person attempts to persuade others to adopt his or her position.
2. Members are obligated to question the rationale of those whose views are different from their own, keeping in mind the rules of relationship: being open, respectful, trusting, honest, and fair, making every effort to communicate concerns in a common language that others can understand, and maintaining unconditional positive regard for one another.
3. Where differences persist, members are expected to debate differences with regard to positions. At no time should there be a blurring between personalities and positions. That is, disagreements should center on ideas, not clashes of personality.
4. Deliberation is most effective when participants are not operating in a "crisis" mode. Therefore, every effort should be made not to rush through the discussion. Participants should be prepared for the process to take some time. Communicative ethics would, therefore, not likely be effective in crisis situations.
5. After all members have had the opportunity to debate issues and dilemmas, the areas of agreement and disagreement should be carefully arrayed.

Negotiation

1. Consensual formulation is the product of the unanimity of views. In the negotiation phase, participants may (*a*) hold on strongly to views that they feel are important, (*b*) may let go of views that seem less important, or (*c*) adopt views about which they have changed their minds because of the convincing arguments of others.
2. Consensus usually ensues as a consequence of reconfiguring one's position. This process involves (*a*) blending opposing views, (*b*) rescinding previous views, or (*c*) appending new views that subsequently transcend proposals made during the information phase.
3. Consensus is achieved by reconciliation of differences through reciprocity. While positions may be changed somewhat, their essential goals do not if true reconciliation is to succeed.
4. What emerge in consensus are proposed resolutions. Nothing is actually solved regarding the issues and dilemmas for the client. Questions and conflicts will only be directly addressed when resolutions are implemented. Decision making only prescribes a plan of action.

It is important to note that all of these elements—concepts, propositions, protocols, and decision making that includes using information, deliberation, and negotiation—are just starting points. The journey toward the resolution of ethical concerns is complex, and in this respect, "doing ethics" takes some time; there is nothing quick about doing ethics. It is not a task either for the impatient or for persons wanting certainty. When one declares, "I hope I made the right decision," there are no guarantees. As Newman and Brown (1996) point out, being ethical does not mean that we have really made the right decision or discovered what is right; it is our best discernment of what is the right thing at a particular point in time and what our part was in the decision-making process. Circumstances might change at any moment, and the decision might be rendered inappropriate or moot. Because of the unpredictable nature of the life course, especially at the end of life, we can never feel comfortable about our expectations of and for one another. It is precisely for this reason that we need one another to be partners in the plan. Family members need to be defined as partners, and paraprofessionals need to become partners with their clients as well as with the professionals with whom they work. In addition, "Professionals compose partnerships with their clients and with their employers in which all parties make ethical decisions" (Kultgen, 1988, p. 6).

In the last analysis, we are all "in it together"—we participate in the community either directly or indirectly when we make decisions. Together, we have a better chance of creating an ethical plan than if we act alone. Even so, there is no guarantee that we have made the right decision. We probably can never be confident that we have made the best choice—the best ethical choice. Maybe this is not what we should expect anyway. Habermas declares that this is not the task of philosophy when he says, "But philosophy cannot arrogate to itself the task of finding answers to substantive questions of justice or of an authentic, unfailed life, for it properly belongs to the participants" (1993, p. 176).

We must acknowledge that those who come to the table as participants with the baggage of their own cultures at a particular time in history cannot be sure that what they negotiate will be the best ethical decision possible. Newman and Brown observe:

We believe that being ethical is more than making good ethical choices regarding isolated incidents or situations. . . . it does not provide a rule book answer to all dilemmas. Rather, being ethical represents the perspective we take on the task we face, the process we use to confront issues, and the guides we use to make decisions. . . . we will not always make the best decision or the best choice, but we will keep trying. (1996, p. 192)

Indeed, we will keep trying. The balanced perspective demands much more of us than we as older adults, family members and friends, paraprofessionals, and professionals may be willing to give. But to approach ethical decision making in any other way, for this writer, is to not really do ethics at all.

18

Ethical Issues in Aging: Synthesis and Prospects for the Twenty-first Century

W. Andrew Achenbaum

Handbooks lay a presumptuous claim to a place for themselves in the scholarly literature. Whereas most publications have limited aims and short shelf lives, works in this genre claim to represent the state of the art—at least as defined by the field's leading practitioners. "One of the few generalizing influences in a world of overspecialization" (*Encyclopaedia Britannica*, 1985, Vol. 21, p. 555), handbooks are designed to render in-depth, topical analyses of nearly all the important facets of a major "problem." Ideally, each chapter should offer themes and facts in a manner accessible to the readers (amateur and expert alike) who rely on the contributors' ability to provide up-to-date, authoritative information. Sometimes historians use successive handbooks to trace how thinking has evolved in a given domain in order to establish a temporal baseline for setting future priorities. In this concluding chapter, therefore, it is appropriate for me, a historian of aging, to put the present volume in context and indicate how its value might be enhanced in future editions.

The first thing to note about this *Handbook on Ethical Issues in Aging* is its timely publication. We have long needed such a volume, but it is unlikely that anyone would have dared to compile such an ambitious compendium even a decade ago. There have, to be sure, been many handbooks devoted to ethics, a branch of moral inquiry that dates back to Plato and Aristotle in Western civilization. Classics by writers as diverse as St. Augustine, Jean-Jacques Rousseau, Immanuel Kant, Karl Marx, Herbert Spencer, and George Santayana still inform contemporary opinions about ethics. For all of their differences, these giants probed the moral attributes and normative meanings of human thought, language, and actions. They sought to establish and evaluate rules for differentiating between good and bad, between right and wrong. Over the centuries, schools of metaethics competed in the marketplace of ideas. Subfields rose and fell. We now have a vast array of utilitarian, deontological, naturalistic, cognitive, and monistic theories that explore what constitutes the good life. This treasure trove from the past enables us to situate changing thoughts and deeds against perduring habits of the heart and everyday experiences.

The formal study of ethics became a highly specialized, factious discipline as leaders in higher education organized knowledge into specialties. Some scholars around the beginning of the twentieth century, revolting against formalism, argued that the great political issues of the era were animated by ethical issues that long had pitted justice against corruption. One camp of philosophers dealing with ethical dilemmas worked to make their field more scientific. Others excoriated the moral relativism inherent in the empirical enterprise (P. Novick, 1988). Many questions that shaped discussions were posed by experts in linguistics and mathematics, who then dominated the field of ethics in universities. The general public took little interest in the scholarly debates of the day, however. "Rarely perhaps has any generation shown so little interest as ours does in any kind of theoretical or systematic ethics. The academic question of a system of ethics seems to be of all questions the most superfluous," wrote Dietrich Bonhoeffer in the early 1940s. "On the contrary it [lack of interest in academic or systematic ethics] arises from the fact that our period, more than any earlier period in the history of the west, is oppressed by a superabounding reality of concrete ethical problems" (Bonhoeffer, 1949, p. 64). The forces of evil violating human dignity, he taught, created a set of sins that were more heinous than others. For such teachings and his opposition to Hitler, Bonhoeffer was sent to Buchenwald; he was hung shortly before the end of the war. The theologian feared that he wrote in vain: "One who is committed to an ethical programme can only waste his forces on the empty air, and even his martyrdom will not be a source of strength for his cause or a serious threat to the wicked" (1949, p. 65).

Bonhoeffer's martyrdom was hardly forgotten, nor would his work prove to be the sole catalyst for the explosion of academic and popular interest in ethical concerns after World War II. The Nuremberg trials and the framing of the United Nations Charter were the first of a series of dramatic occasions that challenged professional ethicists and ordinary citizens to think anew about the meanings of human rights and, more boldly, to imagine the scope and limits of what it means to be an integral part of an interdependent world community. Episode after episode of ethnic cleansings in Africa, Southeast Asia, and Europe demanded political responses to fundamental questions of right and wrong. The proliferation of nuclear arsenals prompted intense debates over the use of technology in controlling human affairs. So, too, did dramatic innovations in genetic technology, the production of synthetic chemicals and drugs, and the adoption of surgical interventions, all of which promised (or threatened) to alter prevailing definitions of life and death.

In recent years, scholars such as John Rawls, Robert Nozick, and Charles Taylor have gained broad audiences for moral philosophy; their competing views concerning the ethics of distributive justice have circulated throughout the academy. Sometimes ethicists' ideas have permeated popular culture. Theologian Joseph Fletcher's formulation of "situation ethics," for instance, seemed to bless all but the most bizarre manifestations of the youth cult of the late 1960s. In retrospect, *Situation Ethics* (1966) may also have set a precedent for age-based treatments of ethical issues: if youth needed its own ethical moorings, so might older age groups. Greenwood Publishing Group probably would not have been interested in this *Handbook on Ethical Issues in Aging*, however, unless specialists and lay readers alike judged that there was a critical mass of concerns to examine. The publication of this volume thus responds to proximate developments in research on aging more than to issues that have evoked perennial controversy in ethics. As Tanya Fusco Johnson stresses in chapter 1, contributors to this volume are responding to the impact of the longevity revolution on people living out their years in a community, for example, the impact on the ways that health care professionals allocate resources in the face of older adults' increasing likelihood of suffering from chronic illness.

Popular notions of old age as a multifaceted "problem" and the conviction that the "subject" was worthy of investigation by experts arose primarily in the twentieth century. The emergence of gerontology as a scientific field of inquiry in Western Europe and the United States paralleled the postwar recrudescence of interest in theoretical and applied ethics. People have pondered the mysteries of senescence for ages, of course, but only since the 1920s have groups of specialists devoted their careers to measuring continuities and changes in the physical, mental, psychological, and socioeconomic dimensions of human growth and development over the life course (Achenbaum, 1995). Demographic forces helped to trigger academic interest in and media presentations about what it signifies to grow older. Increasing numbers of elderly people caused various sectors in society to formulate new theories, institutional solutions, and public policy initiatives. For example, legislative precedents in Europe and North America for retirement and health care provisions for the elderly date back to early modern times. Nonetheless, the state's current, sizable investment in the so-called old-age welfare state did not become a controversial political issue until the contemporary era. Now, in an era in which the public sector is being downsized, efforts to reduce commitments to the aged are generating a novel set of ethical questions about whether justice is served by perpetuating age-based entitlements, especially those that mainly benefit class-bound segments of the older population. Many liberals, moderates, and conservatives would prefer to return to a system of public assistance dependent on "need," not "age." Similarly, in an era marked by considerable gains in adult longevity, scholars, lawyers, and physicians have essayed to frame theories and applications of bioethics appropriate for an aging society. The imputed worth of added years to aging individuals, gerontologists increasingly stress, brings both opportunities and challenges to maturing societies (Pifer & Bronte, 1986).

Many of the issues addressed in this handbook, therefore, have been percolating for several decades. John Dewey, after all, made a stirring plea for taking account of ethics in his Introduction to Edmund Vincent Cowdry's *Problems of Ageing* (1939), arguably the first gerontologic compendium produced in the United States. The eminent philosopher urged researchers to link the natural sciences, social sciences, medical sciences, and humanistic perspectives in studying the dimensions of aging. "Science and philosophy meet on common ground in their joint interest in discovering the processes of normal growth and in the institution of conditions which will favor and support ever continued growth," he observed (p. xxvii). Dewey hypothesized that the environment humans created probably had greater influence on adult development than biological dictates. "We cannot separate the processes of maturing from those of ageing even though the two are not identical. The split that now exists between the two, in terms both of individual activity and happiness and of social usefulness, would appear to be socially or culturally produced" (Dewey, 1939, p. xxv). Ethical issues in aging, in Dewey's scheme of things, had profound theoretical consequences for doing science. In addition, ethics had immediate relevance for both individual growth and institution building. Besides linking science and politics, ethics gave people's lives meaning as they aged: "There is urgent need for a philosophy of personal and institutional life that is consequent with present knowledge" (Dewey, 1939, p. xxvi).

Theologians and philosophers since 1940 have echoed many of Dewey's themes. Exploring the frontiers of aging from vantage points of various ethical perspectives, Paul Maves (1949) (and a generation later, Barbara Payne, 1975) encouraged colleagues to explore religious aspects of growing older. Bioethicists often delighted in the 1970s in turning conventional gerontologic wisdom on its head: Arthur Caplan (1981) pointedly likened aging to a disease. More recently, ethicist Daniel Callahan (1987) provoked considerable controversy in gerontologic circles with his argument for stringently limiting health care to older people. Harry R. Moody's *Ethics in an Aging Society* (1992) represents an important contribution to the literature by a philosopher who has spent most of his career in gerontological centers.

Experts in the humanities are not the only scholars who spoke or wrote about ethical choices confronting the elderly and younger cohorts in an aging society (Cole, Kastenbaum, & Van Tassel, 1992). Convinced that politics and ethics are inextricably connected, physicians, lawyers, and psychologists, as well as natural and social scientists, have made important contributions to the gerontological literature dealing with ethical problems. Robert Butler's Pulitzer Prize–winning *Why Survive?* (1975) abounds in moral indictments of the ways that Americans treat their elders. Political scientist Robert Binstock has coedited several books on health care ethics; so have sociologists Carroll Estes and Mary Minkler. More than any other academic tribe, gerontologists have succeeded in exposing the ethical flaws that surround the so-called generational-equity debate. Other researchers on aging have concerned themselves with the moral ramifications of technological innovations for the elderly (Maddox, 1987, 1995). None of these works intended to survey all ethical issues in aging. Still, considered as a whole, they provide the setting for understanding many of the dilemmas and issues covered in this volume.

In her introductory chapter to this *Handbook on Ethical Issues in Aging*, Tanya Fusco Johnson seeks to identify common threads that run through the volume without diminishing the diversity of viewpoints she deems essential for critical analysis. Johnson identifies seven major values: autonomy, privacy, beneficence, justice, nonmaleficence, fidelity, and accountability. My reading of the gerontologic literature indicates that she has made reasonable selections. Her colleagues apparently agree, because they all amplify the nuances and ambiguities that are embedded in the meanings of these terms in the chapters that follow chapter 1. It is important to note, however, that these seven clusters do not in themselves constitute a "unified terminological framework" for this *Handbook on Ethical Issues in Aging*. Instead, they provide multiple starting points: they "infer the potential for a conflict of interest—the competing demands of the specializations of medicine, mental health, religious tenets, legal mandates, and social care, whether provided by the professional or the family, along with the discipline-specific leverage the contributor may exert in working through his or her own ethical reasoning on the subject matter." Johnson and her collaborators fortunately go beyond arid exegeses of philosophical principles. In so doing, they emulate the position of colleagues in bioethics who nowadays get beyond the limitations of principlism by offering concrete examples of specific moral tenets in action.

One of the strengths of this handbook is that it acknowledges that the study of ethics rests on more than the elucidation of fundamental principles. "While each contributor is 'in the same church,' each is not necessarily 'in the same pew,' " Johnson notes toward the end of chapter 1. "They have launched their ideas about their topics in the context of ethics in aging with a sense of urgency, immediacy, and uncompromising honesty." It is instructive to note that scholars at the Hastings Center and the Park Ridge Center (neither of which has yet established a major gerontologic focus in its portfolio) increasingly turn to phenomenology, casuistry, and narrative ethics to explore the normative foundations of decision making and social interactions (Dubose, Hamel, & O'Connell, 1994). With few exceptions, the chapters in *Handbook on Ethical Issues in Aging* offer case studies, and several of them refer to names and events recounted in the newspapers, such as the latest twists in the campaign by Dr. Jack Kevorkian to assist people who wish to commit suicide.

The case studies help Johnson and her colleagues achieve the stated objectives of this *Handbook on Ethical Issues in Aging*: to focus on the individual and community, to demystify the field of ethics, to provide a common working vocabulary, and to look at contexts. Juxtaposing three case studies, for instance, gives Lawrence Heintz in chapter 8 an opportunity to document that judgment impairment is a matter of degree that comes in many forms. Heintz establishes a broad context for the case studies, which in turn stirs interest in a whole spectrum of moral questions that otherwise would have been ignored. "Only recently have we come to see that we must critically examine the sociocultural context if we are to understand [that] . . . by stressing the autonomy and rights of individuals, other significant considerations (for example, community and common good, duties and responsibilities) have been neglected, as have critical philosophical questions concerning the value of medical progress and personal and public health in communal life" (ten Have, 1994, p. 32). Insofar as they broaden the framework in which the analytic narrative unfolds, case studies engage readers: they encourage reflexivity in a way precluded by didactic expositions. Clusters of ideas blend together more fluidly than if they were dissected in a vacuum.

These case studies also enable readers to recognize that multiple perspectives usually recast the dynamics in every situation in which ethical decisions must be made. Very often these realities cannot be neatly finessed in an antiseptic laboratory necessary for conducting scientific experiments. Nor can conflicted opinions be easily reconciled. This is especially evident in chapter 5 on ethical issues in medical care by Back and Pearlman. By disentangling clinical issues and ethical principles, the physician-authors make it very apparent that caregivers must transform general notions when they apply them to specific instances. The act of modifying principles, moreover, requires health care professionals to sort out options on several dimensions. (Indeed, the ethical activity may be even more complicated than Back and Pearlman state: at several points in their discussion, I wondered whether lawyers would stipulate the same critical issues the physicians indicated.) We need not " 'reduce' the superstructure of speech, law, or morality to a simple result of the substructure but rather in order to understand how choices are constrained in the real world," Moody points out. Instead, we "need to shift our attention away from abstract rights and from isolated individuals to look instead at the social setting in which communication takes place" (Moody, 1992, p. 247).

By encouraging contributors to provide chapter-length treatments of issues such as personal safety (chapter 10) and to cross domains in analyzing various health care problems, this handbook manages to consider the pertinence of some fresh terms with which to ponder ethical considerations. I was delighted by McCullough, Wilson, Rhymes, and Teasdale's description of a "preventive-ethics approach" to long-term-care decision making process in chapter 16. The phrase explicitly plays on the "language of management of ambiguity" that is essential in dealing with aging clients, who present the accumulated assets and deficits acquired in the course of living long lives. Furthermore, I was struck by the parallels that Beth Virnig, Robert Morgan, and Carolee DeVito drew in chapter 15 between the ethical principles of health care and the principles of research ethics. By teasing out similarities in the ways that investigators and researchers use keywords—voluntarism, nonmaleficence, beneficence, utility, and justice—the authors succeeded in getting us behind participants' views of reality to see commonalities in disparate domains.

One of the most original formulations of the ethical implications of preventive care comes in chapter 9 by Martha Holstein and David McCurdy, "Ethical Issues in Mental Health Care." They map out issues across individual, social, and cultural levels on normative and historical planes. Stressing that a broad social strategy is a "critical vector" within a larger theory of human good, Holstein and McCurdy conclude that "the stronger the evidence about causation, the more compelling the case for intervention; the case becomes even more compelling if the roots are socially remedial."

Such efforts to expose and combine facets of ethical issues in this handbook bring to mind a closing line of T. S. Eliot's *Four Quartets* (1962), composed while Bonhoeffer was writing his thoughts on ethics in jail: "When the tongues of flame are in-folded." To the extent that Eliot's verses speak to gerontologists, the message seems to be as follows: Despite differences of kind, there ultimately may be a unifying force behind ethical issues in aging. The search will not advance by refining statements of principles through an endless investigation of case studies. Rather, by taking account of multiple perspectives in a few selected examples well chosen, it should become possible to see essential complementarities in seemingly disparate entities that fold into a constructive, positive view of reality for young and old alike.

Eliot envisioned ultimate unity through spiritual growth. So did Bonhoeffer: "It is not by astuteness, by knowing the tricks, but simply by simple steadfastness in the truth of God, by training the eye upon the truth until it is simple and wise, that there comes the experience and the knowledge of the ethical reality" (Bonhoeffer, 1949, p. 65). Several contributors to this volume seem to elaborate the position articulated by Eliot and Bonhoeffer insofar as they stress "ethical issues in a religiously diverse society" (chapter 3) and "ethical issues in spiritual care" (chapter 4). On balance, however, the prevailing tone of the *Handbook on Ethical Issues in Aging* is secular realism. Such a stance quite appropriately reflects the posture of most academic ethicists these days. Her unwillingness to preempt the search for commonalities without due concern for process may explain why Tanya Fusco Johnson chose in chapter 17 to illustrate an application of Jürgen Habermas's "communicative ethics" in decision making. Focusing on process enabled Johnson to be true to her discipline-engrained thinking as a sociologist. Johnson could think in terms of interactive dynamics and reciprocal relations, satisfy her multidisciplinary predilections by tapping her interest in theology, and respect the "democratic" political orientation evident in her role as volume editor.

Since Johnson commissioned chapters to illuminate the salience of seven values in thinking about ethical issues in aging, let us revisit the volume by focusing on keywords. As I read this volume, I kept going back to Anthony Cortese's assertion in chapter 2 that "the most fundamental social problems regarding health care are ultimately issues of power and justice." I believe that Cortese is correct. Indeed, power conflicts and power decisions implicitly or explicitly pervade nearly all of the chapters. The aged, nurses, and other parties with a stake in the ethical issue at hand wish to be empowered. Their efforts can be thwarted or facilitated by the power of professions, the decisions of the courts, or the influence of public opinion or the power that inheres in commonplace wisdom. That noted, what more can be said?

Were I to revise this handbook in a subsequent edition, I would continue to discuss the individual and societal ramifications of the seven value dimensions set forth at the outset. I would encourage contributors to make an even greater effort to integrate all seven of the values in their respective analyses, noting which of them seem to predominate in the domain under consideration. Johnson or someone else designated to render the last word might then survey the various pacesetters, indicating that "justice" is of greater importance than, say, "fidelity." Onto this schema I would then impose a conception of democracy, capitalism, and the state that revolves around a worldview of "power." To identify the conflicts, consensus, and contradictions over the use of power reinforces a central theme in the *Handbook on Ethical Issues in Aging*: interactions among divergent groups with differing perspectives matter. Linking ethics and politics through the medium of power attests to "differences of interest and of the possibility of organizing to realize those interests in, through, or against . . . the autonomy of institutions, strategic alliances, and contingent actions in situations" (Alford & Friedland, 1985, p. 408). Stressing the difference principle in the context of power conflicts, moreover, provides a segue from interpreting keywords to wrestling with another analytic element in this volume that merits great attention: do ethical issues in aging transcend national boundaries?

Although some effort was made to report developments in other parts of the world that might shed light on what is happening in America, the focus of most chapters in this handbook is on the situation of the elderly in the United States. Conditions in this country surely are distinctive: the growth in the aged population in the United States has been less dramatic or sudden than in many countries in the Pacific basin; this nation has not had to cope with rising numbers of elders as it tries to meet the needs of large numbers of children and youth. Yet do demographic particularities per se make the American case (or that in any other country) exceptional, much less unique? Even if we limit comparisons to Western Europe, which most resembles the United States in values and public policies, are there not general principles that seem to operate across national boundaries? Does it matter that older people in Great Britain are routinely denied kidney dialysis, or that there is a growing trend in England and other industrialized nations to deny some health care on grounds of age? Are Americans to view Dutch tolerance of euthanasia as somehow more barbaric or enlightened than sentiment here?

Over the past decade, I have had an opportunity to participate in several international conferences in which ethical issues in aging were paramount. I was struck by the importance of national context: physicians in the Balkans, making not much more than compatriots who drove taxis, simply did not have the resources to effect high-tech interventions that surgeons in Sweden could deploy. But despite ideological disagreements and markedly different national backgrounds, most participants readily understood the keywords that are deployed in this handbook, and occasionally they could reach consensus: for instance, Daniel Callahan and colleagues at the Institute for Bio-Ethics in Maastricht, the Netherlands, assembled a group of nearly two dozen experts for a three-year project to discuss future ways of allocating health care resources in an aging society. With remarkably little difficulty, they rejected utilitarian cost-benefit calculations (ter Meulen, Topinkova, & Callahan, 1994). The international team realized, however, that implementing standards for promoting quality of life was more difficult because they had to take account of variations within countries.

Indeed, in virtually every nation-state, there exists a wide range of experiences and ecological settings that make it hard to implement state policies in a consistent manner. Officials very often cannot bridge the gulf between rich and poor, between urban and rural, between educated and illiterate, or between religious factions and ethnic clans. In the United States, which prides itself on its middle-class mores, racial divisions, primarily between (and within) African American communities and white enclaves, afford people at advanced ages differential access to health care and social services. The categories multiply when we think of the differences between the values espoused by an adolescent male who is a Black Muslim and his grandmother who attends the African Methodist Church and, in another ghetto, the Orthodox Jewish physician who lives next door to an atheist banker from France. Public policy shifts add new wrinkles: In the wake of new immigration and welfare laws, it is already evident that older people who are not citizens are going to be denied benefits that they expected. I hope that in future editions of this handbook, contributors will give greater emphasis to racial differences.

In this same vein, I wish that gender differences had received fuller attention. Gerontologists have reported for several decades that men and women face different disability and mortality risks as they age. Caregiving varies by gender. Even psychologists such as David Gutmann, who posit greater expressions of androgyny in later years, acknowledge different styles and attitudes. Sex and gender thus must be taken seriously in studying aging issues. Most of the contributors in fact offered a good mix of male and female case studies, but I expected more consideration of the possibility that "women's way of knowing" would color perceptions of the value dimensions that affect ethical issues in aging. Of course, to accentuate the differences that exist within national boundaries, as I am doing, insisting that differences by race and gender be accentuated will diminish the chances of cross-cultural comparisons. Few other nations must confront our legacy of slavery and segregation in dealing with people of color. Established traditions make for distinctive women's cultures everywhere.

In the face of these seemingly endless twists and variations, I would take my cue from Helen Luke, a wise old lady who in her seventh decade noted that "the discrimination of levels is the very reverse of living our lives in compartments" (1992, p. 155). To view values as mixed in a kaleidoscope is to perceive in the differences certain connecting patterns. The seven values that Johnson has identified do indeed provide a basis for discriminating discussion that need not reify people's positions or compartmentalize their viewpoints. So do questions of how to evaluate outcomes, which figure in several chapters. McCullough and his colleagues in chapter 16 offer a stepwise strategy for dealing with competing value domains. Similarly, Anetzberger in chapter 10 establishes a hierarchy of principles for adult protective services that puts greatest emphasis on autonomy. Such efforts to prioritize serve to break down our tendency to compartmentalize issues.

Perhaps even more galvanizing are contemplations of the future of aging itself. Given the range of public policies explicitly directed to the elderly and given our national penchant for treating different age groups as if they were distinctive, it was an entirely appropriate decision to compile a *Handbook on Ethical Issues in Aging* that dealt primarily with older people. That said, given the fluidity of the life cycle and the tendency in recent history to expand or contract age barriers in light of prevailing conditions, I was delighted to see links made between the aged and the aging. If ethicists are to discriminate among hierarchial rankings of values, then it is important to see whether the same logic that governs care for the oldest of the old also applies to prenatal care—an issue raised in several chapters. More problematic, given the field of gerontology, and thus worthy of serious consideration is the relationship between the vulnerable aged and the disabled middle-aged. We see intimations of the tension in this volume. Gari Lesnoff-Caravaglia, knowing full well the animus against age in so many stereotypic notions, reminds us in chapter 14 that the elderly (even those whose world is shrinking) are not handicapped. Yet as Jennifer Solomon points out in chapter 12, parents who care for their developmentally disabled 50-year-old children often must cope with infirmities of their own. A *Handbook on Ethical Issues in Aging* is a wonderful place to discriminate, without compartmentalizing, between the worlds of aging and the realms of disability.

Tanya Fusco Johnson and her colleagues deserve our thanks for compiling this useful compendium. This *Handbook on Ethical Issues in Aging* deals with many important problems. In the years ahead, as ethical questions become even more important to gerontologists, it will be important to build on this analysis as we seek to establish a hierarchy of values that can be adapted in very different, historically fluid situations.

References

Abramson, M. (1985a). The autonomy-paternalism dilemma in social work practice. *Social Casework: The Journal of Contemporary Social Work, 66*(September), 387–393.

Abramson, M. (1985b). Caught in the middle. *Generations, 10*(2), 35–37.

Abramson, M. (1989). Autonomy vs. paternalistic beneficence: Practice strategies. *Social Casework: The Journal of Contemporary Social Work, 70*(February), 101–105.

Abramson, M. (1991). Ethical assessment of the use of influence in adult protective services. *Journal of Gerontological Social Work, 16*(1/2), 125–135.

Achenbaum, W. A. (1978). *Old age in the new land: The American experience since 1790.* Baltimore: Johns Hopkins University Press.

Achenbaum, W. A. (1985). Religion in the lives of the elderly: Contemporary and historical perspective. In Gari Lesnoff-Caravaglia (Ed.), *Values, ethics, and aging* (pp. 98–116). New York: Human Sciences Press.

Achenbaum, W. A. (1995). *Crossing frontiers.* New York: Cambridge University Press.

Agich, G. J. (1993). *Autonomy and long-term care.* New York: Oxford University Press.

Agich, G. J. (1995). Actual autonomy and long-term care decision making. In L. B. McCullough & N. L. Wilson (Eds.), *Long-term care decisions: Ethical and conceptual dimensions* (pp. 113–136). Baltimore: Johns Hopkins University Press.

Agus, J. B. (1967). Jewish ethics. In J. Macquarrie (Ed.), *Dictionary of Christian ethics* (pp. 177–180). Philadelphia: Westminster Press.

Ahmed, I., & Takeshita, J. (1996–1997). Late-life depression. *Generations, 20*(Winter), 17–21.

Alford, R. R., & Friedland, R. (1985). *Powers of theory.* New York: Cambridge University Press.

Ambrogia, D., & London, C. (1985). Elder abuse laws: Their implications for caregivers. *Generations, 9,* 37–39.

American Association of Retired Persons (AARP). (1990). *Ethics committees: Allies in long-term care—A guidebook to forming an ethics committee.* Washington, DC: American Association of Homes for the Aging and AARP.

American Bar Association. (1981). *Model code of professional responsibility.* Chicago: Author.

American Bar Association. (1983). *Model rules of professional conduct.* Chicago: Author.

American Bar Association. (1995). A lawyer's responsibility. *Rules of professional conduct.* Chicago: Author.

American College of Physicians. (1989). Cognitively impaired subjects. *Annals of Internal Medicine, 111,* 843–848.

American Medical Association. (1847). Code of medical ethics. *Transactions of the National Medical Convention, 1846–1847,* 83–106.

American Medical Association. (1989). *Physician and public attitudes on health care.* Chicago: Author.

American Medical Association. (1996–1997). Principles of medical ethics. *Code of medical ethics: Current opinions with annotations.* Washington, DC: Author.

American Medical Association Council on Ethical and Judicial Affairs. (1995). Ethical issues in managed care. *JAMA, 273,* 331–335.

American Nurses' Association. (1985). *Code for nurses with interpretive statements.* Washington DC: Author.

American Nurses' Association. (1987). *Standards and scope of gerontological nursing practice.* Washington, DC: Author.

American Psychiatric Association. (1994). *PSM-IV.* Washington, DC: Author.

American Psychological Association. *Ethical principles of psychologists and code of conduct.* Washington, DC: Author, pp. 3–4.

Analects. (1982). In N. Smart & R. D. Hecht (Eds.), *Sacred texts of the world: A universal anthology* (p. 309). New York: Crossroad.

Anatore, B., & Loya, F. (1973). *An analysis of minority and white suicide rates in Denver.* Paper presented at the Annual Meeting of the Rocky Mountain Psychological Association, Las Vegas.

Anderson, H. (1990). The congregation as a healing resource. In D. S. Browning, T. Jobe, & I. S. Evison (Eds.), *Religious and ethical factors in psychological practice* (pp. 264–286). Chicago: Nelson-Hall.

Andrews, J. (1989). *Poverty and poor health among elderly Hispanic Americans.* Baltimore: Commonwealth Fund Commission on Elderly People Living Alone.

Anetzberger, G. J. (1987). *The etiology of elder abuse by adult offspring.* Springfield, IL: Charles C. Thomas.

Anetzberger, G. J. (1995). Protective services and long term care. In Z. Harel & R. Dunkle (Eds.), *Matching people with services in long-term care* (pp. 261–281). New York: Springer.

Anetzberger, G. J. (1996). Protective services in the context of long-term care. In *Silent Suffering: Elder Abuse in America* (pp. 106–111). Long Beach, CA: Archstone Foundation.

Anetzberger, G. J., Dayton, C., and McMonagle, P. (1997). A community dialogue series on ethics and elder abuse: Guidelines for decision-making. *Journal of Elder Abuse & Neglect, 9*(1), 33–50.

Anetzberger, G. J., Lachs, M. S., O'Brien, J. G., O'Brien, S., Pillemer, K. A., & Tomita, S. K. (1993). Elder mistreatment: A call for help. *Patient Care, 27*(11), 93–130.

Anetzberger, G. J., & Miller, C. A. (1995). Impaired psychological functioning: Elder abuse and neglect. In C. A. Miller (Ed.), *Nursing care of older adults: Theory and practice* (pp. 518–552). (2nd ed.). Philadelphia: Lippincott.

Annas, G., & Glantz, L. (1980). Brief *amicus curiae (Spring)* on behalf of the American Society of Law and Medicine, Inc., p. 5. Cited in A. E. Buchanan & D. W. Brock (Eds.), *Deciding for others: The ethics of surrogate decision making*. Cambridge: Cambridge University Press.

Anonymous. (1834). Editorial. *London Times*.

Archea, C., Whittington, F., & Strasser, D. (1995). *Restraint use in nursing homes*. Paper presented at the Annual Scientific Meeting of the Gerontological Society of America, Los Angeles, CA.

Aristotle. (1985). *Nichomachean ethics* (T. Irwin, Trans.). Indianapolis: Hackett.

Arras, J. D. (1984). Toward an ethic of ambiguity. *Hastings Center Report, 14*(5), 25–33.

Arras, J. D. (1995). Conflicting interests in long-term care decision making: Acknowledging, dissolving, and resolving conflicts. In L. McCullough & N. Wilson (Eds.), *Long-term care decisions: Ethical and conceptual dimensions* (pp. 197–217). Baltimore: Johns Hopkins University Press.

Arras, J. D., & Dubler, N. N. (1994). Bringing the hospital home: Ethical and social implications of high-tech home care. *Hastings Center Report, 24*(5), S19–S28.

Asch, D. A., & Christakis, N. A. (1995). Physician characteristics associated with decisions to withdraw life support. *American Journal of Public Health, 85*(3), 367–372.

Asian wave is changing U.S. scene. (1990, November 8). *Honolulu Star-Bulletin*, p. A-3.

Atkinson, R. M., Ganzini, L., & Bernstein, M. J. (1992). Alcohol and substance-use disorders in the elderly. In J. A. Birren, W. Schaie, R. B. Sloan, & G. D. Cohen (Eds.), *Handbook of mental health and aging* (2nd ed.) (pp. 515–555). New York: Academic Press.

Bachman, R. (1992). *Elderly victims: Bureau of Justice Statistics special report*. Washington, DC: U.S. Department of Justice.

Back, A. L., Wallace, J. I., Starks, H. E., & Pearlman, R. A. (1996). Physician-assisted suicide and euthanasia in Washington State: Patient requests and physician responses. *JAMA, 275*(12), 919–925.

Baier, A. (1985). *Postures of the mind*. Minneapolis: University of Minnesota Press.

Baier, A. C. (1987). The need for more than justice. In M. Hanen & K. Nielsen (Eds.), *Science, morality, and feminist theory*. Calgary, Alberta: University of Calgary Press.

Bandman, E. L. (1994). Tough calls: Making ethical decisions in the care of older patients. *Geriatrics, 49*(12), 46–53.

Barnes, A. P. (1992). Beyond guardianship reform: A re-evaluation of autonomy and beneficence for a system of principled decision-making in long term care. *Emory Law Journal, 41*, 633–760.

Barthalis, P. L. (1995). Why nursing homes should sponsor ethics committees. *BENO Newsletter, 4*(1), 7–10.

Battin, M. (1992). Assisted suicide: Can we learn from Germany? *Hastings Center Report, 22* (March–April), 44–51.

Bayles, M. D., & High, D. M. (Eds.). (1978). *Medical treatment of the dying: Moral issues*. Cambridge, MA: G. K. Hall & Company.

Beauchamp, T. L. (1991). *Philosophical ethics: An introduction to moral philosophy* (2nd ed.). New York: McGraw-Hill.
Beauchamp, T. L., & Childress, J. F. (1994). *Principles of biomedical ethics* (4th ed.). New York: Oxford University Press.
Beauchamp, T. L., & Perlin, S. (Eds.). (1978). *Ethical issues in death and dying.* Englewood Cliffs, NJ: Prentice-Hall.
Beauvoir, S. de. (1972). *The coming of age.* New York: G. P. Putnam's Sons.
Beck, P. (1982). Two successful interventions in nursing homes: The therapeutic effects of cognitive activity. *Gerontologist, 22,* 378–383.
Beck, R. W., & Beck, S. H. (1989). The incidence of extended households among middle-aged black and white women: Estimates from a 15-year panel study. *Journal of Family Issues, 10,* 147–168.
Bedford, V. H. (1989). Understanding the value of siblings in old age. *American Behavioral Scientist, 33,* 33–44.
Bedford, V. H. (1995). Sibling relationships in middle and old age. In R. Blieszner & V. H. Bedford (Eds.), *Handbook of aging and the family* (pp. 201–222). Westport, CT: Greenwood Press.
Beecher, H. K. (1966). Ethics and clinical research. *New England Journal of Medicine, 274,* 1354–1360.
Beitler, D. (1990). *Secured units, dilemma #1: Resident protection or confinement?* Paper presented at the Annual Conference of the Alzheimer's Association, Chicago.
Bengtson, V. C., Cuellar, J. B., & Ragan, P. K. (1977). Stratum contrasts and similarities in attitudes toward death. *Journal of Gerontology, 32,* 76–88.
Bengtson, V. C., Rosenthal, C. J., & Burton, L. (1990). Families and aging: Diversity and heterogeneity. In R. H. Binstock & L. K. George (Eds.), *Handbook of aging and the social sciences* (3rd ed.) (pp. 263–287). New York: Academic Press.
Benjamin, A. E. (1992). An overview of in-home health and supportive services for older persons. In M. G. Ory & A. P. Duncker (Eds.), *In-home care for older people: Health and supportive services* (pp. 9–52). Newbury Park, CA: Sage Publications.
Bentham, J. (1970). *An introduction to the principles of morals and legislation* (J. H. Burns & H. L. A. Hart, Eds.). London, England: Athlone. (Original work published 1789)
Berrin, S. (1995). When we are blessed with time. *Sh'ma: A Journal of Jewish Responsibility, 26*(497), September 15, 1995, pp. 1–2.
Berry, J. T. (1990, April). *Information memorandum AoA-IM-90-14: Report to Congress on long-term care ombudsman activities for FY 1988.* Washington, DC: U.S. Department of Health and Human Services, Administration on Aging.
Bianchi, E. C. (1982). *Aging as a spiritual journey.* New York: Crossroad.
Billings, I., Goldfield, N., Havighurst, C. C., Minogue, W. F., Waxman, H. A., & Shrager, D. S. (1990). *Medical quality and the law.* Washington, DC: Roscoe Pound Foundation.
Binney, E., & Swan, J. (1991). The political economy of mental health care for the elderly. In M. Minkler & C. Estes (Eds.), *Critical perspectives on aging: The political and moral economy of growing old* (pp. 165–188). Amityville, NY: Baywood.
Binstock, R. H. (1995). Policies on aging in the post–cold war era. In W. Crotty (Ed.), *Post-cold war policy: The domestic and social context.* Chicago: Nelson-Hall.

References

Blackhall, L. J., Murphy, S. T., Frank, G., Michel, V., & Azen, S. (1995). Ethnicity and attitudes toward patient autonomy. *JAMA, 274*(10), 820–825.

Blakeslee, J., Goldman, B., & Papougenis, D. (1990). Untying the elderly: Kendal's restraint-free program at Longwood & Crosslands. *Generations, 14*(Suppl.), 79–80.

Blanton, P. G. (1989). Zen and the art of adult protective services: In search of a unified view. *Journal of Elder Abuse and Neglect, 1*(1), 27–34.

Blauner, R. (1966). Death and social structure. *Psychiatry, 29*, 378–394.

Blazer, D. (1991). Spirituality and aging well. *Generations, 15*(Winter), 61–65.

Blenkner, M., Bloom, M., Nielson, M., & Weber, R. (1974). *Final report: Protective services for older people: findings from the Benjamin Rose Institute Study.* Cleveland, OH: Benjamin Rose Institute.

Block, S. D., & Billings, J. A. (1994). Patient requests to hasten death: Evaluation and management in terminal care. *Archives of Internal Medicine, 154*(18), 2039–2047.

Blustein, J. (1982). *Parents and children: The ethics of the family.* New York: Oxford University Press.

Bond, J., & Coleman, P. (1993). Ageing into the twenty-first century. In J. Bond, P. Coleman, & S. Peace (Eds.), *Ageing in society: An introduction to social gerontology* (2nd ed.). Thousand Oaks, CA: Sage Publications.

Bond, J., Coleman, P., & Peace, S. (Eds.). (1993). *Ageing in society: An introduction to social gerontology* (2nd ed.). Thousand Oaks, CA: Sage Publications.

Bonhoeffer, D. (1949). *Ethics* (Neville Horton Smith, Trans.) London: Fontana Library.

Bookin, D. (Ed.). (1992). *Working with impaired elders in the community: A guide to the decision-making process and legal interventions.* Cleveland, OH: Federation for Community Planning.

Borowitz, E. (1995). We cannot know for certain what lies beyond death. In J. Lyden (Ed.), *Enduring issues in religion* (pp. 227–244). San Diego: Greenhaven Press.

Boston, G., Nitzberg, R., & Kravitz, M. (1979). *Criminal justice and the elderly: A selected bibliography.* Rockville, MD: National Institute of Law Enforcement and Criminal Justice.

Boyajian, J. A. (1991). Sacrificing the old and other health care goals. In N. Jecker (Ed.), *Aging and ethics: Philosophical problems in gerontology* (pp. 307–338). Totowa, NJ: Humana Press.

Boyle, P., & Callahan, D. (Eds.). (1995). *What price mental health? The ethics and politics of setting priorities.* Washington, DC: Georgetown University Press.

Braithwaite, V. (1992). Caregiving burden: Making the concept scientifically useful and policy relevant. *Research on Aging, 14*, 3–27.

Brakman, S. V. (1995). Filial responsibility and long-term care decision making. In L. B. McCullough & N. L. Wilson (Eds.), *Long-term care decisions: Ethical and conceptual dimensions* (pp. 181–196). Baltimore: Johns Hopkins University Press.

Brock, D. W. (1992). Voluntary active euthanasia. *Hastings Center Report, 22*(2), 10–22.

Brody, E. M. (1981). Women in the middle and family help to older people. *Gerontologist, 21*, 471–480.

Brody, E. M. (1985). Parent care as a normative family stress. *Gerontologist, 25*, 19–29.

Brody, H. (1992). *The healer's power.* New Haven: Yale University Press.

Brooks, D. D., Smith, D. R., & Anderson, R. J. (1991). Medical apartheid: An American perspective. *JAMA, 266*, 2746–2749.

Brower, H. T. (1992). Physical restraints: A potential form of abuse. *Journal of Elder Abuse and Neglect, 4*(4), 47–58.

Brown, B. A., Miles, S., & Aroskar, M. A. (1987). The prevalence and design of ethics committees in nursing homes. *Journal of the American Geriatrics Society, 35*, 1028–1033.

Brown, S. A. (1958). Spirituals. In L. Hughes & A. Bontemps (Eds.), *The Book of Negro folklore* (pp. 279–311). New York: Dodd, Mead.

Browning, D. (1991). Introduction. In D. S. Browning & I. S. Evison (Eds.), *Does psychiatry need a public philosophy?* (pp. 1–12). Chicago: Nelson-Hall.

Buchanan, A. E., & Brock, D. W. (1989). *Deciding for others: The ethics of surrogate decision making*. Cambridge: Cambridge University Press.

Burstein, B. (1988). Involuntary aged clients: Ethical and treatment issues. *Social Casework: The Journal of Contemporary Social Work, 69*, 518–524.

Burton, L. A. (Ed.). (1992). *Religion and the family: When God helps*. New York: Haworth Pastoral Press.

Burton, L. M. (1991). Black grandparents rearing grandchildren of drug-addicted parents: Stressors, outcomes, and social services needs. *Gerontologist, 32*, 744–751.

Burton, L. M., & Bengtson, V. (1985). Black grandmothers: Issues of timing and continuity of roles. In V. Bengtson & J. Robertson (Eds.), *Grandparenthood* (pp. 61–78). Beverly Hills, CA: Sage.

Butler, R. N. (1969). Age-ism: Another form of bigotry. *Gerontologist, 9*, 243–246.

Butler, R. N. (1975). *Why survive? Being old in America*. New York: Harper & Row.

Butler, R. N. (1989). Dispelling age-ism: The cross-cutting intervention. *Annals of the Academy of Political and Social Science, 503*, 138–147.

Callahan, D. (1987). *Setting limits: Medical goals in an aging society*. New York: Simon & Schuster.

Callahan, D. (1991a). Families as caregivers: The limits of morality. In N. Jecker (Ed.), *Aging and ethics: Philosophical problems in gerontology* (pp. 155–169). Totowa, NJ: Humana Press.

Callahan, D. (1991b). Medical futility, medical necessity: The-problem-without-a-name. *Hastings Center Report, 21*(4), 30–35.

Callahan, D. (1994). Bioethics: Private choice and common good. *Hastings Center Report, 24*(May–June), 28–31.

Callahan, D. (1995). Terminating life-sustaining treatment of the demented. *Hastings Center Report, 25*(November–December), 25–31.

Callahan, J. C. (1988). *Ethical issues in professional life*. New York: Oxford University Press.

Callahan, J. J., Jr. (1982). Elder abuse programming: Will it help the elderly? *Urban and Social Change Review, 15*(2), 15–16.

Callahan, J. J., Jr. (1988). Elder abuse: Some questions for policymakers. *Gerontologist, 28*(4), 453–458.

Callender, W. D., Jr. (1982). *Improving protective services for older Americans: National Law and Social Work Seminar*. Portland: University of Southern Maine.

Campion, E. W. (1985). Ethical issues in the care of the patient involved in Alzheimer's research. In V. L. Melnick & N. N. Dubler (Eds.), *Alzheimer's dementia: Dilemmas in clinical research* (pp. 71–78). Clifton, NJ: Humana Press.

Cantor, M. (1991). Family and community: Changing roles in an aging society. *Gerontologist, 31*, 337–346.

Cantor, M. (1994). Family caregiving: Social care. In M. Cantor (Ed.), *Family caregiving: Agenda for the future* (pp. 1–9). San Francisco: American Society on Aging.

Capezuti, E., Brush, B. L., and Lawson, W. T. (1997). Reporting elder mistreatment. *Journal of Gerontological Nursing, 23*(7), 24–32.

Caplan, A. L. (1981). *Ethics in hard times*. New York: Plenum Press.

Caplan, A. L. (1990). The morality of the mundane: Ethical issues arising in the daily lives of nursing home residents. In R. A. Kane & A. L. Caplan (Eds.), *Everyday ethics: Resolving dilemmas in nursing home life* (pp. 37–50). New York: Springer.

Carrese, J. A., & Rhodes, L. A. (1995). Western bioethics on the Navajo reservation: Benefit or harm? *JAMA, 274*(10), 826–829.

Cassileth, B. R., & Berlyne, D. (1989). Counseling the cancer patient who wants to try unorthodox or questionable therapies. *Oncology, 3*(4), 29–33.

Cassileth, B. R., Lusk, E. J., Strouse, T. B., & Bodenheimer, B. J. (1984). Contemporary unorthodox treatments in cancer medicine. *Annals of Internal Medicine, 101*, 105–112.

Chervenak, F. A., & McCullough, L. B. (1991). Clinical guides to preventing ethical conflicts between pregnant women and their physicians. *American Journal of Obstetrics and Gynecology, 162*, 303–307.

Childress, J. F. (1982). *Who should decide? Paternalism in health care*. Oxford: Oxford University Press.

Chrisman, N. J., & Kleinman, A. (1980). Health beliefs and practices among American ethnic groups. In S. Thernstrom (Ed.), *Harvard encyclopedia of American ethnic groups* (pp. 452–462). Cambridge, MA: Harvard University Press.

Churchill, L. R. (1985). The ethics of hospice care. In G. W. Davidson (Ed.), *The hospice: Development and administration* (2nd ed.) (pp. 163–179). Washington, DC: Hemisphere Publishing Corporation.

Cicirelli, V. G., Coward, R. T., & Dwyer, J. W. (1992). Siblings as caregivers for impaired elders. *Research on Aging, 14*(3), 331–350.

Clark-Daniels, C. L., Daniels, R. S., & Baumhover, L. A. (1990). Abuse and neglect of the elderly: Are emergency department personnel aware of mandatory reporting laws? *Annals of Emergency Medicine, 19*, 970–977.

Clough, R. (Ed.). (1996). *The abuse of care in residential institutions*. Concord, MA: Paul & Company.

Cohen, A. (1955). *Delinquent boys*. Glencoe, IL: Free Press.

Cohen, C. B. (1988). *Casebook on the termination of life-sustaining treatment and the care of the dying*. Bloomington: Indiana University Press.

Cohen, E. S. (1988). The elderly mystique: Constraints on the autonomy of the elderly with disabilities. *Gerontologist, 28*(Suppl.), 24–31.

Cohen, E. S. (1992). What is independence? *Generations, 16*(1), 49–52.

Cohen, E. S. (1996). Resolving ethical dilemmas arising from diminished decision-making capacity of the elderly. In M. Smyer, K. W. Schaie, and M. B. Kapp (Eds.), *Older adults' decision-making and the law* (pp. 162–174). New York: Springer.

Cohen, G. (1993). Comprehensive assessment: Capturing strengths, not just weaknesses. *Generations, 17*(Winter/Spring), 47–50.

Cohen, J. S., Fihn, S. D., Boyko, E. J., Jonsen, A. R., & Wood, R. W. (1994). Attitudes toward assisted suicide and euthanasia among physicians in Washington State. *New England Journal of Medicine, 331*, 89–94.

Cole, E. B., & Coultrap-McQuin, S. (Eds.). (1992). *Explorations in feminist ethics: Theory and practice*. Bloomington: Indiana University Press.

Cole, T. R. (1997). Ethics and aging: What difference do the humanities make? In M. Holstein (Ed.), *Ethical Currents, 48* (Winter), 10–11.

Cole, T. R., Kastenbaum, R., & Van Tassel, D. (1992). *Handbook of the humanities and aging*. New York: Springer.

Cole, T. R., & Winkler, M. G. (Eds.). (1994). *The Oxford book of aging*. New York: Oxford University Press.

Collett, T. S. (1994, March). The ethics of intergenerational representation. *Fordham Law Review, 62*(5), 1453–1501.

Collins, M. (1982). *Improving protective services for older Americans: Social worker role*. Portland: University of Southern Maine.

Collopy, B. J. (1988). Autonomy in long-term care: Some crucial distinctions. *Gerontologist, 28*(Suppl.), 10–17.

Collopy, B. J. (1993). The burden of beneficence. In R. A. Kane & A. L. Caplan (Eds.), *Ethical conflicts in the management of home care: The case manager's dilemma* (pp. 93–100). New York: Springer.

Collopy, B. J. (1994). Frail but still autonomous: Self-determination of the elder in long-term care. In *Making ethical decisions in long-term care: A collection of monographs and white papers produced for the AAHSA Commission on Ethics in Long-Term Care* (pp. 1–33). Washington, DC: American Association of Homes and Services for the Aging.

Collopy, B. J. (1995). Safety and independence: Rethinking some basic concepts in long-term care. In L. McCullough & N. Wilson (Eds.), *Long-term care decisions: Ethical and conceptual dimensions* (pp. 137–152). Baltimore: Johns Hopkins University Press.

Collopy, B. J., & Bial, M. C. (1994). Social work and bioethics: Ethical issues in long-term-care practice. In I. A. Gutheil (Ed.), *Work with older people: Challenges and opportunities* (pp. 109–138). New York: Fordham University Press.

Collopy, B. J., Dubler, N., & Zuckerman, C. (1990). The ethics of home care: Autonomy and accommodation. *Hastings Center Report, 20*(2), 1–16.

Conrad, N. (1985). Spiritual support for the dying. *Nursing Clinics of North America, 20*(2), 415–426.

Cook, F. L., Skogan, W. G., Cook, T. D., & Antunes, G. E. (1978). Criminal victimization of the elderly: The physical and economic consequences. *Gerontologist, 18*, 338–349.

Cook, T. D. (1978). Research revisited: Crime against the old. *APA Monitor, 9*, 1–11.

Cook, T. D., & Campbell, D. T. (1979). *Quasi-experimentation: Design and analysis issues for field settings*. Boston: Houghton Mifflin.

Cooke, R. E. (1994). Vulnerable children. In M. A. Grodin & L. H. Glantz (Eds.), *Children as research subjects: Science, ethics, and law* (pp. 193–214). New York: Oxford University Press.

Corless, I. B. (1994). Dying well: Symptom control within hospice care. In J. J. Fitzpatrick & J. S. Stevenson (Eds.), *Annual review of nursing research* (pp. 125–146). New York: Springer.

Cortese, A. J. (1980). *Ethnic ethics: Subjective choice and inference in Chicano and black children*. Doctoral dissertation, University of Notre Dame, Department of Sociology and Anthropology.

Cortese, A. J. (1982a). A comparative analysis of ethnicity and moral judgment. *Colorado Association for Chicano Research Review, 1*, 2–101.

Cortese, A. J. (1982b). Moral development in Chicano and Anglo children. *Hispanic Journal of Behavioral Sciences, 4*, 353–366.

Cortese, A. J. (1984a). Moral judgment in Chicano, black, and white young adults. *Sociological Focus, 17*, 189–199.

Cortese, A. J. (1984b). Standard issue scoring of moral reasoning: A critique. *Merrill-Palmer Quarterly, 30*, 227–246.

Cortese, A. J. (1985). The sociology of moral judgment: Social and ethnic factors. *Mid-American Review of Sociology, 9*, 109–124.

Cortese, A. J. (1986). Habermas and Kohlberg: Morality, justice, and rationality. In J. Wilson & S. McNall (Eds.), *Current perspectives in social theory* (pp. 141–156). Greenwich, CT: JAI Press.

Cortese, A. J. (1986b). The inception, evolution, and current state of the moral development school of Lawrence Kohlberg. In R. Monk (Ed.), *Structures of knowing* (pp. 327–346). Lanham, MD: University Press of America.

Cortese, A. J. (1987). The internal consistency of moral reasoning: A multitrait-multimethod analysis. *Journal of Psychology, 121*, 373–386.

Cortese, A. J. (1989a). Beyond justice and legitimation: Interpersonal and communicative morality. *New Observations, 72*, 20–23.

Cortese, A. J. (1989b). The interpersonal approach to morality: A gender and cultural analysis. *Journal of Social Psychology, 129*, 429–442.

Cortese, A. J. (1989c). Structural consistency in moral judgement. *British Journal of Social Psychology, 28*, 279–281.

Cortese, A. J. (1990). *Ethnic ethics: The restructuring of moral theory*. Albany: State University of New York Press.

Cortese, A. J. (1996). A comparative analysis of Japanese religion and ethics: Implications for the West. *Journal of Comparative Sociology and Ethics, 23*, 1–26.

Cortese, A. J., & Mestrovic, S. G. (1990). From Durkheim to Habermas: The role of language in moral theory. In J. Wilson (Ed.), *Current perspectives in social theory* (pp. 63–91). Greenwich, CT: JAI Press.

Covert, A. B., Rodrigues, T., & Solomon, K. (1977). The use of mechanical and chemical restraints in nursing homes. *Journal of the American Geriatrics Society, 25*, 85–89.

Covey, H. C. (1988). Historical terminology used to represent older people. *Gerontologist, 28*(3), 291–297.

Coy, J. A. (1989). Philosophic aspects of patient noncompliance: A critical analysis. *Topics in Geriatric Rehabilitation, 4*(3), 52–60.

Coyne, A. C. (1991). The relationship between cognitive impairment and elder abuse. In T. Tatara, M. M. Rittman, & K. J. Kaufer Flores (Eds.), *Findings of five elder abuse studies* (pp. 3–20). Washington, DC: National Aging Resource Center on Elder Abuse.

Coyne, A. C., Petenza, M., and Berbig, L. J. (1996). Abuse in families coping with dementia. *Aging, 367*, 93–95.

Cranford, R. E., & Doudera, A. E. (1984). *Institutional ethics committees and health care decision making*. Ann Arbor: Health Administration Press.

Cravedi, K. G. (1986). Elder abuse: The evolution of federal and state policy reform. *Pride Institute Journal of Long Term Home Health Care, 5*(4), 4–9.

Crawford, K. F. (1994). How ethical dilemmas are resolved. *Journal of Long-Term Care Administration, 22*(3), 24–28.

Crawford, S. C. (1982). *The evolution of Hindu ethical ideals.* Honolulu: University Press of Hawaii.

Crosby, E. M., & Leff, I. M. (1994, March). Ethical considerations in Medicaid estate planning: An analysis of the ABA Model Rules of Professional Conduct. *Fordham Law Review, 62*(5), 1503–1516.

Cruzan v. Director, 497 U.S. 261 (1990).

Cruzan v. Harmon, 760 S.W.2d 408 (1988).

Crystal, S. (1987). Elder abuse: The latest "crisis." *Public Interest, 88,* 56–66.

Crystal, S. (1996). Social policy and elder abuse. In K. A. Pillemer & R. S. Wolf (Eds.), *Elder abuse: Conflict in the family* (pp. 331–340). Doven, MA: Auburn House.

Cubillos, H. L., & Prieto, M. M. (1987). *The Hispanic elderly: A demographic profile.* Washington, DC: National Council of La Raza.

Curtis, J. R., Park, D. R., Krone, M. R., & Pearlman, R. A. (1995). Use of the medical futility rationale in do-not-attempt-resuscitation orders. *JAMA, 273*(2), 124–128.

Cutler, S. J., & Tisdale, W. A. (1992). Ethical issues in working with self-neglect. In E. Rathbone-McCuan & D. R. Fabian (Eds.), *Self-neglecting elders: A clinical dilemma.* New York: Auburn House.

Daar, J. F. (1995). Medical futility and implications for physician autonomy. *American Journal of Law and Medicine, 21*(2/3), 221–240.

Daniels, N. (1988). *Am I my parents' keeper? An essay on justice between the young and the old.* New York: Oxford University Press.

Daniels, R. S., Baumhover, L. A., & Clark-Daniels, C. L. (1989). Physicians' mandatory reporting of elder abuse. *Gerontologist, 29*(3), 321–327.

Danis, M., Southerland, L. I., Garrett, J. M., Smith, J. L., Hielema, F., Pickard, C. G., Egner, D. M., & Patrick, D. L. (1991). A prospective study of advance directives for life-sustaining care. *New England Journal of Medicine, 324*(13), 882–888.

Davidson, G. W. (Ed.). (1985). *The hospice: Development and administration* (2nd ed.). Washington, DC: Hemisphere Publishing Corporation.

Davis, M. C. (1992). The client's right to self-determination. *Caring, 11*(6), 26–32.

Declaration of Helsinki: Recommendations guiding medical doctors in biomedical research involving human subjects. (1964). Adopted by the 18th World Medical Assembly, Helsinki, Finland, 1964. *New England Journal of Medicine, 271,* 473–474.

Department of Health and Rehabilitative Services, Dade County Public Health Unit. (1990). *Final report of the Study to Assess Falls among the Elderly (SAFE).* Submitted to the Centers for Disease Control. Dade County, FL. Unpublished.

Dewey, J. (1939). Introduction. In E. V. Cowdry (Ed.), *Problems of ageing* (pp. XXIII–XXVIII). Baltimore: Williams & Wilkins.

The Dhammapada (P. Lal, Trans.). (1972). New York: Farrar, Straus & Giroux.

Dietz, M. (1985). Citizenship with a feminist face: The problem with maternal thinking. *Political Theory, 13,* 19–37.

Donegan, A. (1977). *The theory of morality.* Chicago: University of Chicago Press.

Donnabedian, A. (1989, Winter). A primer of quality assurance and monitoring in medical care. *University of Toledo Law Review, 20*(2), 401–453.

Doty, P. (1988). Long-term care in international perspective. *Health Care Financing Review, 10*(1) (Annual Suppl.), 145–155.

Doty, P. (1990, June). A comparison of long-term care financing in the U.S. and other nations: Dispelling some myths. *Ageing International,* pp. 10–14.

References

Downie, R. S., & Telfer, E. (1969). *Respect for persons.* London: George Allen & Unwin.
Drane, J. (1991). Doctors as priests: Providing a social ethics for a secular culture. In D. S. Browning & I. S. Evison (Eds.), *Does psychiatry need a public philosophy?* (pp. 40–60). Chicago: Nelson-Hall.
Dresser, R. S. (1992). Wanted: single, white male for medical research. *Hastings Center Report, 22*(1), 24–29.
Dresser, R. S. (1994). Advance directives: Implications for policy. *Hastings Center Report, 24*(6), S2–S5.
Dresser, R. S. (1995). Dworkin on dementia: Elegant theory, questionable policy. *Hastings Center Report, 25*(6), 32–38.
Dresser, R. S., & Robertson, J. A. (1989). Quality of life and non-treatment decisions for incompetent patients: A critique of the orthodox approach. *Law, Medicine, and Health Care, 17,* 234–244.
Dubin, B. A., Lelong, J., & Smith, B. K. (1988). *Faces of neglect.* Austin: University of Texas, Hogg Foundation for Mental Health.
Dubler, N. N. (1985). Legal issues in research on institutionalized demented patients. In V. L. Melnick & N. N. Dubler (Eds.) *Alzheimer's dementia: Dilemmas in clinical research* (pp. 149–173). Clifton, NJ: Humana Press.
Dubler, N. N. (1990). Autonomy and accommodation: Mediating individual choice in the home setting. *Generations, 14*(Suppl.), 29–31.
Dubose, E. R., Hamel, R., & O'Connell, L. J. (Eds.). (1994). *A matter of principles?* Valley Forge, PA: Trinity Press International.
Dugan, E., & Kivett, V. R. (1994). The importance of emotional and social isolation to loneliness among very old rural adults. *Gerontologist, 34*(3), 340–346.
Duke, J. (1991). A national study of self-neglecting adult protective services clients. In T. Tatara, M. M. Rittman, & K. J. Flores (Eds.), *Findings of five elder abuse studies* (pp. 22–50). Washington, DC: National Aging Resource Center on Elder Abuse.
Duke, J. (1993). *A national study of involuntary protective services to adult protective services clients.* Richmond, VA: National Association of Adult Protective Services Administrators and Virginia Department of Social Services.
Dunham, H. W. (1976). Comment. In J. Westermeyer (Ed.), *Anthropology and mental health* (pp. 35–36). The Hague: Mouton.
Dunkle, R. E. (1984). An historical perspective on social service delivery to the elderly. *Journal of Gerontological Social Work, 7*(3), 5–18.
Durkheim, E. (1951). *Suicide* (J. A. Spaulding & G. Simpson, Trans.). Glencoe, IL: Free Press.
Durkheim, E. (1961). *Moral Education* (E. K. Wilson & H. Schnurer, Trans.). Glencoe, IL: Free Press.
Durnbaugh, T. (1988). *Maneuvering in the health care system* (J. Rogers, Ed.) Scottdale, PA: Herald Press.
Dworkin, R. (1977). *Taking rights seriously.* Cambridge, MA: Harvard University Press.
Earl, L. L., & Stoller, E. P. (1983). Help with activities of everyday life: Sources of support for the noninstitutionalized elderly. *Gerontologist, 23,* 64–70.
Ehrenreich, B. (1990, December 10). Our health-care disgrace. *Time,* p. 112.
Eichrodt, W. (1949). *What is the social meaning of the Old Testament?* New York: World Council of Churches.
Eisenberg, D. M., Kessler, R. C., Foster, C., Norlock, F. E., Calkins, D. R., & Delbanco,

T. L. (1993). Unconventional medicine in the United States: Prevalence, costs, and patterns of use. *New England Journal of Medicine, 328*(4), 246–252.

Eliot, T. S. (1943). *Four quartets*. New York: Harvest Books.

Eliot, T. S. (1962). *The complete poems and plays*. New York: Harcourt, Brace & World.

Elman, C. (1995). An age-based mobilisation: The emergence of old age in American politics. *Ageing and Society, 15*, 299–324.

Emanuel, E. J. (1995). Medical ethics in the era of managed care: The need for institutional structures instead of principles for individual cases. *Journal of Clinical Ethics, 6*(4), 335–338.

Emanuel, E. J., & Emanuel, L. L. (1992). Four models of the physician-patient relationship. *JAMA, 267*(16), 2221–2226.

Emanuel, L. L., Barry, M. J., Stoeckle, J. D., Ettelson, L. M., & Emanuel, E. J. (1991). Advance directives for medical care: A case for greater use. *New England Journal of Medicine, 324*, 889–895.

Emanuel, L. L., & Emanuel, E. J. (1989). The medical directive: A new comprehensive advance care document. *JAMA, 261*(22), 3288–3293.

Enck, R. E. (1994). *The medical care of terminally ill patients*. Baltimore: Johns Hopkins University Press.

Encyclopaedia Britannica. (1985). Chicago: Encyclopedia Britannica.

Engel, G. (1980). The clinical application of biopsychosocial models. *American Journal of Psychiatry, 137*, 535–544.

Engelhardt, K. G. (1989). Health and human service robotics: Multi-dimensional perspectives. *International Journal of Technology and Aging, 1*(2), 6–41.

Estes, C. L., & Binney, E. A. (1991). The biomedicalization of aging: Dangers and dilemmas. In M. Minkler & C. L. Estes (Eds.), *Critical perspectives in aging: The political and moral economy of growing old* (pp. 117–134). Amityville, NY: Baywood.

Eustis, N. N., & Fischer, L. R. (1992). Relationships between home care clients and their workers: Implications for quality of care. *Gerontologist, 31*(4), 447–456.

Evans, M., & Welge, C. (1991). Trends in the spatial dimensions of the long-term care delivery system. *Social Science and Medicine, 33*(4), 477–487.

Fabian, D. R., & Rathbone-McCuan, E. (1992). Elder self-neglect: A blurred concept. In E. Rathbone-McCuan & D. R. Fabian (Eds.), *Self-neglecting elders: A clinical dilemma* (pp. 3–12). New York: Auburn House.

Faden, R., & Beauchamp, T. L. (1986). *A history and theory of informed consent*. New York: Oxford University Press.

Fahey, C. J. (1992). Ethics comes out of the closet. *Aging Today, 13*(6), 3.

Fahey, C. J. (1994). Religion and spirituality: Key elements to health promotion among older adults. *Perspectives in Health Promotion and Aging, 9*(3), 1–8.

Fahey, C. J., & Holstein, M. (1993). Toward a philosophy of the third age. In T. R. Cole, R. Kastenbaum, & P. Jakobi (Eds.), *Voices and visions of aging: Toward a critical gerontology* (pp. 241–256). New York: Springer.

Farris, B. E., & Glenn, N. D. (1976). Fatalism and familism among Anglos and Mexican Americans in San Antonio. *Sociology and Social Research, 60*, 390–402.

Faulkner, L. R. (1982). Mandating the reporting of suspected cases of elder abuse: An inappropriate, ineffective, and ageist response to the abuse of older adults. *Family Law Quarterly, 16*(1), 64–91.

Featherstone, M., & Hepworth, M. (1990). Images of ageing. In J. Bond & P. Coleman (Eds.), *Ageing in society: An introduction to social gerontology*. London: Sage.

Feinberg, J. (1973). *Social philosophy*. Englewood Cliffs, NJ: Prentice-Hall.

Feinberg, J. (1984). *Harm to others*. Vol. 1. In *The moral limits of the criminal law*. Oxford: Oxford University Press.

Feldman, D. M. (1986). *Health and medicine in the Jewish tradition*. New York: Crossroad.

Ferguson, E. J. (1978). *Protecting the vulnerable adult: A perspective on policy and program issues in adult protective services*. Ann Arbor: University of Michigan, Institute of Gerontology.

Ferraro, K. F., LaGrange, R. L., & McReady, W. C. (1990). *Are older people afraid of crime? Examining risk, fear, and constrained behavior: Final report to the AARP Andrus Foundation*. Dekalb: Northern Illinois University.

Ficarra, B. I. (1989). Medicolegal and bioethical responsibilities in triage. In C. H. Wecht (Ed.), *Legal medicine, 10*, 201–219.

Fiegener, J. J., Fiegener, M., & Meszaros, J. (1989). Policy implications of a statewide survey on elder abuse. *Journal of Elder Abuse and Neglect, 1*(2), 39–58.

Finkel, S. (1993). Mental health and aging. A decade of progress. *Generations, 17*(Winter/Spring), 25–30.

Finkelstein, J. A. (1995). Quality of asthma care. *Pediatrics, 95*(3), 389–394.

Finley, G. E. (1983). Fear of crime in the elderly. In J. I. Kosberg (Ed.), *Abuse and maltreatment of the elderly: Causes and interventions* (pp. 21–39). Boston: John Wright.

Finley, N. J. (1989). Theories of family labor as applied to gender differences in caregiving for elderly parents. *Journal of Marriage and the Family, 51*, 79–89.

Fins, J. J., & Bacchetta, M. D. (1995). Framing the physician-assisted suicide and voluntary active euthanasia debate: The role of deontology, consequentialism, and clinical pragmatism. *Journal of the American Geriatrics Society, 43*(5), 563–568.

Fischer, D. H. (1978). *Growing old in America*. Oxford: Oxford University Press.

Fischer, M. M. (1969). *Negro slave songs in the United States*. New York: Citadel.

Fitting, M. D. (1986). Ethical dilemmas in counseling elderly adults. *Journal of Counseling and Development, 64*, 325–327.

Fletcher, J. (1966). *Situation ethics*. Philadelphia: Westminster Press.

Foley, K. M. (1991). The relationship of pain and symptom management to patient requests for physician-assisted suicide. *Journal of Pain and Symptom Management, 6*(5), 289–297.

Folstein, M. F., Folstein, S. E., & McHugh, P. R. (1975). Mini-mental state: A practical method for grading the cognitive state of patients for the clinician. *Journal of Psychiatric Research, 12*, 189–198.

Forrow, L., Arnold, R. M., & Parker, L. S. (1993). Preventive ethics: Expanding the horizons of clinical ethics. *Journal of Clinical Ethics, 4*, 287–294.

Foster, S. E., & Brizius, J. A. (1993). Caring too much? American women and the nation's caregiving crisis. In J. Allen & A. Pifer (Eds.), *Women on the front lines: Meeting the challenge of an aging America* (pp. 47–73). Washington DC: Urban Institute Press.

Frankel, T. (1983). Fiduciary law. *California Law Review, 71*, 795–836.

Frankena, W. K. (1980). *Thinking about morality*. Ann Arbor: University of Michigan Press.

Frankl, V. E. (1992). *Man's search for meaning*. Boston: Beacon Press.
Freedman, B. (1981). Competence, marginal and otherwise. *International Journal of Law and Psychiatry, 4,* 53–72.
Friedan, B. (1993). *The fountain of age*. New York: Simon & Schuster.
Friend, R. A. (1991). Older lesbian and gay people: A theory of successful aging. *Journal of Homosexuality, 20,* 99–118.
Frodi, A. M. (1981). Contribution of infant characteristics to child abuse. *American Journal of Mental Deficiency, 85*(4), 341–349.
Frolik, L. A. (1981). Plenary guardianship: An analysis, a critique, and a proposal for reform. *Arizona Law Review, 23,* 599–660.
Fulmer, T., and Anetzberger, G. J. (1995). Knowledge about family violence interventions in the field of elder abuse. Background paper for the Committee on the Assessment of Family Violence Interventions of the National Research Council and Institute of Medicine.
Fulmer, T. T., & O'Malley, T. A. (1987). *Inadequate care of the elderly: A health care perspective on abuse and neglect*. New York: Springer.
Gallup, G., & Newport, F. (1991). Mirror of America: Fear of dying. *Gallup Poll News Service, 55,* 3–5.
Gamble, E. R., McDonald, P. J., & Lichstein, P. R. (1991). Knowledge, attitudes, and behavior of elderly persons regarding living wills. *Archives of Internal Medicine, 151,* 277–280.
Gardner, P., & Hudson, B. L. (1996). Advance report of final mortality statistics, 1993. *Monthly Vital Statistics Report, 44*(7, Suppl.). Hyattsville, MD: National Center for Health Statistics.
Gatsonis, G. A., Epstein, A. M., & McNeil, B. J. (1995). Variations in the utilization of coronary angiography for elderly patients with an acute myocardial infarction: An analysis using hierarchical logistic regression. *Medical Care, 33*(6), 625–642.
Gaylin, W. (1994). Knowing good and doing good. *Hastings Center Report, 24* (May–June), 36–41.
Gelfand, D. E. (1988). *The aging network: Programs and services* (3rd ed.). New York: Springer.
George, L. K. (1993). Depressive disorders and symptoms in later life. *Generations, 17* (Winter/Spring), 35–38.
Gerber, L. S. (1995). Ethics and caring: Cornerstones of nursing geriatric case management. *Journal of Gerontological Nursing, 21*(12), 15–19.
Gibson, J. M. (1990). National values history project. *Generations,* 14(Suppl.), 51–64.
Gibson, J. M. (1994). Mediation for ethics committees: A promising process. *Generations, 18*(Winter), 58–60.
Gibson, J. M., & Kushner, T. K. (1986). Will the "conscience of an institution" become society's servant? *Hastings Center Report, 16*(3), 9–11.
Gilbert, D. A. (1986). The ethics of mandatory elder abuse reporting statutes. *Advances in Nursing Science, 8*(2), 51–62.
Gilbert, J. P. (Ed.). (1986). *Guidebook book one: Spiritual life, spiritual hunger, transformation, discipline*. Nashville: Graded Press.
Gilligan, C. (1982). *In a different voice: Psychological theory and women's development*. Cambridge, MA: Harvard University Press.
Gilligan, C. (1984). The conquistador and the dark continent: Reflections on the psychology of love. *Daedalus, 113,* 75–95.

Gold, D. T. (1989). Generational solidarity. *American Behavioral Scientist, 33*, 19–32.

Goldenberg, R. L., Bronstein, J. M., & Haywood, J. L. (1995). Access to neonatal intensive care for low-birthweight infants: The role of maternal characteristics. *American Journal of Public Health, 85*(3), 357–361.

Goldscheider, C. (1971). *Population, modernization, and social structure.* Boston: Little, Brown.

Goldsmith, J., & Goldsmith, S. S. (1976). Crime and the elderly: An overview. In J. Goldsmith & S. S. Goldsmith (Eds.), *Crime and the elderly: Challenge and response* (pp. 1–6). Lexington, MA: Lexington Books.

Gordon, M. M. (1964). *Assimilation in American life.* New York: Oxford University Press.

Gottlich, V. (1994). Beyond granny bashing: Elder abuse in the 1990s. *Clearinghouse Review, 28*, 371–381.

Graber, G. C., Beasley, A. D., & Eaddy, J. A. (1985). *Ethical analysis of clinical medicine: A guide to self-evaluation.* Baltimore: Urban & Schwarzenberg.

Green, B. A., & Coleman, N. (1994, March). Foreword to special issue: Ethical issues in representing older clients. *Fordham Law Review, 62*(5), 961–986.

Greenberg, J., & Cohen, R. L. (Eds.). (1982). *Equity and justice in social behavior.* New York: Academic Press.

Greenfield, J. (1993). Hope, battles, pain, and love. *New Choices for Retirement Living, 33*(3), 62–67.

Griffin, J. (1986) *Well-being.* Oxford: Oxford University Press.

Grob, G. (1983). *Mental illness and American society, 1875–1940.* Princeton, NJ: Princeton University Press.

Gubrium, J. F. (1975). *Living and dying at Murray Manor.* New York: St. Martin's Press.

Gubrium, J. F., & Holstein, J. A. (1990). *What is family?* Mountain View, CA: Mayfield.

Guccione, A. A. (1988). Compliance and patient autonomy: Ethical and legal limits to professional dominance. *Topics in Geriatric Rehabilitation, 3*(3), 62–73.

Gurian, B., & Goisman, R. (1993). Anxiety disorders in the elderly. *Generations, 17* (Winter/Spring), 39–42.

Gurwitz, J. H., Col, N. F., & Avorn, J. (1992). The exclusion of the elderly and women from clinical trials in acute myocardial infarction. *JAMA, 268*, 1417–1422.

Gutmann, D. (1980). Observations on culture and mental health in later life. In J. Birren & R. B. Sloan (Eds.), *Handbook of mental health and aging* (pp. 429–447). Englewood Cliffs, NJ: Prentice-Hall.

Gutmann, D. (1992). Culture and mental health: Later life revisited. In J. E. Birren, R. B. Sloan, & G. D. Cohen (Eds.), *Handbook of mental health and aging* (2nd ed.) (pp. 75–97). New York: Academic Press.

Haber, C. (1983). *Beyond sixty-five: The dilemma of old age in America is past.* New York: Cambridge University Press.

Habermas, J. (1984). *The theory of communicative action.* Vol. 1, *Reason and the rationalization of society* (T. McCarthy, Trans.). Boston: Beacon Press.

Habermas, J. (1990). *Moral consciousness and communicative action* (Christian Lenhardt & Shierry Weber Nicholsen, Trans.). Cambridge, MA: MIT Press.

Habermas, J. (1993). *Justification and application: Remarks on discourse ethics.* Cambridge, MA: MIT Press.

Habermas, J. (1996). Postscript to between facts and norms. In M. Deflem (Ed.), *Ha-*

bermas, modernity, and law (pp. 135–150). Thousand Oaks, CA: Sage Publications.

Haddad, A. M. (1989). Ethical issues in home care: An overview. *Caring,* 8(3), 6–8.

Halamandaris, V. J. (1983). Fraud and abuse in nursing homes. In J. I. Kosberg (Ed.), *Abuse and maltreatment of the elderly: Causes and interventions* (pp. 104–114). Boston: John Wright.

Hamann, A. A. (1993). Family surrogate laws: A necessary supplement to living wills and durable powers of attorney. *Villanova Law Review, 38,* 103–176.

Hanks, R. S., & Settles, B. H. (1988–1989). Theoretical questions and ethical issues in a family caregiving relationship. *Journal of Applied Social Sciences, 13*(1), 9–39.

Hare, R. M. (1981). *Moral thinking: Its levels, methods, and point.* Oxford: Clarendon Press.

Harmon, L. (1990). Falling off the vine: Legal fictions and doctrine of substituted judgment. *Yale Law Journal, 100,* 1–71.

Harris, D. K., & Benson, M. L. (1996, July/August). Theft in nursing homes: An invisible problem. *Aging Today,* p. 17.

Harris, L., & Associates. (1975). *The myth and reality of aging in America.* Washington, DC: National Council on the Aging.

Harsanyi, J. C. (1982). Morality and the theory of rational behavior. In A. Sen & B. Williams (Eds.), *Utilitarianism and beyond* (pp. 39–62). Cambridge: Cambridge University Press.

Hartwell, S. (1943). Mental disease of the aged. In G. Lawton (Ed.), *New goals for old age* (pp. 132–143). New York: Columbia University Press. Reprint. New York: Arno Press, 1972.

Harvey, L. K., and Shubat, S. K. (1989). *Physician and public attitudes on health care.* Chicago: American Medical Association.

Hatcher, C., & Hatcher, D. (1975). Ethnic group suicide: An analysis of Mexican American and Anglo suicide rates for El Paso, Texas. *Crisis Intervention, 6,* 2–9.

Hauerwas, S., with Bendi, Richard, & Burrell, D. (1977). From system to story: An alternative pattern for rationality in ethics. In S. Hauerwas (Ed.), *Truthfulness and tragedy: Further investigations in Christian ethics.* Notre Dame, IN: University of Notre Dame Press.

Havighurst, R. J. (1976). The relative importance of social class and ethnicity in human development. *Human Development, 19,* 56–65.

Hawkins, A. F., & Kildee, D. E. (1990). *Older Americans Act: Administration on Aging does not approve intrastate funding formulas* (HRD-90-85). Washington, DC: U.S. General Accounting Office.

Hayes, C., & Spring, J. C. (1988). Professional judgment and clients' rights. *Public Welfare, 46*(2), 22–28.

Health Care Financing Administration. (1988). *Medicare/Medicaid nursing home information, 1987–1988.* Washington, DC: U.S. Government Printing Office.

Hegland, A. (1992, February). Mixing the good with the bad: Abuse Registry irregularities threaten aides' rights. *Contemporary Long Term Care,* pp. 52, 55, 78.

Heintz, L. L. (1988). Legislative hazard: Keeping patients living against their wills. *Journal of Medical Ethics, 14*(2), 82–87.

Heintz, L. L. (1997). Efficacy of advance directives in a general hospital. *Hawaii Medical Journal, 58,* 203–207.

References

Hennessy, C. H. (1989). Autonomy and risk: The role of client wishes in community-based long-term care. *Gerontologist, 29*(5), 633–639.
Henshel, R. L. (1990). *Thinking about social problems.* New York: Harcourt Brace Jovanovich.
Herskovits, M. J. (1941). *The myth of the negro past.* New York: Harper.
Herskovits, M. J. (1972). *Cultural relativism: Perspectives in cultural pluralism* (Frances Herskovits, Ed.). New York: Random House.
Hiatt, E. H., & Dell, R. (1993). The special burden of mental illness. *New Conversations, 15*(Summer), 32–34.
High, D. M. (1978). Is "natural death" an illusion? *Hastings Center Report, 8*(4), 37–42.
High, D. M. (1988). All in the family: Extended autonomy and expectations in surrogate health care decision making. *Gerontologist, 28*, 46–51.
High, D. M. (1989). Standards for surrogate decision making: What the elderly want. *Journal of Long Term Care Administration, 17*, 8–13.
High, D. M. (1990). Who will make health care decisions for me when I can't? *Journal of Aging and Health, 2*, 291–309.
High, D. M. (1991). A new myth about families of older people? *Gerontologist, 31*(5), 611–618.
High, D. M. (1992). Research with Alzheimer's disease subjects: Informed consent and proxy decision making. *Journal of the American Geriatrics Society, 40*, 950–957.
High, D. M. (1993). Advance directives and the elderly: A study of intervention strategies to increase use. *Gerontologist, 33*, 342–349.
High, D. M. (1994a). Families' roles in advance directives. *Hastings Center Report, 24*(6) (Special Supplement), S16–S18.
High, D. M. (1994b). Surrogate decision making: Who will make decisions for me when I can't? *Clinics in Geriatric Medicine, 10*, 445–462.
High, D. M., & Turner, H. B. (1987). Surrogate decision-making: The elderly's familial expectations. *Theoretical Medicine, 8*, 303–320.
Hill, T. P. (1996). Health care: A social contract in transition. *Social Science and Medicine, 43*, 783–789.
Hirschel, A. E. (1996). Setting the stage: The advocates' struggle to address gross neglect in Philadelphia nursing homes. *Journal of Elder Abuse & Neglect, 8*(3), 5–20.
Hobbs, L. (1976). Adult protective services: A new program approach. *Public Welfare, 33*, 28–37.
Hofland, B. F. (1990). Introduction. *Generations, 14*(Suppl.), 5–8.
Hofland, B. F. (1994). When capacity fades and autonomy is constricted: A client-centered approach to residential care. *Generations, 18*(4), 31–36.
Hofland, B. F., & David, D. (1990). Autonomy and long-term-care practice: Conclusions and next steps. *Generations, 14*(Suppl.), 91–94.
Hogstel, M. O., & Gaul, A. L. (1991). Safety or autonomy: An ethical issue for clinical gerontological nurses. *Journal of Gerontological Nursing, 17*(3), 6–11.
Holstein, M. (1995). Multidisciplinary ethical decision-making: Uniting differing professional perspectives. In T. F. Johnson (Ed.), *Elder mistreatment: Ethical issues, dilemmas, and decisions* (pp. 169–182). Binghamton, NY: Haworth Press.
Holstein, M. (1996). *Negotiating disease: Senile dementia and Alzheimer's disease, 1900–1980.* Unpublished doctoral dissertation, University of Texas Medical Branch, Institute for the Medical Humanities, Galveston.
Holstein, M. (1999). Women and productive aging: Troubling implications. In M. Mink-

ler & C. Estes (Eds.), *Critical gerontology: Perspectives from political and moral economy* (pp. 359–373). Amityville, NY: Baywood.

Holstein, M., & Cole, T. R. (1995). Long-term care: A historical reflection. In L. B. McCullough & N. L. Wilson (Eds.), *Long-term care decisions: Ethical and conceptual dimensions* (pp. 15–34). Baltimore: Johns Hopkins University Press.

Holstein, M., & Cole, T. R. (1996). The evolution of long-term care in America. In R. Binstock, L. Cluff, & O. Von Mering (Eds.), *The future of long-term care: Social and policy issues* (pp. 19–47). Baltimore: Johns Hopkins University Press.

The Holy Bible, containing the Old and New Testaments: Revised Standard Version. (1953). New York: Thomas Nelson & Sons.

Holzberg, C. S. (1982). Ethnicity and aging: Anthropological perspectives on more than just the minority elderly. *Gerontologist, 22*, 249–257.

Honegger, H. (1991). Avoiding futility: Assessment of cancer patients in intensive care units. *Annals of Oncology, 2*, 530–531.

Hooyman, N. R., & Kiyak, H. A. (1996). *Social gerontology: A multidisciplinary perspective* (4th ed.). Boston: Allyn & Bacon.

Hoppe, S. K., & Martin, H. W. (1978). *Changing patterns of suicidal behavior among Mexican Americans, 1960–1970.* Paper presented at the Annual Meeting of the Society for Applied Anthropology, Merida, Mexico.

Horowitz, A., & Dobrof, R. (1982). *The role of families in providing long-term care to the frail and chronically ill elderly living in the community: Final report submitted to the Health Care Financing Administration.* New York: Brookdale Center on Aging.

Horowitz, G., & Estes, C. (1971). *Protective services for the aged.* Washington, DC: U.S. Department of Health, Education, and Welfare.

Horstman, P. (1975). Protective services for the elderly: The limits of "parens patriae." *Missouri Law Review, 40*, 215.

Horwitz, A. V., & Reinhard, S. C. (1995). Ethnic differences in caregiving duties and burdens among parents and siblings of persons with severe mental illnesses. *Journal of Health and Social Behavior, 36*, 138–150.

Hospers, J. (1961). *Human conduct: An introduction to the problems of ethics.* New York: Harcourt, Brace & World.

Howe, N. (1995). Why the graying of the welfare state threatens to flatten the American dream—or worse. *Generations, 19*(3), 15–19.

Hudson, R. B. (1989). The "graying" of the federal budget and its consequences for old age policy. In I. C. Colby (Ed.), *Social welfare policy: Perspectives, patterns, and insights* (pp. 261–283). Chicago: Dorsey Press.

Hudson, R. B. (1995). The history and place of age-based public policy. *Generations, 19*(3), 5–10.

Hudson, R. B. (1997). The history and place of age-based public policy. In R. B. Hudson (Ed.), *The future of age-based public policy* (pp. 1–22). Baltimore: Johns Hopkins University Press.

Hughes, C. (1909). Normal senility and dementia senilis: The therapeutic staying of old age. *Alienist and Neurologist, 30*, 63–76.

Hughes, M. M. (1995). Strategies to promote ethical awareness. *Caring, 14*(9), 6–11.

Hull, J. (Chairman). (1993). *National uniformity for paraprofessional title, qualifications, and supervision.* Home Care Aide Association of America.

Hume, D. (1963). *"Of Suicide", essays: Moral, political and literary.* Oxford: Oxford University Press.

Humphry, D. (1991). *Final exit: The practicalities of self-deliverance and assisted suicide for the dying.* Eugene, OR: Hemlock Society.
Hunt, A. D., Crotty, M. T., & Crotty, R. B. (1991). *Ethics of world religions.* San Diego: Greenhaven Press.
Hunt, S. S. (1989). *Working through ethical dilemmas in ombudsman practice.* Washington, DC: National Center for State Long Term Ombudsman Resources.
Iga, M., & Tatai, K. (1975). Characteristics of suicides and attitudes toward suicide in Japan. In N. L. Farberow (Ed.), *Suicide in different cultures* (pp. 255–280). Baltimore: University Park Press.
Ignatieff, M. (1986). *The needs of strangers.* New York: Penguin Books.
In the Matter of Karen Quinlan. (1975). Arlington, VA: University Publications of America.
In re O'Connor, 72 N.Y.2d 517, 531 N.E.2d 607, 534 N.Y.S.2d 886 (1988).
In re Quinlan, 355A. 2nd 647 (N.J. 1976).
In re Wanglie, No. PX-91-283 (Minn. 4th Dist. CT. Hennepin County July 1, 1991) p. 217.
Iozzio, M. J. (1992). Ethical decision-making in home care. *Caring, 11*(6), 51–52.
Jackson, J. J. (1972). Comparative life styles of family and friend relationships among older black women. *Family Coordinator, 21,* 477–485.
Jackson, J. J. (1985). Race, national origin, ethnicity, and aging. In R. H. Binstock & E. Shanas (Eds.), *Handbook of aging and the social sciences* (2nd ed.) (pp. 264–303). New York: Van Nostrand Reinhold.
Jameton, A. (1988). In the borderlands of autonomy: Responsibility in long term care facilities. *Gerontologist, 28*(Suppl.), 18–23.
Jamison, J. E. (1995). Spirituality and medical ethics. *American Journal of Hospice and Palliative Care, 12*(3), 41–45.
Jecker, N. S. (Ed.). (1991). *Aging and ethics: Philosophical problems in gerontology.* Totowa, NJ: Humana Press.
Jecker, N. S. (1995). What do husbands and wives owe each other in old age? In L. B. McCullough & N. L. Wilson (Eds.), *Long-term care decisions: Ethical and conceptual dimensions* (pp. 155–180). Baltimore: Johns Hopkins University Press.
Jecker, N. S., Carrese, J. A., & Pearlman, R. A. (1995). Caring for patients in cross-cultural settings. *Hastings Center Report, 25*(1), 6–14.
Jennings, B. (1986, September–October). Community bioethics: Votes on a new movement. *Federation Reports,* 18–21.
Jennings, J. (1987). Elderly parents as caregivers for their adult dependent children. *Social Work, 32,* 430–433.
Job, S., & Anema, M. G. (1988). Elder care: Ethical dimensions. *Journal of Gerontological Nursing, 14*(12), 16–19.
Johnson, C. L. (1978). Family support systems of elderly Italian Americans. *Journal of Minority Aging, 3–4,* 34–41.
Johnson, C. L. (1985). *Growing up and growing old in Italian American families.* New Brunswick, NJ: Rutgers University Press.
Johnson, C. L., & Catalano, D. J. (1981). Childless elderly and their family supports. *Gerontologist, 21,* 610–618.
Johnson, S. H. (1990). The fear of liability and the use of restraints in nursing homes. *Law, Medicine, and Health Care, 18,* 263–273.
Johnson, T. F. (1991). *An empirical study of the voluntary befriending programs for the*

socially isolated older adults in four towns. Newcastle-upon-Tyne, England: Age Concern England.
Johnson, T. F. (1995a). Aging well in contemporary society. *American Behavioral Scientist, 39*(2), 120–130.
Johnson, T. F. (1995b). Ethics and elder mistreatment: Uniting protocol with practice. In T. F. Johnson (Ed.), *Elder mistreatment: Ethical issues, dilemmas, and decisions.* Binghamton, NY: Haworth Press.
Jones, J. S. (1994). Elder abuse and neglect: Responding to a national problem. *Annals of Emergency Medicine, 23,* 845–848.
Jonsen, A. R., Siegler, M., & Winslade, W. (1982). *Clinical ethics: A practical approach to ethical decisions in clinical medicine.* New York: Macmillan.
Jonsen, A. R., & Toulmin, S. (1988). *The abuse of casuistry: A history of moral reasoning.* Berkeley: University of California Press.
Jost, T. S. (1989). Regulatory approaches to problems in the quality of medical care: Diagnosis and prescription. *University of California, Davis, Law Review, 22,* 573–608.
Kalb, P. E. (1996). Controlling health care costs by controlling technology: A private contractual approach. *Yale Law Journal, 99,* 1108–1126.
Kalish, R. A. (1968, December). Suicide: An ethnic comparison in Hawaii. *Bulletin of Suicidology,* pp. 37–43.
Kalish, R. A. (1979). The new ageism and the failure models: A polemic. *Gerontologist, 15,* 486–492.
Kalish, R. A. (1985). The social context of death and dying. In R. H. Binstock & E. Shanas (Eds.), *Handbook of aging and the social sciences* (2nd ed.) (pp. 149–170). New York: Van Nostrand Reinhold.
Kalish, R. A., & Reynolds, D. K. (1976). *Death and ethnicity: A psychocultural study.* Los Angeles: University of Southern California Press.
Kamasutra (Sir R B, Trans.). (1963). Bombay: Jaico Publishing House.
Kamisar, Y. (1978). Euthanasia legislation: Some nonreligious objections. In T. L. Beauchamp & S. Perlin (Eds.), *Ethical issues in death and dying* (pp. 220–231). Englewood Cliffs, NJ: Prentice-Hall.
Kane, R. A. (1993a). Ethical and legal issues in long-term care: Food for futuristic thought. *Journal of Long-term Care Administration, 21*(3), 66–74.
Kane, R. A. (1993b). Uses and abuses of confidentiality. In R. A. Kane & A. L. Caplan (Eds.), *Ethical conflicts in the management of home care: The case managers' dilemma* (pp. 147–157). New York: Springer.
Kane, R. A. (1994). Ethics and long-term care: Everyday considerations. *Clinics in Geriatric Medicine, 10*(3), 489–499.
Kane, R. A. (1995). Decision making, care plans, and life plans in long-term care: Can case managers take account of clients' values and preferences? In L. B. McCullough & N. L. Wilson (Eds.), *Long-term care decisions: Ethical and conceptual dimensions* (pp. 87–109). Baltimore: Johns Hopkins University Press.
Kane, R. A., & Caplan, A. L. (Eds.). (1990). *Everyday ethics: Resolving dilemmas in nursing home life.* New York: Springer.
Kane, R. A., & Caplan, A. L. (Eds.). (1993). *Ethical conflicts in the management of home care: The case manager's dilemma.* New York: Springer.
Kane, R. A., Freeman, I. C., Caplan, A. L., Aroskar, M. A., & Urv-Wong, E. K. (1990). Everyday autonomy in nursing homes. *Generations, 14*(Suppl.), 69–71.

Kane, R. A., & Kane, R. L. (1987). *Long-term care: Principles, programs, and policies.* New York: Springer.

Kane, R. A., Penrod, J. D., & Kivnick, H. Q. (1993). Ethics and case management: Preliminary results of an empirical study. In R. A. Kane & A. L. Caplan (Eds.), *Ethical conflicts in the management of home care: The case manager's dilemma* (pp. 7–25). New York: Springer.

Kane, R. L., & Kane, R. A. (1990). Healthcare for older people: Organizational and policy issues. In R. H. Binstock & L. K. George (Eds.), *Handbook of aging and the social sciences* (3rd ed.) (pp. 415–437). San Diego: Academic Press.

Kant, I. (1938). *Fundamental principles of the metaphysics of ethics.* New York: Appleton-Century Company.

Kant, I. (1949). *Immanuel Kant's critique of practical reason and other writings in moral philosophy* (L. W. Beck, Trans. and Ed.). Chicago: University of Chicago Press.

Kant, I. (1950). *Immanuel Kant's critique of pure reason* (N. K. Smith, Trans.). New York: Humanities Press.

Kant, I. (1956). *Critique of practical reason* (L. W. Beck, Trans.). New York: Liberal Arts Press. (Original work published 1788).

Kant, I. (1959). *Foundations of the metaphysics of morals* (C. W. Beck, Trans.). New York: Liberal Arts Press.

Kant, I. (1963). *Lectures on Ethics* (L. Infield, Trans., L. W. Beck, Ed.). New York: Harper & Row.

Kant, I. (1964). *Groundwork of the metaphysic of morals* (H. J. Paton, Trans.). New York: Harper & Row.

Kapp, M. B. (1991). Legal and ethical issues in family caregiving and the role of public policy. *Home Health Care Services Quarterly, 12*(4), 5–28.

Kapp, M. B. (1995a). Elder mistreatment: Legal interventions and policy uncertainties. *Behavioral Sciences and the Law, 13*, 365–380.

Kapp, M. B. (1995b). Aging and the law. In R. H. Binstock & L. K. George (Eds.), *Handbook of aging and the social sciences* (4th ed.) (pp. 467–479). San Diego: Academic Press.

Kapp, M. B. (1997). Should older persons be able to give assets to family members without affecting Medicaid eligibility? In A. E. Scharlach & L. W. Kaye (Eds.), *Controversial issues in aging* (pp. 160–172). Boston: Allyn & Bacon.

Kapp, M. B., & Bigot, A. (1985). *Geriatrics and the law: Patient rights and professional responsibilities.* New York: Springer.

Kapp, M. B., Pies, H. E., Jr., & Doudera, A. E. (Eds.). (1985). *Legal and ethical aspects in health care for the elderly.* Westport, CT: Greenwood Press.

Kart, C. S., & Dunkle, R. E. (1995). Institutional settings: Programs and services. In Z. Harel & R. E. Dunkle (Eds.), *Matching people with services in long-term care* (pp. 221–284). New York: Springer.

Kasper, J. F., Mulley, A. G., Jr., & Wennberg, J. E. (1992). Developing shared decision-making programs to improve the quality of health care. *Quality Review Bulletin, 18*, 183–190.

Kass, L. R. (1985). *Toward a more natural science: Biology and human affairs.* New York: Free Press.

Kassler, J. (1994). *Bitter medicine: Greed and chaos in American health care.* New York: Carol Publishing Group.

Kastenbaum, R. J. (1977). *Death, society, and human experience.* St. Louis, MO: C. V. Mosby.

Kaufman, S. R., and Becker, G. (1996). Frailty, risk, and choice: Cultural discourses and the question of responsibility. In M. Smyer, K. W. Schaie, & M. B. Kapp (Eds.), *Older adults' decision-making and the law* (pp. 48–70). New York: Springer.

Kavesh, W. (1996–1997). The practice of geriatric medicine: How geriatricians think. In P. Blanchette (Ed.), *Progress in geriatrics: A clinical care update. Generations, 20*(Winter), 54–59.

Kaye, L. W., & Applegate, J. S. (1990). *Men as caregivers to the elderly: Understanding and aiding unrecognized family support.* Lexington, MA: Lexington Books.

Kelly, T., & Kropf, N. (1995). Stigmatized and perpetual parents: Older parents caring for adult children with life-long disabilities. *Journal of Gerontological Social Work, 24,* 3–16.

Kelman, H. C., & Warwick, D. P. (1978). The ethics of social intervention: Goals, means, and consequences. In G. Bermant, H. C. Kelman, & D. P. Warwick (Eds.), *The ethics of social intervention* (pp. 3–33). Washington, DC: Hemisphere Publishing Corporation.

Kiefer, C. W. (1974a). *Changing cultures, changing lives: An ethnographic study of three generations of Japanese Americans.* San Francisco: Jossey-Bass.

Kiefer, C. W. (1974b). Lessons from the issei. In J. F. Gubrium (Ed.), *Late life: Communities and environmental policy* (pp. 167–197). Springfield, IL: Charles C. Thomas.

Kimboko, P., & Jewell, E. (1994). A beginner's guide to ethical awareness in long-term care services. *Activities, Adaptation, and Aging, 18*(3/4), 5–26.

King, P. A. (1991). The authority of families to make medical decisions for incompetent patients after the Cruzan decision, *Law, Medicine, and Health Care, 19,* 76–79.

Kitchener, K. S. (1984). Intuition, critical evaluation, and ethical principles: The foundation for ethical decisions in counseling psychology. *Counseling Psychologist, 12*(3), 43–56.

Kitwood, T. (1997). *Dementia reconsidered.* Buckingham, England: Open University Press.

Kivnick, H. Q. (1993). Everyday mental health: A guide to assessing life strengths. *Generations, 17*(Winter/Spring), 13–20.

Klosterman, E. (1994). *Social worker reliance on the NASW Code of Ethics.* Paper presented at the Annual Conference of the National Association of Social Workers, Ohio Chapter, Akron.

Kluckhohn, C. (Ed.). (1962). *Culture and behavior.* New York: Free Press.

Knight, J. A. (1994). Ethics of care in caring for the elderly. *Southern Medical Journal, 87*(9), 909–917.

Koenig, H. G. (1995). Religion and health in later life. In M. A. Kimble, S. H. McFadden, J. W. Ellor, & J. J. Seeber (Eds.), *Aging, spirituality, and religion: A handbook* (pp. 9–29). Minneapolis: Fortress Press.

Koenig, H. G., Cohen, H. J., Blazer, D. G., Kudler, H. S. Krishnan, K., & Sibert, T. (1995). Religious coping and cognitive symptoms of depression in elderly medical patients. *Psychosomatics, 36*(4), 369–375.

Koenig, H. G., Cohen, H. J., Blazer, D. G., Pieper, C., Meador, K. G., Shelp, F., Goli, V., & DiPasquale, R. (1992). Religious coping and depression among elderly hospitalized medically ill men. *American Journal of Psychiatry, 149,* 1693–1700.

Koenig, H. G., George, L., & Schneider, R. (1994). Mental health care for older adults in the year 2020: A dangerous and avoided topic. *Gerontologist, 34*, 674–679.

Koenig, R., Goldner, N. S., Kresojevich, R., & Lockwood, G. (1971). Ideas about illness of elderly black and white in an urban hospital. *Aging and Human Development, 2*, 217–225.

Kohlberg, L. (1969). Stage and sequence: The cognitive-developmental approach to socialization. In D. Goslin (Ed.), *Handbook of socialization theory and research* (pp. 347–480). Chicago: Rand McNally.

Kohlberg, L. (1981). *Essays on moral development.* Vol. 1, *The philosophy of moral development.* New York: Harper & Row.

Kohlberg, L. (1984). *Essays on moral development.* Vol. 2, *The psychology of moral development.* New York: Harper & Row.

Korbin, J. E., Anetzberger, G. J., & Eckert, J. K. (1989). Elder abuse and child abuse: A consideration of similarities and differences in intergenerational family violence. *Journal of Elder Abuse and Neglect, 1*(4), 1–14.

Korte, A. O. (1981). Theoretical perspectives in mental health and the Mexicano elders. In M. Miranda & R. A. Ruiz (Eds.), *Chicano aging and mental health* (pp. 1–37). Washington, DC: U.S. Government Printing Office.

Kosterlitz, J. (1992, February 15). A sick system. *National Journal*, pp. 376–388.

Kotulak, R. (1997, May 19). Scientists find new wrinkles in Americans' aging process. *Chicago Tribune*, pp. 1, 8.

Kraft, F. (1991). As Christians we must talk about it. *Church and Society* 81(January–February), 2–5.

Kripalani, A. (1993, July). Health care: Prema Mathai-Davis. *Indian American*, p. 14.

Kultgen, J. (1988). *Ethics and professionalism.* Philadelphia: University of Pennsylvania Press.

Kunitz, S. J., & Levy, J. E. (1981). Navajos. In A. Harwood (Ed.), *Ethnicity and medical care* (pp. 337–396). Cambridge, MA: Harvard University Press.

Labouvie-Vief, G., DeVoe, M., & Bulka, D. (1989). Speaking about feelings: Conceptions of emotion across the life-span. *Psychology and Aging, 4*(4), 425–437.

Lachs, M. S., Berkman, L., Fulmer, T., and Horwitz, R. I. (1994). A prospective community-based pilot study of risk factors for the investigation of elder mistreatment. *Journal of the American Geriatrics Society, 42*, 169–173.

Ladd, J. (Ed.). (1979). *Ethical issues relating to life and death.* New York: Oxford University Press.

LaGrange, R. L., & Ferraro, K. F. (1987). The elderly's fear of crime: A critical examination of the research. *Research on Aging, 9*(3), 372–391.

Lamm, R. D. (1989). *The brave new world of health care.* Unpublished paper.

Lammers, W. W. (1983). *Public policy and the aging.* Washington, DC: CQ Press.

Lantos, J., Miles, S., Silverstein, M., & Stocking, C. (1988). Survival after cardiopulmonary resuscitation in babies of very low birth weight: Is CPR futile therapy? *New England Journal of Medicine, 318*, 91–95.

Lantos, J., Singer, P., Walker, R., Gramelspacher, G., Shapiro, G., Sanchez-Gonzalez, M., Stocking, C., Miles, S., & Siegler, M. (1989). The illusion of futility in clinical practice. *American Journal of Medicine, 87*, 81–84.

Lapidus, I. M. (1978). Adulthood in Islam: Religious maturity in the Islamic tradition. In E. Erikson (Ed.), *Adulthood* (pp. 97–112). New York: Norton.

Latimer, E. (1991). Caring for seriously ill and dying patients: The philosophy and ethics. *Canadian Medical Association Journal, 144*(7), 859–864.

Lawton, M. P. (1980). Do elderly research subjects need special protection? Psychological vulnerability. *IRB: A Review of Human Subjects Research, 2*(8), 5–7.

Lawton, M. P., & Yaffe, S. (1980). Victimization and fear of crime in elderly public housing tenants. *Journal of Gerontology, 35*(5), 768–779.

Lebowitz, B. D. (1978, January 31). *Statement before the U.S. House Committee on Science and Technology, Subcommittee on Domestic and International Scientific Planning, Analysis, and Cooperation*. Washington, DC: U.S. Government Printing Office.

Lebowitz, B. D., & Niederehe, G. (1992). Concepts and issues in mental health and aging. In J. E. Birren, R. B. Sloane, & G. D. Cohen (Eds.), *Handbook of mental health and aging* (2nd ed.) (pp. 3–26). New York: Academic Press.

Lee, M. A., Nelson, H. D., Tilden, V. P., Ganzini, L., Schmidt, T. A., & Tolle, S. W. (1996). Legalizing assisted suicide: Views of physicians in Oregon. *New England Journal of Medicine, 334*, 310–315.

Lehmann, P. (1992). Ethical decision making and woman abuse in social work. *Social Worker, 60*(3), 133–137.

Lesnoff-Caravaglia, G. (Ed.). (1985). *Values, ethics, and aging*. New York: Human Sciences Press.

Lesnoff-Caravaglia, G. (1988). Aging in a technological society. In G. Lesnoff-Caravaglia (Ed.), *Aging in a technological society* (pp. 272–283). New York: Human Sciences Press.

Lesnoff-Caravaglia, G., & Klys, M. (1987). Lifestyle and longevity. In G. Lesnoff-Caravaglia (Ed.), *Realistic expectations for long life* (pp. 35–38). New York: Human Sciences Press.

Levin, J. S., & Tobin, S. S. (1995). Religion and psychological well-being. In M. A. Kimble, S. H. McFadden, J. W. Ellor, & J. J. Seeber (Eds.), *Aging, spirituality, and religion: A handbook* (pp. 30–46). Minneapolis: Fortress Press.

Levine, C. (1988). Has AIDS changed the ethics of human subjects research? *Law, Medicine, and Health Care, 16*, 167–173.

Lewis, H. (1971). Blackways of Kent: Religion and salvation. In H. M. Nelsen, R. Yokley, & A. K. Nelsen (Eds.), *The black church in America* (pp. 100–118). New York: Basic Books.

Lidz, C. W., & Arnold, R. M. (1990). Institutional constraints on autonomy. *Generations, 14*(Suppl.), 65–68.

Lidz, C. W., Fischer, L., & Arnold, R. M. (1992). *The erosion of autonomy in long-term care*. New York: Oxford University Press.

Lieb, I. C. (1991). *Past, present, and future: A philosophical essay about time*. Urbana: University of Illinois Press.

Lippy, S. K. (1995). Ethics committees in long term care: A realistic endorsement. *BENO Newsletter, 4*(1), 5–6.

Llewellyn, K. N. (1931). Some realism about realism. *Harvard Law Review, 44*, 1222–1264.

Localio, A. R., Lawthers, A. G., & Bengtson, J. M. (1993). Relationship between malpractice claims and cesarean delivery. *JAMA, 269*(3), 366–373.

Locke, J. (1960). *Two treatises of government*. Cambridge: Cambridge University Press.

Loewy, E. H. (1996). Guidelines, managed care, and ethics. *Archives of Internal Medicine, 156*(18), 2038–2040.

Lofgren, R. P., MacPherson, D. S., Granieri, R., Myllenbeck, S., & Sprafka, J. M. (1989). Mechanical restraints on the medical wards: Are protective devices safe? *American Journal of Public Health, 79*, 735–738.

Logstrup, K. E. (1971). *The ethical demand*. Philadelphia: Fortress Press.

Logue, B. J. (1994). When hospice fails: The limits of palliative care. *Omega, 29*, 291–301.

Long, J. B. (1975). The death that ends death in Hinduism and Buddhism. In E. Kubler-Ross (Ed.), *Death: The final stage of growth* (pp. 52–74). Englewood Cliffs, NJ: Prentice-Hall.

Longres, J. F. (1993). *Self-neglect among the elderly*. Unpublished manuscript, University of Wisconsin, Madison.

Longres, J. F. (1994). Self-neglect and social control: A modest test of an issue. *Journal of Gerontological Social Work, 22*(3–4), 3–20.

Lopez, C., & Aguilera, E. (1991). *On the sidelines: Hispanic elderly and the continuum of care*. Washington, DC: Policy Analysis Center and Office of Institutional Development, National Council of La Raza.

Lopez, G. P. (1996, Summer). An aversion to clients: Loving humanity and hating human beings. *Harvard Civil Rights–Civil Liberties Law Review, 31*(2), 315–323.

Luke, H. M. (1992). *Kaleidoscope*. New York: Parabola Books.

Lustbader, W. (1996). Self-neglect: A practitioner's view. *Aging, 367*, 51–61.

Lynn, J. (1991). Why I don't have a living will. *Law, Medicine, and Health Care, 19*(1–2), 101–104.

Lynn, J., Johnson, J., & Levine, R. J. (1994). The ethical conduct of health services research: A case study of 55 institutions' applications to the SUPPORT project. *Clinical Research, 42*, 3–10.

MacAdam, M. (1993). Home care reimbursement and effects on personnel. *Gerontologist, 33*(1), 55–63.

MacIntyre, A. (1981). *After virtue*. South Bend, IN: University of Notre Dame Press.

Macionis, J. J. (1996). *Society: The basics* (3rd ed.). New York: Prentice Hall.

Mackie, J. L. (1977). *Ethics: Inventing right and wrong*. New York: Penguin.

MacNamara, R. D. (1988). *Freedom from abuse in organized care settings for the elderly and handicapped*. Springfield, IL: Charles C. Thomas.

Maddox, G. (Ed.). (1987). *Encyclopedia of aging*. New York: Springer.

Maddox, G. (Ed.). (1995). *Encyclopedia of aging* (2nd ed.). New York: Springer.

Madsen, W. (1969). Mexican Americans and Anglo Americans: A comparative study of mental health in Texas. In S. C. Plog & R. B. Edgerton (Eds.), *Changing perspectives in mental illness* (pp. 217–247). New York: Holt, Rinehart & Winston.

Magee, J. J. (1988). *A professional's guide to older adults' life review: Releasing the peace within*. Lexington, MA: Lexington Books.

Maldonaldo, D. (1975). The Chicano aged. *Social Work, 20*, 213–216.

Mandelbaum, D. (1959). Social uses of funeral rites. In H. Feifel (Ed.), *The meaning of death* (pp. 189–217). New York: McGraw-Hill.

Mannheim, K. (1971). *Ideology and utopia* (L. Wirth & E. Shils, Trans.). New York: Harcourt, Brace, Jovanovich.

Manning, R. (1992). Just caring. In E. Browning-Cole & S. Coultrap-McQuin (Eds.),

Explorations in feminist ethics: Theory and practice (pp. 45–54). Bloomington: Indiana University Press.

Manthorpe, J. (1993). Elder abuse and key areas in social work. In P. Decalmer & F. Glendenning (Eds.), *The mistreatment of elderly people* (pp. 88–101). London: Sage.

Manton, K. G. (1980). Sex and race. Specific mortality differentials in multiple cause of death data. *Gerontologist, 20*, 480–493.

Mappes, T. A., & Zembaty, J. S. (Eds.). (1986). *Biomedical ethics* (2nd ed.). New York: McGraw-Hill.

Margulies, P. (1994, March). Access, connection, and voice: A contextual approach to representing senior citizens of questionable capacity. *Fordham Law Review, 62*(5), 1073–1099.

Mariner, W. K. (1995). Business vs. medical ethics: Conflicting standards for managed care. *Journal of Law, Medicine, and Ethics, 23*(3), 236–246.

Markides, K. S. (1982). Ethnicity and aging: A comment. *Gerontologist, 22*, 467–472.

Markides, K. S., & Machalek, R. (1984). Selective survival, aging, and society. *Archives of Gerontology and Geriatrics, 3*, 207–222.

Markides, K. S., & Mindel, C. H. (1987). *Aging and Ethnicity*. Newbury Park, CA: Sage.

Martin, M. W. (1995). *Everyday morality: An introduction to applied ethics* (2nd ed.). Belmont, CA: Wadsworth.

Marty, M. (1987). Foreword. In L. E. Sullivan (Ed.), *Healing and restoring* (pp. ix–xiii). New York: Macmillan.

Maslow, A. (1968). *Toward a psychology of being* (2nd ed.). New York: Van Nostrand Reinhold.

Matlaw, J. R., & Mayer, J. B. (1986). Elder abuse: Ethical and practical dilemmas for social work. *Health and Social Work, 11*, 85–94.

Maves, P. (1949). *Older people and the church*. New York: Abingdon-Cokesbury.

May, W. F. (1983). *The physician's covenant: Images of the healer in medical ethics*. Philadelphia: Westminster Press.

McCarthy, T. (1978). *The critical theory of Jürgen Habermas*. Cambridge, MA: MIT Press.

McCormick, R. A. (1974). To save or let die: The dilemma of modern medicine. *JAMA, 229*, 172–176.

McCormick, R. A. (1987). *Health and medicine in the Catholic tradition*. New York: Crossroad.

McCulloh, E. B. (1990). Aging as a spiritual journey. *Generations, 14*(Fall), 56–60.

McCullough, L. B., & Chervenak, F. A. (1994). *Ethics in obstetrics and gynecology*. New York: Oxford University Press.

McCullough, L. B., & Wear, S. S. (1985). Respect for autonomy and medical paternalism reconsidered. *Theoretical Medicine, 6*, 295–308.

McCullough, L. B., & Wilson, N. L. (Eds.). (1995). *Long-term care decisions: Ethical and conceptual dimensions*. Baltimore: Johns Hopkins University Press.

McCullough, L. B., Wilson, N. L., Rhymes, J. A., & Teasdale, T. A. (1995). Managing the conceptual and ethical dimensions of long-term care decision making: A preventive ethics approach. In L. B. McCullough & N. L. Wilson (Eds.), *Long-term care decisions: Ethical and conceptual dimensions* (pp. 221–240). Baltimore: Johns Hopkins University Press.

McCullough, L. B., Wilson, N. L., Teasdale, T. A., Kolpakchi, A. L., & Skelly, J. R. (1993). Mapping personal, familial, and professional values in long-term care decisions. *Gerontologist, 33*(3), 324–332.

McDermott, C. J. (1989). Empowering the elderly nursing home resident: The resident rights campaign. *Social Work, 34* (March), 155–157.

McDonald, M. J. (1973). The management of grief: A study of black funeral practices. *Omega, 4,* 139–148.

McFadden, S., & Gerl, R. R. (1990). Approaches to understanding spirituality in the second half of life. *Generations, 14*(Fall), 35–38.

McGinnis, L. S. (1991). Therapies, 1990: An overview. *Cancer, 67*(6 Suppl.), 1788–1792.

McIntosh, J., & Santos, J. F. (1981a). Suicide among minority elderly: A preliminary investigation. *Suicide and Life-threatening Behavior, 11,* 151–166.

McIntosh, J., & Santos, J. F. (1981b). Suicide among Native Americans: A compilation of findings. *Omega, 11,* 303–316.

McLaughlin, C. (1988). Doing good: A worker's perspective. *Public Welfare, 46*(2), 29–32.

Meagher, M. S. (1993). Legal and legislative dimensions. In B. Byers & J. E. Hendricks (Eds.), *Adult protective services: Research and practice* (pp. 87–107). Springfield, IL: Charles C. Thomas Publisher.

Meddaugh, D. I. (1993). Covert elder abuse in the nursing home. *Journal of Elder Abuse and Neglect, 5*(3), 21–37.

Meisel, A. (1989). *The right to die.* New York: John Wiley & Sons.

Melden, A. I. (1981). Are there welfare rights? In P. G. Brown, C. Johnson, & P. Vernier (Eds.), *Income support: Conceptual and policy issues* (pp. 259–278). Totowa, NJ: Rowman & Littlefield.

Mendelson, M. A. (1974). *Tender loving greed: How the incredibly lucrative nursing home "industry" is exploiting America's old people and defrauding us all.* New York: Alfred A. Knopf.

Meyers, B. (1984). Minority group: An ideological formulation. *Social Problems, 31,* 1–15.

Michels, R. (1995). Priority setting in mental health. In P. J. Boyle & D. Callahan (Eds.), *What price mental health? The ethics and politics of setting priorities* (pp. 193–197). Washington, DC: Georgetown University Press.

Miles, S. H. (1994). Physicians and their patients' suicides. *JAMA, 271*(22), 1786–1788.

Miles, S. H., & Koepp, R. (1996). Comments on the AMA report "Ethical issues in managed care." *Journal of Clinical Ethics, 6*(4), 306–310.

Miles, S. H., & Meyers, R. (1994). Untying the elderly: 1989–1993 update. *Clinics in Geriatric Medicine, 10,* 513–526.

Mill, J. S. (1969). *Utilitarianism.* In *Collected works of John Stuart Mill.* Vol. 10. Toronto: University of Toronto Press.

Mill, J. S. (1979). *Utilitarianism.* Indianapolis: Hackett.

Miller, B., & Cafasso, L. (1992). Gender differences in caregiving: Fact or artifact? *Gerontologist, 32,* 498–507.

Miller, F. G., Quill, T. E., Brody, H., Fletcher, J. C., Gostin, L. O., & Meier, D. E. (1994). Regulating physician-assisted death. *New England Journal of Medicine, 331*(2), 119–123.

Miller, R. W. (1992). Moral realism. In L. C. Becker & C. B. Becker (Eds.), *Encyclopedia of ethics* (pp. 847–852). New York: Garland.

Miller, S. J. (1986). Conceptualizing interpersonal relationships. *Generations, 10*(4), 6–9.

Mills, D. Q. (1987). *Not like our parents: How the baby boom generation is changing America.* New York: William Morrow.

Minkler, M. (1994). Grandparents as parents: The American experience. *Ageing International, 21*, 24–28.

Minkler, M., & Roe, K. M. (1993). *Grandmothers as caregivers: Raising children of the crack cocaine epidemic.* Newbury Park, CA: Sage Publications.

Minkler, M., & Roe, K. M. (1996). Grandparents as surrogate parents. *Generations, 20*(1), 34–38.

Minkler, M., Roe, K. M., & Price, M. (1992). The physical and emotional health of grandmothers raising grandchildren in the crack cocaine epidemic. *Gerontologist, 32*, 752–761.

Mixson, P. M. (1995). An adult protective services perspective. *Journal of Elder Abuse and Neglect, 7*(2/3), 69–87.

Mixson, P. M. (1996). How adult protective services evolved, and obstacles to ethical casework. *Aging, 367*, 14–17.

Moberg, D. O. (1990). Spiritual maturity and wholeness in the later years. In J. J. Seeber (Ed.), *Spiritual maturity in the later years* (pp. 5–18). New York: Haworth Press.

Molis, D. B. (1992, August). Choice: It's the resident's right. *Provider*, pp. 19–29.

Mondragon, D. (1987). U.S. physicians' perceptions of malpractice liability factors in aggressive treatment of dying patients. *Medicine and Law: An International Journal, 6*, 441–447.

Moody, H. R. (1988). From informed consent to negotiated consent. *Gerontologist, 28*(Suppl.), 64–70.

Moody, H. R. (1990). The Islamic vision of aging and death. *Generations, 14*(Fall), 15–18.

Moody, H. R. (1992). *Ethics in an aging society.* Baltimore: Johns Hopkins University Press.

Moody, H. R. (1994, Fall). Simplicity. *Aging and the Human Spirit, 4*(2), 5.

Moore, J. W. (1970). The death culture of Mexico and Mexican Americans. *Omega, 1*, 271–291.

Morison, R. S. (1971). Death: Process or event? *Science, 173*, 694–698.

Morris, R. (1994). Public policy for the elderly: Are priorities shifting? Unfamiliar choices for advocates in the 1990s. *Journal of Aging and Social Policy, 6*(1/2), 1–8.

Morrison, R. S., Olson, E., Mertz, K. R., & Meier, D. E. (1995). The inaccessibility of advance directives on transfer from ambulatory to acute care settings. *JAMA, 274*(6), 478–482.

Moss, A. H. (1994). Dialysis decisions and the elderly. In G. A. Sachs & C. K. Cassel (Eds.), *Clinics in geriatric medicine: Clinical ethics* (pp. 463–473). Philadelphia: W. B. Saunders.

Mudd, E. (1981). Spiritual needs of terminally ill patients. *Bulletin of the American Protestant Hospital Association, 45*(3), 1–5.

Muilenburg, J. (1952). The ethics of the Prophet. In R. N. Anshen (Ed.), *Moral principles of action* (pp. 527–542). New York: Harper & Brothers.

Mumford, L. (1963). *Technics and civilization*. New York: Harcourt, Brace & World.

Murtaugh, C., Kemper, P., & Spillman, B. C. (1990). The risk of nursing home use in later life. *Medical Care, 28*(10), 952–962.

National Association of Social Workers. (1996). Ethical principles. In *The NASW code of ethics*. Washington, DC: Author.

National Center for Health Statistics. (1980). Final mortality statistics, 1978. *Monthly Vital Statistics Report, 29*(6, Suppl.).

National Center for Health Statistics. (1985). *Vital statistics of the United States, 1980* (Vol. 2). Washington, DC: U.S. Government Printing Office.

National Center for Health Statistics. (1996). *The National Home and Hospice Care Survey: 1993 summary*. Washington, DC: U.S. Government Printing Office.

National Center for Health Statistics. (1997). *Health, United States, 1996*. Washington, DC: U.S. Government Printing Office.

National Commission for the Protection of Human Subjects of Biomedical and Behavioral Research. (1978). *The Belmont report: Ethical principles and guidelines for the protection of human subjects of research*. DHEW (OS) 78-0014, Bethesda, MD.

National Health Lawyers Association. (1995). *Colloquium report on legal issues related to clinical practice guidelines*. Washington, DC: Author.

Newman, D. L., & Brown, R. D. (1996). *Applied ethics for program evaluation*. Thousand Oaks, CA: Sage Publications.

Noddings, N. (1984). *Caring: A feminine approach to ethics and moral education*. Berkeley: University of California Press.

Novick, A. (1991). Clinical trials with vulnerable or disrespected subjects. *AIDS and Public Policy Journal, 4*, 125–130.

Novick, P. (1988). *That noble dream*. New York: Cambridge University Press.

Noyes, L. E., & Silva, M. C. (1993). The ethics of locked special care units for persons with Alzheimer's disease. *American Journal of Alzheimer's Care and Related Disorders and Research, 8*(4), 12–15.

Nozick, R. (1977). *Anarchy, state and utopia*. New York: Basic Books.

O'Bryant, S. L. (1988). Sibling support and older widows' well-being. *Journal of Marriage and the Family, 50*, 173–183.

O'Connell, L. J. (1994). Health care reform: An act of faith? *Centerline: A Newsletter of the Park Ridge Center for the Study of Health, Faith, and Ethics, 3*(1),1.

Office of Technology Assessment. (1990). *Unconventional cancer treatments*. Washington, DC: U.S. Government Printing Office.

Office of Technology Assessment. (1992). *Special care units for people with Alzheimer's and other dementias: Consumer education, research, regulatory, and reimbursement issues*. Washington, DC: U.S. Government Printing Office.

Ogden, M., Spector, M. I., & Hill, C. (1970). Suicides and homicides among American Indians. *Public Health Reports, 85*, 75–80.

Older Women's League. (1989, May). *Failing America's caregivers: A status report on women who care*. Washington, DC: Older Women's League.

Olsen, D. P. (1993). Populations vulnerable to the ethics of caring. *Journal of Advanced Nursing, 18*, 1696–1700.

O'Malley, P. E. (1996). Group work with older people who are developmentally disabled and their caregivers. *Journal of Gerontological Social Work, 25*, 105–119.

Opler, M. E. (1946). Reaction to death among Mescalero Apache. *Southwestern Journal of Anthropology, 2*, 454–467.

Orgren, R. A. (1995). Personal communication.

Osgood, N. J. (1995). Assisted suicide and older people—a deadly combination: Ethical problems in permitting assisted suicide. *Issues in Law and Medicine, 10*, 415–435.

Ostfeld, A. M. (1980). Older research subjects: Not homogeneous, not especially vulnerable. *IRB: A Review of Human Subjects Research, 2*(8), 7–8.

Outhwaite, W. (1994). *Habermas: A critical introduction.* Stanford, CA: Stanford University Press.

Palgi, P., & Abramovitch, H. (1984). Death: A cross-cultural perspective. *Annual Review of Anthropology, 13*, 385–417.

Papougenis, D. (1991). Facilities continue to report restraint free status. *Untie the Elderly, 3*(1), 2.

Passel, J. S., & Robinson, J. G. (1984). *Revised estimates of the coverage of the population in the 1980 census based on demographic analysis: A report on work in progress.* Paper presented at the Annual Meeting of the American Statistical Association, Washington, DC.

Paton, R. N., Huber, R., & Netting, F. E. (1994). The long-term care ombudsman program and complaints of abuse and neglect: What have we learned? *Journal of Elder Abuse and Neglect, 6*(1), 97–115.

Paveza, G. J., Cohen, D., Eisdorfer, C., Freels, S., Todd, S., Ashford, J. W., Gorelick, P., Hirschman, Luchins, D., & Levy, P. (1992). Severe family violence and Alzheimer's disease: Prevalence and risk factors. *Gerontologist, 32*(4), 493–497.

Payne, B. (1975). *Love in the later years.* New York: Association Press.

Payne, B. K., & Cikovic, R. (1995). An empirical examination of the characteristics, consequences, and causes of elder abuse in nursing homes. *Journal of Elder Abuse and Neglect, 7*(4), 61–74.

Paz, O. (1961). *The labyrinth of solitude.* New York: Grove.

Pearce, R. G. (1994, March). Family values and legal ethics: Competing approaches to conflicts in representing spouses. *Fordham Law Review, 62*(5), 1253–1318.

Pearlman, R. A. (1994). Ethical issues in geriatric care. In W. R. Hazzard, E. Bierman, J. Blass, W. Ettinger, and J. Halter (Eds.), *Principles of geriatric medicine and gerontology* (pp. 397–408). New York: McGraw-Hill.

Pearlman, R. A., Cain, K. C., Patrick, D. L., Appelbaum-Maizel, M., Starks, H. E., Jecker, N. S., & Uhlmann, R. F. (1993). Insights pertaining to patient assessments of states worse than death. *Journal of Clinical Ethics, 4*(1), 33–41.

Pearlman, R. A., Cole, W., Patrick, D., Starks, H., & Cain, K. (1995). Advance care planning: Eliciting patient preferences for life-sustaining treatment. *Patient Education and Counseling, 26*, 353–361.

Perez-Tamayo, R. (1977). On death. *Advances in Thanatology, 4*(1), 82–97.

Peters, G. R., Hoyt, D. R., Babchuk, N., Kaiser, M., & Ijima, Y. (1987). Primary-group support systems of the aged. *Research on Aging, 9*(3), 392–416.

Piaget, J. (1965). *The moral judgment of the child* (2nd ed.). New York: Free Press.

Pifer, A., & Bronte, L. (Eds.). (1986). *Our aging society.* New York: W. W. Norton.

Pillemer, K. A. (1986). Risk factors in elder abuse: Results from a case-control study. In

K. A. Pillemer & R. S. Wolf (Eds.), *Elder abuse: Conflict in the family* (pp. 239–263). Dover, MA: Auburn House.

Pillemer, K., & Moore, D. W. (1989). Abuse of patients in nursing homes: Findings from a survey of staff. *Gerontologist, 29*(3), 314–320.

Plassman, B. L., & Breitner, J. C. (1996). Recent advances in the genetics of Alzheimer's disease and vascular dementia with an emphasis on gene-environment interactions. *Journal of the American Geriatrics Society, 44*(10), 1242–1250.

Pokorski, R. J. (1997). Insurance underwriting in the genetic era. *American Journal of Human Genetics, 60*(1), 205–216.

Poll: Seventy-nine percent support letting terminally ill refuse treatment. (1990, June 7). *Lexington Herald-Leader*, p. 3.

Post, S. G. (1992). Aging and meaning: The Christian tradition. In T. Cole, D. D. Van Tassel, & R. Kastenbaum (Eds.), *Handbook of the humanities and aging* (pp. 127–146). New York: Springer.

Post, S. G. (1994). Genetics, ethics, and Alzheimer disease. *Journal of the American Geriatrics Society, 42*(7), 782–786.

Post, S. G., & Whitehouse, P. J. (1995). Fairhill guidelines on ethics of the care of people with Alzheimer's disease: A clinical summary. *Journal of the American Geriatrics Society, 43*, 1423–1429.

Potter, J. F., & Jameton, A. (1986). Respecting the choices of neglected elders: Autonomy or abuse. In M. W. Galbraith (Ed.), *Elder abuse: Perspectives on an emerging crisis* (pp. 95–109). Kansas City, KS: Mid-America Congress on Aging.

Powell, B. V., & Link, R. C. (1994, March). The sense of a client: Confidentiality issues in representing the elderly. *Fordham Law Review, 62*(5), 1197–1251.

President's Commission for the Study of Ethical Problems in Medicine and Biomedical and Behavioral Research. (1982). *Making health care decisions* (Vols. 1–3). Washington, DC: U.S. Government Printing Office.

President's Commission for the Study of Ethical Problems in Medicine and Biomedical and Behavioral Research. (1983). *Deciding to forego life-sustaining treatment* (pp. 121–196). Washington, DC: U.S. Government Printing Office.

Price, R. (1948). *A review of the principal questions in morals* (3rd ed.). Oxford: Oxford University Press. (Reprint of 1787 edition)

Public Law No. 101–508 (1990).

Public professionals differ on ethics of health care reform. (1993). *Medical Ethics Advisor, 9*(12), 154–158.

Purtilo, R. B. (1991). Rehabilitation and technology: Ethical considerations. *International Journal of Technology and Aging, 4*(2), 163–170.

Quam, J. K., & Whitford, G. (1992). Adaptation and age-related expectations of older gay and lesbian adults. *Gerontologist, 32*, 367–374.

Quay, H. C., Johnson, V. S., & McClelland, K. (1980). *The economic, social, and psychological impacts on the elderly resulting from criminal victimization*. Paper presented at the Annual Meeting of the American Society of Criminology, San Francisco.

Quill, T. E. (1991). Death and dignity: A case of individualized decision making. *New England Journal of Medicine, 324*, 691–694.

Quill, T. E., Cassel, C. K., & Meier, D. E. (1992). Care of the hopelessly ill: Proposed clinical criteria for physician-assisted suicide. *New England Journal of Medicine, 327*, 1380–1384.

Quinn, M. J. (1985). Elder abuse and neglect: Raise new dilemmas. *Generations, 10*(2), 22–25.
Quinn, M. J., & Tomita, S. K. (1997). *Elder abuse and neglect: Causes, diagnosis, and intervention strategies* (2nd ed.). New York: Springer.
Rader, J. (1987). A comprehensive staff approach to problem wandering. *Gerontologist, 27*(6), 756–760.
Ramsey, P. (1973). *Health care and changing values*. Keynote presentation at the Institute of Medicine Conference, Washington, DC.
Rathbone-McCuan, E., & Whalen, M. C. (1992). Geriatric protective services and self-neglect. In E. Rathbone-McCuan & D. R. Fabian (Eds.), *Self-neglecting elders: A clinical dilemma* (pp. 144–160). New York: Auburn House.
Ratzan, R. M. (1980). "Being old makes you different": The ethics of research with elderly subjects. *Hastings Center Report, 10*(5), 32–42.
Rawls, J. (1971). *A theory of justice*. Cambridge, MA: Belknap Press of Harvard University Press.
Regan, J. J. (1981). Protecting the elderly: The new paternalism. *Hastings Law Journal, 32*(5), 1111–1132.
Regan, J. J. (1990). *The aged client and the law*. New York: Columbia University Press.
Regan, J.S.D. (1985). *The discovery of elder abuse: Learning to live in the brave new world of mandatory reporting, protective services, and public guardianship*. Paper presented at the Elder Abuse Prevention and Intervention Policy Conference, Chicago.
Rein, J. E. (1994, March). Clients with destructive and socially harmful choices—What's an attorney to do? Within and beyond the competency construct. *Fordham Law Review, 62*(5), 1101–1176.
Reinhardt, U. E. (1994). Managed competition in health care reform: Just another American dream, or the perfect solution? *Journal of Law, Medicine, and Ethics, 22*(2), 106–120.
Report from the Secretary's Task Force on Elder Abuse. (1992). Washington, DC: U.S. Department of Health and Human Services.
Reynolds, D. K., & Kalish, R. A. (1974). Anticipation of futurity as a function of ethnicity and age. *Journal of Gerontology, 29*, 224–231.
Reynolds, D. K., Kalish, R. A., & Farberow, N. L. (1975). A cross-ethnic study of suicide attitudes and expectations in the United States. In N. L. Farberow (Ed.), *Suicide in different cultures* (pp. 35–50). Baltimore: University Park Press.
Rhoden, N. K. (1988). Litigating life and death. *Harvard Law Review, 102*, 375–446.
Rhodes, M. L. (1991). *Ethical dilemmas in social work practice*. Milwaukee, WI: Family Service America.
Rhymes, J. (1990). Hospice care in America. *JAMA, 264*, 369–372.
Richardson, J. L., Solis, J. M., & Hisserich, J. C. (1984). Place of death of Hispanic persons in Los Angeles County. *Hispanic Journal of Behavioral Sciences, 6*, 161–168.
Roberts, A. R. (1990). *Helping crime victims: Research, policy, and practice*. Newbury Park, CA: Sage.
Roca, R. P. (1994, March). Determining decisional capacity: A medical perspective. *Fordham Law Review, 62*(5), 1177–1196.
Rollins, J. (1985). *Between women: Domestics and their employers*. Philadelphia: Temple University Press.

Romano, M. (1994, April). Unshackling the elderly. *Contemporary Long Term Care*, pp. 38–42.
Roof, W. C. (1994). *A generation of seekers: The spiritual journeys of the baby boom generation*. New York: HarperCollins.
Rooney, A. L. (1997). Everyday ethics and home health care challenges. *Home Health Care Management & Practice, 9*(6), 31–37.
Rosenthal, C. J. (1983). Aging, ethnicity and the family: Beyond the modernization thesis. *Canadian Ethnic Studies, 15*(3), 1–16.
Rosenthal, C. J. (1986). Family supports in later life: Does ethnicity make a difference? *Gerontologist, 26*, 19–24.
Ross, W. D. (1930). *The right and the good*. Oxford: Clarendon Press.
Roth, L. H., Meisel A., & Lidz, C. W. (1977). Tests of competency to consent to treatment. *American Journal of Psychiatry, 134*, 279–284.
Rothenberg, K. H. (1996). The Institute of Medicine's Report on Women and Health Research: Implications for IRBs and the research community. *IRB: A Review of Human Subjects Research, 18*, 1–3.
Rothman, D. J. (1991). *Strangers at the bedside*. New York: Basic Books.
Rubenstein, L. Z. (1996–1997). Update on preventive medicine for older people. *Generations, 20*(Winter), 47–53.
Rubin, B. L. (1985). Refusal of life-sustaining treatment for terminally ill incompetent patients: Court orders and an alternative. *Columbia Journal of Law and Social Problems, 19*, 47–68.
Ruddick, S. (1986). Maternal thinking. In M. Pearsall (Ed.), *Women and values* (pp. 340–351). Belmont, CA: Wadsworth.
Russell, C. (1993). The master trend. *American Demographics, 15*(10), 28–37.
Russell, C. (1995). The baby boom turns 50. *American Demographics, 17*(12), 22–33.
Sabatino, C. (1990). Client rights, regulations, and the autonomy of home-care consumers. *Generations, 14*(Suppl.), 21–24.
Sabin, J. E. (1995). General psychiatry and the ethics of managed care. *General Hospital Psychiatry, 17*(4), 293–298.
Sabin, J. E., & Daniels, N. (1994). Determining "medical necessity" in mental health practice. *Hastings Center Report, 24*(November–December), 5–13.
Sachs, G. A. (1994). Advance consent for dementia research. *Alzheimer Disease and Associated Disorders, 8*(Suppl. 4), 19–27.
Sachs, G. A., Rhymes, J., & Cassel, C. K. (1993). Biomedical and behavioral research in nursing homes: Guidelines for ethical investigations. *Journal of the American Geriatrics Society, 41*, 771–777.
Sadler, J., Wiggins, O., & Schwartz, M. (Eds.). (1994). *Philosophical perspectives on psychiatric diagnostic classification*. Baltimore: Johns Hopkins University Press.
Sage, W. M., Hastings, K. E., & Berenson, R. A. (1994). Enterprise liability for medical malpractice and health care quality improvement. *American Journal of Law and Medicine, 20*(1–2), 1–28.
Salend, E., Kane, R. A., Satz, M., & Pynoos, J. (1984). Elder abuse reporting: Limitations of statutes. *Gerontologist, 24*(1), 61–69.
Samuelson, R. J. (1990, October 29). Pampering the elderly. *Newsweek*, p. 61.
Sandel, M. (1982). *Liberalism and the limits of justice*. Cambridge: Cambridge University Press.

Sandrick, K. M. (1996, June 26). AMA opposes physician assisted suicide. *Medical Tribune News*, p. 1.
Sapp, S. (1995). Ethical perspectives. In M. Kimble, S. McFadden, J. Ellor, & J. Seeber (Eds.), *Aging, spirituality, and religion* (pp. 187–196). Minneapolis: Fortress Press.
Sarton, M. (1973). *As we are now*. New York: W. W. Norton.
Sartorius, R. (Ed.). (1983). *Paternalism*. Minneapolis: University of Minnesota Press.
Sattin, R. W., Rodriguez, J. G., DeVito, C. A., Lambert-Humber, D., & Stevens, J. A. (1991). The epidemiology of fall-related injuries among older persons. In R. Weindruch, E. C. Hadley., & M. G. Ory (Eds.), *Reducing frailty and falls in older persons* (pp. 44–56). Springfield, IL: Charles C. Thomas.
Saunders, C., & Baines, M. (1989). *Living with dying: The management of terminal disease*. Oxford: Oxford University Press.
Scallet, L. J., & Havel, J. T. (1995). Who will set priorities for mental health? In P. J. Boyle & D. Callahan (Eds.), *What price mental health? The ethics and politics of setting priorities* (pp. 69–80). Washington, DC: Georgetown University Press.
Schieber, G., Pollier, J., & Greenwald, L. (1991). Health care systems in twenty-four countries. *Health Affairs, 10*(3), 22–38.
Schmidt, W. C., Jr. (1995). *Guardianship: Court of last resort for the elderly and disabled*. Durham, NC: Carolina Academic Press.
Schneiderman, L. J., Faber-Langendoen, K., & Jecker, N. S. (1994). Beyond futility to an ethic of care. *American Journal of Medicine, 96*(2), 110–114.
Schneiderman, L. J., Jecker, N. S., & Jonsen, A. R. (1990). Medical futility: Its meaning and ethical implications. *Annals of Internal Medicine, 112*, 949–954.
Schneiderman, L. J., Kaplan, R. M., Pearlman, R. A., & Teetzel, H. (1993). Do physicians' own preferences for life-sustaining treatment influence their perceptions of patients' preferences? *Journal of Clinical Ethics, 4*(1), 28–33.
Schulz, R. (1976). Effects of control and predictability on the physical and psychological well-being of the institutionalized aged. *Journal of Personality and Social Psychology, 33*, 563–573.
Scott, J. P. (1983). Siblings and other kin. In T. H. Brubaker (Ed.), *Family relationships in later life* (pp. 47–62). Beverly Hills, CA: Sage.
Seckler, A. B., Meier, D. E., Mulvihill, M., & Paris, B. E. (1991). Substituted judgment: How accurate are proxy predictions? *Annals of Internal Medicine, 115*, 92–98.
Sehgal, A., Galbraith, A., Chesney, M., Schoenfeld, P., Charles, G., & Lo, B. (1992). How strictly do dialysis patients want their advance directives followed? *JAMA, 267*(1), 59–63.
Seicol, Rabbi. (1997). Limited by theological language. *Aging and Spirituality: Newsletter of American Society on Aging's Forum on Religion, Spirituality, and Aging, 9*(1), 1–8.
Seiden, R. H. (1970). We're driving young blacks to suicide. *Psychology Today, 4*(3), 24–28.
Seiden, R. H. (1981). Mellowing with age: Factors influencing the nonwhite suicide rate. *International Journal of Aging and Human Development, 13*, 265–282.
Selig, S., Tomlinson, T., & Hickey, T. (1991). Ethical dimensions of intergenerational reciprocity: Implications for practice. *Gerontologist, 31*(5), 624–630.
Sengstock, M. C., Hwalek, M., & Petrone, S. (1989). Services for aged abuse victims: Service types and related factors. *Journal of Elder Abuse and Neglect, 1*(4), 37–56.

Sengstock, M. C., McFarland, M. R., & Hwalek, M. (1990). Identification of elder abuse in institutional settings: Required changes in existing protocols. *Journal of Elder Abuse and Neglect, 2*(1/2), 31–50.

Sharpe, A. (1997, January 24). More states turn over mental-health care to the private sector. *Wall Street Journal*, pp. A1, A11.

Sherman, E. (1993). Mental health and successful adaptation in later life. *Generations, 17*(Winter/Spring), 43–46.

Sherman, E., Newman, E. S., Nelson, A., & Van Buren, D. (1975). *Crimes against the elderly in public housing: Policy alternatives.* Albany: State University of New York, School of Social Welfare.

Showstack, J., Lurie, N., Leatherman, S., Fisher, E., & Inui, T. (1996). Health of the public: The private-sector challenge. *JAMA, 276*(13), 1071–1074.

Shue, H. (1980). *Basic rights: Subsistence, affluence, and U.S. foreign policy.* Princeton, NJ: Princeton University Press.

Siegel, B., & Silverstein, S. (1994). *What about me? Growing up with a developmentally disabled sibling.* New York: Insight Books/Plenum.

Sievertsen, D., & Brown, K. (1996, November 19). Interview, Good Samaritan Hospital, Downers Grove, IL.

Silverstein, M., & Waite, L. (1993). Are blacks more likely than whites to receive and provide social support in middle and old age? Yes, no, and maybe so. *Journals of Gerontology, 48*(4), S212–S222.

Simmons, J. L. (1993). *67 ways to protect seniors from crime.* New York: Henry Holt.

Simmons, M. G. (1990). *The dilemma of secured units and the use of restraints.* Paper presented at the Annual Public Forum of the Alzheimer's Association, Washington, DC.

Simonsick, E. M., Lafferty, M., Phillips, C. L., Mendes de Leon, C., Kasl, S. V., Seeman, T. E., Fillenbaum, G., Hebert, P., & Lemke, J. (1993). Risk due to inactivity in physically capable older adults. *American Journal of Public Health, 83*, 1443–1450.

Simpson, E. L. (1974). Moral development research: A case study of scientific cultural bias. *Human Development, 17*, 81–106.

Singer, P. (Ed.) (1986). *Applied ethics.* Oxford: Oxford University Press.

Singer, P. (Ed.). (1994). *Ethics.* Oxford: Oxford University Press.

Smart, N., & Hecht, R. D. (Eds.). (1982). *Sacred texts of the world: A universal anthology.* New York: Crossroad.

Smith, G. P., II. (1996). *Legal and healthcare ethics for the elderly.* Washington, DC: Taylor & Francis.

Smith, L. (1989, March 27). What do we owe to the elderly? *Fortune*, pp. 54–62.

Smith, L. R., Milano, C. A., Molter, B. S, Elbeery, J. R., Sabiston, D. C., Jr., & Smith, P. K. (1994). Preoperative determinants of postoperative costs associated with coronary artery bypass graft surgery. *Circulation, 90*(5, Pt.2), 124–128.

Solomon, J. C., & Marx, J. (1995). To grandmother's house we go: Health and school adjustment of children raised solely by grandparents. *Gerontologist, 35*(3), 386–394.

Sorum, P. C. (1996). Ethical decision making in managed care. *Archives of Internal Medicine, 156*(18), 2041–2045.

Sowell, T. (1995). *The vision of the anointed: Self-congratulation as a basis for social policy.* New York: Basic Books.

Speare, A., & Avery, R. (1993). Who helps whom in older parent-child families? *Journals of Gerontology, 48*(2), S64–S73.
Speas, K., & Obenshain, B. (1995). *AARP: Images of aging in America: Final report.* Chapel Hill, NC: FGI Integrated Marketing.
Spencer, C. (1995). *Rights and responsibilities: Excerpts from a national workshop on ethical dilemmas in abuse and neglect cases involving older adults.* Paper presented at the Annual Scientific Meeting of the Gerontological Society of America, Los Angeles.
Spencer, C. (1996). Abuse and neglect of older adults: An examination of ethical dilemmas and a model for ethical decision-making. Paper presented at the Annual Scientific Meeting of the Gerontological Society of America, Washington, DC.
Spiegel, D., Bloom, J. R., Kraemer, H. C., & Gottheil, E. (1989). Effect of psychosocial treatment on survival of patients with metastatic breast cancer. *Lancet, 2*(8668), 888–891.
Stacey-Konnert, C. (1993). Preventive interventions for older adults. *Generations, 17*(Winter-Spring), 77–78.
Stacks, J. F. (1995–1996). Good Newt, bad Newt: Is the Gingrich vision of a brighter future worth the risk of a radically new direction in American governance? *Time, 146*(26), 90–95.
Stafford, R. S. (1991). The impact of nonclinical factors on repeat cesarean section. *JAMA, 265*(1), 59–63.
Stannard, C. I. (1973). Old folks and dirty work: The social conditions for patient abuse in a nursing home. *Social Problems, 20*(3), 329–342.
Steering Committee of the Physicians' Health Study Research Group. (1989). Final report on the aspirin component of the ongoing Physicians' Health Study. *New England Journal of Medicine, 321*(3), 129–135.
Stein, K. F. (1991). A national agenda for elder abuse and neglect research: Issues and recommendations. *Journal of Elder Abuse & Neglect, 3*(3), 91–108.
Steinmetz, S. K. (1981). Elder abuse. *Aging, 315/316*, 6–10.
Steinmetz, S. K. (1988). *Duty bound: Elder abuse and family care.* Newbury Park, CA: Sage.
Stone, D. (1988). *Policy paradox and political reason.* Glenview, IL: Scott, Foresman/Little, Brown College Division.
Stone, R., Cafferata, G. L., & Sangl, J. (1987). Caregivers of the frail elderly: A national profile. *Gerontologist, 27*(5), 616–626.
Straus, M. A., Gelles, R. J., & Steinmetz, S. (1980). *Behind closed doors: Violence in the American family.* Garden City, NY: Anchor Books.
Strauss, W., & Howe, N. (1991). *Generations: The history of America's future, 1584 to 2069.* New York: William Morrow.
Sullivan, L. W. (1989). *Keynote address and remarks.* Presented at the American Association of Retired Persons Minority Affairs Initiative Conference, Washington, DC.
Sung, K. T. (1990). A new look at filial piety. *Gerontologist, 30*(5), 610–617.
Superintendent of Belchertown State Sch. v. Saikewicz. 370 N.E. 2nd 417 (Mass. 1977).
Symer, M. (Ed.). (1993). Progress and prospects in mental health. *Generations, 17*(Winter-Spring).
Tatara, T. (1993). Understanding the nature and scope of domestic elder abuse with the use of state aggregate data: Summaries of the key findings of a national survey

of state APS and aging agencies. *Journal of Elder Abuse and Neglect, 5*(4), 35–57.
Tatara, T. (1995). *An analysis of state laws addressing elder abuse, neglect, and exploitation.* Washington, DC: National Center on Elder Abuse.
Tatara, T. (1996). *Elder abuse: Questions and answers* (6th ed.). Washington, DC: National Center on Elder Abuse.
Taylor, A. G., & Haussmann, G. M. (1988). Meaning and measurement of quality nursing care. *Applied Nursing Research, 1*(2), 84–88.
Taylor, C. (1989). *Sources of the self: The making of the modern identity.* Cambridge, MA: Harvard University Press.
ten Have, H. (1994). Principlism: A Western European appraisal. In E. DuBose, R. Hamel, & L. O'Connell (Eds.), *A matter of principles: Ferment in U.S. bioethics.* Valley Forge, PA: Trinity Press International.
ten Have, H.A.M.J. (1995). Medical technology assessment and ethics: Ambivalent relations. *Hastings Center Report, 25*(September–October), 13–19.
Tennstedt, S. L., Crawford, S., & McKinlay, J. (1993). Determining the pattern of community care: Is coresidence more important than caregiver relationships? *Journals of Gerontology, 48*(2), S74–S83.
Teno, J., Nelson, H. L., & Lynn, J. (Eds.). (1994). *Hastings Center Report, 24*(6) (Special Supplement), 31–36.
ter Meulen, R. (1996). Apolipoprotein E genotyping in Alzheimer's disease: National Institute on Aging/Alzheimer's Association Working Group. *Lancet, 347*(9008), 1091–1095.
ter Meulen, R., Topinkova, E., & Callahan, D. (1994). What do we owe the elderly? *Hastings Center Report, 24*, Special Report.
Thobaben, M. (1989). State elder/adult abuse and protection laws. In R. Filinson & S. R. Ingman (Eds.), *Elder abuse: Practice and policy* (pp. 138–152). New York: Human Sciences Press.
Tilak, S. (1989). *Religion and aging in the Indian tradition.* Albany: State University of New York Press.
Tillich, P. (1957). *The dynamics of faith.* New York: Harper & Brothers.
Tinetti, M. E., Liu, W. L., Marottoli, R. A., & Ginter, S. F. (1991). Mechanical restraint use among residents of skilled nursing facilities. *JAMA, 265*, 468–471.
Toffler, A., & Toffler, H. (1995). *Creating a new civilization: The politics of the third wave.* Atlanta: Turner.
Torres-Gil, F. (1994, October 14). Increased focus on crimes against the elderly is priority. *Older American Report*, p. 345.
Townsend, C. (1971). *Old age: The last segregation.* New York: Grossman.
Traxler, A. J. (1986). Elder abuse laws: A survey of state statues. In M. W. Galbraith (Ed.), *Elder abuse: Perspectives on an emerging crisis* (pp. 139–167). Kansas City, KS: Mid-America Congress on Aging.
Tremblay, P. R. (1994, March). Impromptu lawyering and de facto guardians. *Fordham Law Review, 62*(5), 1429–1445.
Truog, R., Brett, A., & Frader, J. (1992). The problem with futility. *New England Journal of Medicine, 326*(23), 1560–1564.
Twycross, R. G. (1974). Clinical experience with diamorphine in advanced malignant disease. *International Journal of Clinical Pharmacology, Therapy, and Toxicology, 7*(3), 184–198.

Uhlmann, R. F., Pearlman, R. A., & Cain, K. C. (1988). Physicians' and spouses' predictions of elderly patients' resuscitation preferences. *Journals of Gerontology, 43*(5), M115–M121.

U.S. Advisory Committee on Human Radiation Experiments. (1996). *Final report of the advisory committee on human radiation experiments.* New York: Oxford University Press.

U.S. Bureau of the Census. (1988). *Statistical abstract of the United States, 1988.* Washington, DC: U.S. Government Printing Office.

U.S. Bureau of the Census. (1989). *Projections of the population of the United States, by age, sex, and race: 1988 to 2080, by Gregory Spencer.* Washington, DC: U.S. Government Printing Office.

U.S. Bureau of the Census. (1990a). *The Hispanic population in the United States, March 1989* (Current Population Reports, Series P-20, No. 444). Washington, DC: U.S. Government Printing Office.

U.S. Bureau of the Census. (1990b). *Marital status and living arrangements, March 1989* (Current Population Reports, Series P-20, No. 445). Washington, DC: U.S. Government Printing Office.

U.S. Bureau of the Census. (1990c). *The need for personal assistance with everyday activities: Recipients and caregivers.* (Current Population Reports, Series P-70, No. 19). Washington, DC: U.S. Government Printing Office.

U.S. Bureau of the Census. (1990d). *Statistical Abstract of the United States, 1990.* Washington, DC: U.S. Government Printing Office.

U.S. Bureau of the Census. (1991, Summer). *The diverse living arrangements of children.* Washington, DC: U.S. Government Printing Office.

U.S. Bureau of the Census & Department of Housing and Urban Development. (1989). *American housing survey for the United States in 1987* (Series H-150–87). Washington, DC: U.S. Government Printing Office.

U.S. Department of Health and Human Services. (1990a). *Income of the population 55 or older, 1988* (Social Security Administration, No. 13-11871). Washington, DC: U.S. Government Printing Office.

U.S. Department of Health and Human Services. (1990b). *Resident abuse in nursing homes. Respondent perceptions of issues.* Washington, DC: U.S. Government Printing Office.

U.S. General Accounting Office. (1987). *Medicare and Medicaid: Stronger enforcement of nursing home requirements needed.* Washington, DC: U.S. General Accounting Office.

U.S. General Accounting Office. (1991). *Elder abuse: Effectiveness of reporting laws and other factors.* Gaithersburg, MD: U.S. General Accounting Office.

U.S. House Select Committee on Aging. (1981). *Elder abuse: An examination of a hidden problem* (Comm. Pub. No. 97–277). Washington, DC: U.S. Government Printing Office.

U.S. House Select Committee on Aging. (1986). *The rights of America's institutionalized aged: Lost in confinement.* Washington, DC: U.S. Government Printing Office.

U.S. House Select Committee on Aging. (1989). *Demographic characteristics of the older Hispanic population* (Comm. Pub. No. 100–696). Washington, DC: U.S. Government Printing Office.

U.S. House Select Committee on Aging. (1990). *Elder abuse: A decade of shame and inaction* (Comm. Pub. No. 101–752). Washington, DC: U.S. Government Printing Office.

References

U.S. Preventive Services Task Force. (1996). *Guide to clinical preventive services* (2nd ed.). Alexandria, VA: International Medical Publishing.

U.S. Senate Special Committee on Aging. (1992). *Aging America: Trends and projections*. Washington, DC: U.S. Government Printing Office.

U.S. Senate Special Committee on Aging, American Association of Retired Persons, Federal Council on the Aging, & U.S. Administration on Aging. (1991). *Aging America: Trends and projections*. Washington, DC: U.S. Department of Health and Human Services.

United States vs. Karl Brandt, Trials of War Criminals before the Nuremberg Military Tribunals Under Control Council Law #10. Volumes 1 & 2. 1948. Washington, DC: U.S. Government Printing Office.

Utech, M. R., & Garrett, R. R. (1992). Elder and child abuse: Conceptual and perceptual parallels. *Journal of Interpersonal Violence, 7*(3), 418–428.

van der Maas, P. J., van Delden, J. J., Pijnenborg, L., & Looman, C. W. (1991). Euthanasia and other medical decisions concerning the end of life. *Lancet, 338*, 669–674.

Venesy, B. A. (1994). A clinician's guide to decision making capacity and ethically sound medical decisions. *American Journal of Physical Medicine and Rehabilitation, 74*(Suppl.), 219–226.

Vinaya, M. (1982). The first sermon. In N. Smart & R. D. Hecht (Eds.), *Sacred texts of the world: A universal anthology* (p. 236). New York: Crossroad.

Vinton, L. (1992). An exploratory study of self-neglectful elderly. *Journal of Gerontological Social Work, 18*(1/2), 55–68.

Vladeck, B. (1980). *Unloving care*. New York: Basic Books.

Walker, M. (1989). Moral understandings: Alternative "epistemology" for a feminist ethics. *Hypatia, 4*(2), 15–28.

Wanzer, S. H., Adelstein, S. J., Cranford, R. E., Federman, D. D., Hook, E., Moertel, C. G., Safar, P., Stone, A., Taussig, H. B., & van Eys, J. (1984). The physician's responsibility toward hopelessly ill patients. *New England Journal of Medicine, 310*, 955–959.

Ward, R. A. (1979). *The aging experience*. New York: J. B. Lippincott.

Watson, M. M., Cesario, T. C., Ziemba, S., & McGovern, P. (1993). Elder abuse in long-term care environments: A pilot study using information from long-term care ombudsman reports in one California county. *Journal of Elder Abuse and Neglect, 5*(4), 95–111.

Waymack, M. H. (1991). Old age and the rationing of scarce health care resources. In N. Jecker (Ed.), *Aging and ethics: Philosophical problems in gerontology*. Totowa, NJ: Humana Press.

Weinstein, W. S., & Khanna, P. (1986). *Depression in the elderly*. New York: Philosophical Library.

Weir, R. F. (1989). *Abating treatment with critically ill patients: Ethical and legal limits to the medical prolongation of life*. New York: Oxford University Press.

Weisgraber, K. H., & Mahley, R. W. (1996). Human apolipoprotein E: The Alzheimer's disease connection. *FASEB Journal, 10*(13), 1485–1494.

Weld, T. D. (1969). *American slavery as it is*. New York: Arno.

Westat, Inc. (1989). *Hispanics. Final report*. Conducted for the Commonwealth Fund, Commission on Elderly People Living Alone. Rockville, MD: Westat, Inc.

Wetle, T. (1985). Ethical issues in long term care of the aged. *Journal of Geriatric Psychiatry, 18*(1), 63–73.

Wetle, T. T. (1987). Age as a risk factor for inadequate treatment. *JAMA, 258*(4), 516.

Wetle, T. T. (1993). Mental health and managed care for the elderly: Issues and options. In M. Smyer (Ed.), *Progress and prospects in mental health. Generations, 17*(Winter/Spring), 69–72.

Wetle, T. T. (1995). Ethical issues and value conflicts facing case managers of frail elderly people living at home. In L. B. McCullough & N. L. Wilson (Eds.), *Long-term care decisions: Ethical and conceptual dimensions* (pp. 63–86). Baltimore: Johns Hopkins University Press.

Wetle, T. T., & Fulmer, T. T. (1995). A medical perspective. In T. F. Johnson (Ed.), *Elder mistreatment: Ethical issues, dilemmas, and decisions* (pp. 31–48). Binghamton, NY: Haworth Press.

Wexler, D. B. (1990). *Therapeutic jurisprudence; The law as a therapeutic agent*. Durham, NC: Carolina Academic Press.

Wexler, D. B., & Winick, B. J. (1991). *Essays in therapeutic jurisprudence*. Durham, NC: Carolina Academic Press.

Whitbeck, C. (1996). Ethics as design: Doing justice to moral problems. *Hastings Center Report, 26*(3), 9–16.

Wiggins, S., Whyte, P., Huggins, M., Adam, S., Theilmann, J., Bloch, M., Sheps, S. B., Schechter, M. T., & Hayden, M. R. (1992). The psychological consequences of predictive testing for Huntington's disease: Canadian Collaborative Study of Predictive Testing. *New England Journal of Medicine, 327*(20), 1401–1405.

Williams, G. (1978). Euthanasia legislation: A rejoinder to nonreligious objections. In T. L. Beauchamp & S. Perlin (Eds.), *Ethical issues in death and dying* (pp. 232–240). Englewood Cliffs, NJ: Prentice-Hall.

Wilson, E. (1986). *The use of physical restraints in nursing homes*. Paper presented at the Annual Conference of the American Association of Homes for the Aging, New York.

Wilson, N. L. (1995). Long-term care in the United States: An overview of the current system. In L. B. McCullough & N. L. Wilson (Eds.), *Long-term care decisions: Ethical and conceptual dimensions* (pp. 35–59). Baltimore: Johns Hopkins University Press.

Wing, S., Manton, K. G., Stallard, E., Harnes, C. G., & Tyroler, H. A. (1985). The black/white mortality crossover: Investigation in a community-based study. *Journal of Gerontology, 40*, 78–84.

Winkler, D. (1983). Paternalism and the mildly retarded. In R. Sartorius (Ed.), *Paternalism* (pp. 83–94). Minneapolis: University of Minnesota Press.

Wolf, R. S. (1995). Current trends in elder abuse research. In *Service provider perspectives on family violence interventions: Proceedings of a workshop* (pp. 52–56). Washington, DC: National Academy Press.

Wood, E., & Karp, N. (1994). Mediation: Reframing care conflicts in nursing homes. *Generations, 18*(4), 54–57.

Working Group on Client Capacity. (1994, March). Report. *Fordham Law Review, 62*(5), 1003–1014.

Working Group on Client Confidentiality. (1994, March). Report. *Fordham Law Review, 62*(5), 1015–1026.

Working Group on Divestment. (1994, March). Report. *Fordham Law Review, 62*(5), 1063–1069.
Working Group on Intergenerational Conflicts. (1994, March). Report. *Fordham Law Review, 62*(5), 1037–1044.
Working Group on Spousal Conflicts. (1994, March). Report. *Fordham Law Review, 62*(5), 1027–1035.
Wydra, H. A. (1994, March). Keeping secrets within the team: Maintaining client confidentiality while offering interdisciplinary services to the elderly client. *Fordham Law Review, 62*(5), 1517–1545.
Wykle, M., & Musil, C. M. (1993). Mental health of older persons: Social and cultural factors. In M. Smyer (Ed.), *Progress and prospects in mental health. Generations, 17*(Winter/Spring), 7–12.
Wylie, F. M. (1971). Attitudes toward aging and the aged among black Americans: Some historical perspectives. *Aging and Human Development, 2*, 66–70.
Yamamoto, J. (1976). Japanese American suicides in Los Angeles. In J. Westermeyer (Ed.), *Anthropology and mental health* (pp. 29–35). The Hague: Mouton.
Yamamoto, J., Okonogi, K., Iwasaki, T., & Yoshimura, S. (1969). Mourning in Japan. *American Journal of Psychiatry, 125*, 1660–1665.
Young, P. A. (1990). Home-care characteristics that shape the exercise of autonomy: A view from the trenches. *Generations, 14*(Suppl.), 17–20.
Youngner, S. (1988). Who defines futility? *JAMA, 260*(14), 2094–2095.
Youngner, S. (1990). Futility in context. *JAMA, 264*(10), 1295–1296.
Zimmerman, J. McK. (Ed.). (1986). *Hospice: Complete care for the terminally ill* (2nd ed.). Baltimore: Urban & Schwarzenberg.
Zoloth-Dorfman, L., & Rubin, S. (1996). The patient as commodity: Managed care and the question of ethics. *Journal of Clinical Ethics, 6*(4), 339–357.
Zuckerman, C. (1994). Clinical ethics in geriatric care settings. *Generations, 18*(4), 9–13.

Author Index

AARP (American Association for Retired Persons), 215
Abramovitch, H., 39
Abramson, M., 17, 199, 205, 215
Achenbaum, W. A., 201, 217, 330, 342
Adam, S., 111
Adelstein, S. J., 128
Agich, G. J., 214, 313, 315, 323, 324
Aguilera, E., 28, 29, 31, 34, 36
Agus, J. B., 64
Ahmed, I., 171, 174, 175, 176, 182
Alford, R. R., 347
Ambrogia, D., 192
American Bar Association, 263
American College of Physicians, 301
American Medical Association, 108, 132, 312
American Psychiatric Association, 175
Anatore, B., 44
Anderson, H., 179, 184
Andrews, J., 29
Anema, M. G., 206
Anetzberger, G. J., 190, 194, 197, 198, 199, 218
Annas, G., 163
Antunes, G., 201, 202
Applebaum-Maizel, M., 103
Applegate, J., 243

Archea, C., 213
Aristotle, 12
Arnold, R. M., 213, 309, 323, 324
Aroskar, M. A., 214
Arras, J. D., 7, 112, 312, 314, 319, 323
Asch, D., 119
Ashford, J. W., 190
Atkinson, R., 176
Avery, R., 243
Azen, S., 99

Babchuk, N., 242
Bacchetta, M. D., 106
Bachman, R., 201, 202
Back, A., 107
Baier, A., 12, 257
Baines, M., 129, 136, 143, 145, 146
Bandman, E., 154
Barnes, A. P., 265
Barry, M. J., 132
Barthalis, P., 214
Battin, M., 106
Baumhover, L. A., 192, 194
Bayles, M. D., 127
Beasley, A. D., 153, 155
Beauchamp, T., 7, 8, 10, 11, 12, 15, 31, 99, 137, 151, 153, 154, 155, 161, 162, 163, 233, 290

Beauvoir, S. de, 211
Beck, P., 215
Beck, R. W., 243
Beck, S. H., 243
Becker, G., 198
Beecher, H., 291
Bengtson, J., 120
Bengtson, V. L., 41, 54, 241, 251
Benjamin, A. E., 309
Benson, M. L., 211
Bentham, J., 11
Berbig, L. J., 192
Berenson, R., 115, 116
Berkman, L., 196
Berlyne, D., 97
Bernstein, M., 176
Berrin, S., 235
Berry, J., 214
Bial, M. C., 199, 206
Bianchi, E., 78, 81, 85
Bigot, A., 198, 210
Billings, J., 107, 116, 117
Binney, E., 170, 334
Binstock, R. H., 216
Blackhall, L., 99
Blakeslee, J., 213
Blanton, P. G., 192, 330
Blauner, R. 39
Blazer, D., 79, 85
Blenkner, M., 197, 216
Bloch, M., 111
Block, S., 107
Bloom, J. R., 97
Bloom, M., 197, 216
Blustein, J., 229
Bodenheimer, B. J., 97
Bond, J., 2, 334
Bonhoeffer, D., 341, 346
Bookin, D., 208
Borowitz, E., 65
Boston, G., 203
Boyko, E. J., 141
Boyle, P., 165, 183
Braithwaite, V., 255
Brakman, S., 314, 315
Breitner, J. C., 110
Brett, A., 96
Brizius, J. A., 243

Brock, D., 106, 151, 153, 154, 155, 161, 162, 163
Brody, E., 206, 242, 243
Brody, H., 106, 141, 142, 311
Bronstein, J., 120
Bronte, L., 342
Brower, H. T., 212, 214
Brown, B., 214
Brown, K., 170–171, 172, 175
Brown, R. D., 11, 16, 339
Brown, S. A., 40
Browning, D., 177, 178
Brush, B. L., 192, 193
Buchanan, A., 151, 153, 154, 155, 161, 162, 163
Bulka, D., 83
Burrell, D., 166
Burstein, B., 199
Burton, L. A., 78
Burton, L. M., 241, 251–252
Butler, R. N., 4, 201, 343

Cafasso, L., 243
Cafferata, G. G., 206, 242
Cain, K C., 101, 103
Calkins, D. R., 97
Callahan, D., 1, 88, 92, 96, 123, 165, 183, 184, 236, 343, 348
Callahan, J. C., 21, 192
Callahan, J. J., Jr., 192, 199
Callender, W. D., Jr., 199
Campbell, D., 295
Campion, E., 298
Cantor, M., 242
Capezuti, E., 192, 193
Caplan, A. L., 1, 214, 324, 343
Carrese, J., 99, 100
Cassel, C. K., 141
Cassileth, B., 97
Catalano, D. J., 243
Cesario, T C., 217
Chardin, T. de, 68
Charles, G., 103
Chervenak, F. A., 309, 313, 321
Chesney, M., 103
Childress, J., 7, 8, 10, 11, 12, 15, 31, 99, 151, 153, 155, 161, 162, 163
Chrisman, N. J., 58

Christakis, N., 119
Christiansen, D., 68
Churchill, L. R., 143
Cicirelli, V. G., 242
Cikovic, R., 211
Clark-Daniels, C. L., 192, 194
Clough, R., 212
Cohen, A., 32
Cohen, D., 190
Cohen, E. S., 199, 206, 223
Cohen, G., 180
Cohen, H. J., 85
Cohen, J. S., 141
Cohen, R. L., 26
Cole, E. B., 257
Cole, T., 80, 183, 316, 343
Cole, W., 101
Coleman, N., 263
Coleman, P., 334
Collett, T. S., 263
Collins, M., 198
Collopy, B. J., 16, 17, 166, 199, 206, 207, 214, 313, 324
Conrad, N., 92
Cook, F. L., 201, 202
Cook, T., 201, 202, 295
Cooke, R., 300
Corless, I. B., 145, 146
Cortese, A. J., 32, 33, 39, 46, 55, 329
Coultrap-McQuin, S., 257
Covert, A., 212
Covey, H., 217
Coward, R. T., 242
Cowdry, E. V., 343
Coy, J. A., 206
Coyne, A. C., 190, 192
Cranford, R. E., 153, 155, 156
Cravedi, K. G., 192
Crawford, K. F., 214
Crawford, S. C., 75
Crawford, S., 242, 243
Crosby, E. M., 263
Crotty, M. T., 13
Crotty, R. B., 13
Crystal, S., 193
Cubillos, H. L., 38
Cuellar, J. B., 41

Curtis, J., 96
Cutler, S. J., 198

Daar, J., 119
Daniels, N., 165, 177, 183, 218
Daniels, R. S., 190, 192, 194
Danis, M., 102
David, D., 214
Davidson, G. W., 142
Davis, M. C., 206, 207
Dayton, C., 218
Declaration of Helsinki: Recommendations guiding medical doctors in biomedical research involving human subjects, 291
Dell, R., 171, 172
Delbanco, T. L., 97
Department of Health and Human Services, Dade County Public Health Unit, 303
DeVito, C., 303
DeVoe, M., 83
Dewey, J., 343
Dietz, M., 257
Dipasquale, R., 85
Dobrof, R., 206
Donegan, A., 12
Donnabedian, A., 115
Doty, P., 311
Doudera, A. E., 1
Downie, R. S., 144
Drane, J., 177
Dresser, R. S., 88, 101, 134
Dubin, B. A., 196
Dubler, N. N., 112, 206, 207, 208, 301, 302
Dubose, E. R., 344
Dugan, E., 230
Duke, J., 196, 197, 199
Dunham, H. W., 52
Dunkle, R. E., 212, 216
Durkheim, E., 33, 42
Durnbaugh T., 89
Dworkin, R., 12
Dwyer, J. W., 242

Eaddy, J. A., 153, 155
Eckert, J. K., 190

Egner, D. M., 102
Ehrenreich, B., 29
Eichrodt, W., 62
Eisdorfer, C., 190
Eisenberg, D., 97
Elbeery, J. R., 120
Eliot, T. S., 81, 346
Elman, C., 218
Emanuel, E. J., 98, 101, 104, 109, 132, 156, 158, 160
Emanuel, L. L., 98, 101, 104, 132, 156, 158, 160
Enck, R. E., 145–146
Engel, G., 318
Engelhardt, K. G., 284
Epstein, A., 121
Estes, C. L., 197, 334
Ettelson, L. M., 132
Eustis, N. N., 224, 225
Evans, M., 212

Faber-Langendoen, K., 97
Fabian, D. R., 196
Faden, R., 151, 153, 154, 155, 290
Fahey, C. J., 14, 80, 84, 173
Farberow, N. L., 44
Farris, B. E., 46
Faulkner, L. R., 192, 199
Featherstone, M., 217
Federman, D. D., 128
Feinberg, J., 12, 258
Feldman, D. M., 65
Ferguson, E. J., 198
Ferraro, K. F., 202
Ficarra, B., 120
Fiegener, J. J., 197
Fiegener, M., 197
Fihn, S. D., 141
Fillenbaum, G., 303
Finkel, S., 171
Finkelstein, J., 120
Finley, G. E., 201, 202
Finley, N. J., 243
Fins, J., 106
Fischer, D. H., 217
Fischer, L., 323–324
Fischer, L. R., 224, 225
Fischer, M. M., 40

Fisher, E., 110
Fitting, M. D., 207
Fletcher, J. C., 106, 141–142, 342
Foley, K. M., 106
Folstein, M., 299
Folstein, S. E., 299
Forrow, L., 309
Foster, C., 97
Foster, S. E., 243
Frader, J., 96
Frank, G., 99
Frankel, T., 264
Frankena, W. K., 12
Frankl, V., 83
Freedman, B., 151, 153, 154
Freels, S., 190
Freeman, I. C., 214
Friedan, B., 84
Friedland, R., 347
Friend, R., 260
Frodi, A. M., 190
Frolik, L. A., 265
Fulmer, T. T., 192, 193–194, 196

Galbraith, R., 103
Gallup, G., 129, 132, 136
Gamble, E. R., 132
Ganzini, L., 141, 176
Gardner, P., 2, 125–126
Garrett, J. M., 102
Garrett, R. R., 190
Gatsonis, C., 121
Gaul, A. L., 205, 206
Gaylin, W., 205
Gelfand, D. E., 203
Gelles, R. A., 190
George, L., 170, 171, 175–176
Gerber, L., 258
Gerl, S. S., 83
Gibson, J. M., 155, 207, 215
Gilbert, D. A., 193
Gilbert, J. P., 82
Gilligan, C., 4, 12, 32, 33, 247, 249, 257, 330
Ginter, S. F., 212
Glantz, L., 163
Glenn, N. D., 46
Goisman, R., 174, 175, 182

Gold, D. T., 243
Goldenberg, R., 120
Goldfield, N., 116, 117
Goldman, B., 213
Goldner, N. S., 42
Goldscheider, C., 39
Goldsmith, J., 201
Goldsmith, S. S., 201
Goli, V., 85
Gordon, M. M., 32
Gorelick, P., 190
Gostin, L. O., 106, 141–142
Gottheil, E., 97
Gottlich, V., 268
Graber, G., 153, 155
Gramelspacher, G., 95
Granieri, R., 212
Green, B. A., 263
Greenberg, J., 26
Greenfield, J., 251
Greenwald, L., 310
Griffin, J., 162
Grob, G., 170, 183
Gubrium, J. F., 133, 211
Guccione, A. A., 206
Gurian, B., 174, 175, 182
Gutmann, D., 180, 183, 348

Habermas, J., 32, 33, 34, 204, 326, 331, 335, 339, 346
Haddad, A. M., 207
Halamandaris, V. J., 211
Hamann, A. A., 134
Hamel, R., 344
Hanks, R. S., 244
Hare, R. M., 11
Harmon, L., 134
Harnes, C. G., 35
Harris, D. K., 211
Harris, L., 201
Harsanyi, J. C., 32
Hartwell, S., 170
Hastings, K. E., 115, 116
Hatcher, C., 44
Hatcher, D., 44
Hauerwas, S., 166
Haussmann, G., 118
Havel, J., 171

Havighurst, C., 116, 117
Havighurst, R. J., 32
Hawkins, A. F., 28, 35
Hayden, M. R., 111
Hayes, C., 198, 199
Haywood, J., 120
Health Care Financing Administration, 213
Hebert, P., 303
Hecht, R. D., 71
Hegland, A., 217
Heintz, L., 156, 158, 160
Hennessy, C. H., 232
Henshel, R. L., 26
Hepworth, M., 217
Herskovits, M. J., 26, 39
Heschel, A. J., 220
Hiatt, E., 171, 172
Hickey, T., 206
Hielema, F., 102
High, D. M., 16, 127, 130, 132, 133, 135, 156, 158, 160, 240, 301, 302
Hill, C., 54
Hill, T. P., 178, 179
Hirschel, A. E., 212
Hisserich, J. C., 45
Hobbs, L., 198
Hofland, B. F., 151, 153, 214, 311
Hogstel, M. O., 205, 206
Holstein, J. A., 133
Holstein, M., 173, 316, 334
Holzberg, C. S., 58
Honegger, H., 96
Hook, E., 128
Hooyman, N., 239, 243, 255
Hoppe, S. K., 44
Horowitz, A., 206
Horowitz, G., 197
Horowitz, R. I., 196
Horstman, P., 198
Horwitz, A., 243
Hospers, J., 20
Howe, N., 218
Hoyt, D. R., 242
Huber, R., 214
Hudson, B. L., 2, 125, 126
Hudson, R. B., 216, 218
Huggins, M., 111

Hughes, M. M., 207
Hume, D., 90
Humphry, D., 106
Hunt, A. D., 13
Hunt, S. S., 215
Hwalek, M., 200, 211

Iga, M., 52
Ignatieff, M., 169, 171, 179, 184
Iijima, Y., 242
In the matter of Karen Quinlan, 127
In re O'Connor, 134
Inui, T., 110
Iozzio, M. J., 207
Iwasaki, T., 47

Jackson, J. J., 35, 40
Jameton, A., 198, 199
Jamison, J., 240
Jecker, N. S., 1, 95, 97, 100, 236, 314, 315
Jennings, B., 121
Jennings, J., 248
Jewell, E., 215
Job, S., 206
Johnson, C. L., 55, 243
Johnson, J., 298
Johnson, S. H., 212
Johnson, T. F., 4, 7, 8, 18, 207, 218, 329–330
Johnson, V. S., 201, 202
Jones, J. S., 193
Jonsen, A. R., 12, 95, 141, 153, 155, 291
Jost, T. S., 116

Kaiser, M., 242
Kalb, P. E., 115, 116
Kalish, R. A., 39, 41, 42, 43, 44, 45, 46, 50, 51, 52, 53
Kamisar, Y., 140
Kane, R. A., 1, 17, 189, 193, 208, 213, 214, 215, 306, 309, 316, 317, 321, 324
Kane, R. L., 189, 306, 309
Kant, I., 11, 32, 33, 254–255, 258, 264
Kaplan, R. M., 103
Kapp, M. B., 1, 192, 198, 203, 210, 240, 241, 259, 270
Karp, N., 216

Kart, C. S., 212
Kasl, S. V., 303
Kasper, J. F., 294
Kass, L. R., 27
Kassler, J., 115, 116, 121
Kastenbaum, R. J., 55, 343
Kaufman, S. R., 198
Kavesh, W., 182
Kaye, L. W., 243
Kelly, T., 248
Kelman, H. C., 56
Kemper, P., 118
Kessler, R. C., 97
Khanna, P., 215
Kiefer, C. W., 51
Kildee, D. E., 28, 35
Kimboko, P., 215
King, P. A., 161, 162
Kitchener, K. S., 15, 195
Kitwood, T., 167
Kivett, V. R., 230
Kivnick, H. Q., 179, 180, 208
Kiyak, H. A., 239, 243, 255
Kleinman, A., 58
Klosterman, E., 208
Kluckhohn, C., 53
Klys, M., 286
Knight, J. A., 246
Koenig, H. G., 84, 85, 170, 176
Koenig, R., 42
Koepp, R., 108
Kohlberg, L., 32–33, 34
Kolpakchi, A. L., 207, 313
Korbin, J. E., 190
Korte, A. O., 55
Kraemer, H. C., 97
Kraft, F., 170
Kravitz, M., 203
Kresojevich, R., 42
Kripalani, A., 59
Krishnan, K., 85
Krone, M. R., 96
Kropf, N. P., 248
Kudler, H. S., 85
Kultgen, J., 339
Kunitz, S. J., 54
Kushner, T. K., 215

Author Index

Labouvie-Vief, G., 83
Lachs, M. S., 196, 218
Ladd, J., 127, 137
Lafferty, M., 303
LaGrange, R. L., 202
Lambert-Humber, D., 303
Lamm, R. D., 118, 121
Lammers, W. W., 216
Lantos, J., 95
Lapidus, I. M., 80
Latimer, E., 246
Lawson, W. T., 192, 193
Lawthers, A. G., 120
Lawton, M. P., 201, 299
Leatherman, S., 110
Lebowitz, B. D., 179, 202
Lee, M. A., 141
Leff, I. M., 263
Lehmann, P., 195
Lelong, J., 196
Lemke J., 303
Lesnoff-Caravaglia, G., 1, 274, 286
Levin, J. S., 173, 179, 182
Levine, C., 303
Levine, R., 298
Levy, J. E., 54
Levy, P., 190
Lewis, H., 42
Lichstein, P. R., 132
Lidz, C. W., 151, 153, 213, 323, 324
Lieb, I. C., 317
Link, R. C., 264
Liu, W. L., 212
Llewellyn, K. N., 270
Localio, A. R., 120
Locke, J., 256
Lockwood, G., 42
Loewy, E.H., 109
Lofgren, R. P., 212
Logstrup, K. E., 332
Logue, B. J., 142
London, C., 192
Long, J. B., 49, 51
Longres, J. F., 196, 199
Looman, C. W., 106
Lopez, C., 28, 29, 31, 34, 36
Lopez, G. P., 264
Loya, F., 44

Luchins, D., 190
Luke, H. M., 349
Lurie, N., 110
Lusk, E. J., 97
Lustbader, W., 196
Lynn J., 101, 132, 298

MacAdam, M., 222
Machalek, R., 35, 42
MacIntyre, A., 99
Macionis, J. J., 31, 32
Mackie, J. L., 11
MacNamara, R. D., 211
MacPherson, D. S., 212
Maddox, G., 343
Madsen, W., 43
Magee, J. J., 81
Mahey, R. W., 111
Maldonado, D., 55, 243
Mandelbaum, D., 39
Mannheim, K., 33
Manning, R., 257
Manthorpe, J., 194
Manton, K. G., 35
Margulies, P., 263
Mariner, W. K., 116
Markides, K. S., 25, 35, 40, 42, 43, 53, 55
Marottoli, R. A., 212
Martin, H. W., 44
Martin, M., 253, 256
Marty, M. W., 60
Marx, J., 251
Maslow, A., 278
Matlaw, J. R., 193
Maves, P., 343
May, W. F., 80, 86, 89, 90
Mayer, J. B., 193
McCarthy, T., 335
McClelland, K., 201, 202
McCormick, R. A., 68, 127
McCulloh, E. B., 82, 83
McCullough, L. B., 1, 14, 207, 307, 309, 312, 313, 314, 317, 321, 330
McDermott, C. J., 215
McDonald, M. J., 42
McDonald, P. J., 132
McFadden, S., 83

McFarland, M. R., 211
McGinnis, L. S., 97
McGovern, P., 217
McHugh, P. R., 299
McIntosh, J., 52, 54
McKinlay, J., 242, 243
McLaughlin, C., 199
McMonagle, P., 218
McNeil, B. J., 121
McReady, W. C., 202
Meador, K. G., 85
Meagher, M. S., 193
Meddaugh, D. I., 211
Meier, D. E., 106, 134, 141–142, 158, 160
Meisel, A., 134, 151, 153
Melden, A. I., 256
Mendelson, M. A., 211
Mertz, K. R., 158, 160
Mestrovic, S. G., 32
Meszaros, J., 197
Meyers, B., 26
Meyers, R., 302
Michel, V., 99
Michels, R., 183
Milano, C. A., 120
Miles, S. H., 95, 106, 108, 214, 302
Mill, J. S., 12, 258
Miller, B., 243
Miller, C. A., 194, 198
Miller, F. G., 106, 141–142
Miller, R. W., 315
Miller, S. J., 221, 231
Mills, D. Q., 218
Mindel, C. H., 25, 35, 40, 42, 43, 53, 55
Minkler, M., 251
Minogue, W. F., 116, 117
Mixson, P. M., 198, 199
Moberg, D. D., 81
Moertel, C. G., 128
Molis, D. B., 215
Molter, B. S., 120
Mondragon, D., 119
Moody, H. R., 1, 16, 80, 81, 86, 93, 118, 204, 208, 218, 315, 335, 343
Moore, D. W., 211
Moore, J. W., 26
Morison, R. S., 136

Morris, R., 218
Morrison, R. S., 158, 160
Moss, A. H., 121
Mudd, E., 92
Muilenburg, J., 62, 63
Mulley, A. G., Jr., 294
Mulvihill, M., 134
Mumford, L., 274
Murphy, S. T., 99
Murtaugh, C., 118
Musil, C. M., 171, 173, 174, 175, 182
Myllenbeck, S., 212

National Center for Health Statistics, 34, 35, 126
Nelson, A., 201
Nelson, H. D., 141
Nelson, H. L., 132
Netting, F. E., 214
Newman, D. L., 11, 16, 339
Newman, E. S., 201
Newport, F., 129, 132, 136
NHLA (National Health Lawyers Association), 117
Niederehe, G., 179
Nielson, M., 197, 216
Nitzberg, R., 203
Noddings, N., 257
Norlock, F. E., 97
Novick, A., 302
Novick, P., 341
Noyes, L. E., 213

Obenshain, B., 206
O'Brien, J. G., 194
O'Brien, S., 194
O'Bryant, S. L., 243
O'Connell, L. J., 124, 344
Office of Technology Assessment, 1990, 189
Office of Technology Assessment, 1992, 213
Ogden, M., 54
Okonogi, K., 47
Older Women's League, 242
Olsen, D. P., 247
Olson, E., 158, 160
O'Malley, P. E., 248, 250

Author Index

O'Malley, T. A., 193–194
Orgren, R. A., 296
Osgood, N. J., 171, 175, 179
Ostfeld, A. M., 298
Outhwaite, W., 335

Palgi, P., 39
Papougenis, D., 213
Paris, B. E., 134
Park, D. R., 96
Parker, L. S., 309
Passel, J. S., 36
Paton, R. N., 214
Patrick, D. L., 101, 102, 103
Paveza, G. J., 190
Payne, B., 343
Payne, B. K., 211
Paz, O., 42
Peace, S., 2
Pearce, R. G., 263
Pearlman, R. A., 85, 86, 96, 100, 101, 103, 107
Penrod, J. D., 208
Perez-Tamayo, R., 43
Perlin, S., 137
Petenza, M., 192
Peters, G. R., 242
Petrone, S., 200
Phillips, C. L., 303
Piaget, J., 32, 33
Pickard, C. G., 102
Pieper, C., 85
Pies, H. E., Jr., 1
Pifer, A., 342
Pijnenborg, L., 106
Pillemer, K. A., 190, 194, 211
Plassman, B. L., 110
Pokorski, R. J., 112
Pollier, J., 310
Post, S. G., 93, 110, 208
Potter, J. F., 198, 199
Powell, B. V., 264
President's Commission for the Study of Ethical Problems in Medicine and Biomedical and Behavioral Research, 127, 133, 137
Price, M., 251
Price, R., 314

Prieto, M. M., 38
Public professionals differ on ethics of health care reform, 122
Purtilo, R. B., 206
Pynoos, J., 193

Quam, J. K., 260
Quay, H. C., 201, 202
Quill, T. E., 106, 141–142
Quinn, M. J., 192, 195, 268

Rader, J., 213
Ragan, P. K., 41
Ramsey, P., 123
Rathbone-McCuan, E., 196, 197
Ratzan, R. M., 301
Rawls, J., 12, 17, 32, 33
Regan, J. J., 192, 193, 218
Regan, J.S.D., 199
Rein, J. E., 264
Reinhard, S. C., 243
Reinhardt, U. E., 115, 116, 119
Report from the Secretary's Task Force on Elder Abuse, 217
Reynolds, D. K., 39, 41, 42, 43, 44, 45, 46, 50, 51, 52, 53
Rhoden, N. K., 134
Rhodes, L. A., 99
Rhodes, M. L., 7, 12, 20, 331
Rhymes, J., 142, 309, 317
Richardson, J. L., 45
Robertson, J. A., 134
Robinson, J. G., 36
Roca, R. P., 263
Rodrigues, T., 212
Rodriguez, J. G., 303
Roe, K. M., 251
Rollins, J., 225
Romano, M., 213
Roof, W. C., 80
Rooney, A. L., 206
Rosenthal, C. J., 54, 55, 241
Ross, W. D., 255
Roth, L. H., 151, 153
Rothenberg, K. H., 291
Rothman, D. J., 299
Rubenstein, L. Z., 181–182
Rubin, B. L., 154

Rubin, S., 109
Russell, C., 218

Sabatino, C., 208
Sabin, J. E., 165, 172, 177, 183
Sabiston, Jr., D. C., 120
Sachs, G. A., 301, 302
Sadler, J., 165
Safar, P., 128
Sage, W. M., 115, 116
Salend, E., 193
Samuelson, R. J., 217
Sanchez-Gonzalez, M., 95
Sandel, M., 12
Sandrick, K. M., 141
Sangl, J., 206, 242
Santos, J. F., 52, 54
Sapp, S., 184
Sarton, M., 211
Sartorius, R., 155
Sattin, R. W., 303
Satz, M., 193
Saunders, C., 129, 136, 143, 145, 146
Scallet, L., 171
Schechter, M. T., 111
Schieber, G., 310
Schmidt, T. A., 141
Schmidt, W. C., Jr., 265
Schneider, R., 170
Schneiderman, L. J., 95, 97, 103
Schoenfeld, P., 103
Schulz, R., 215
Schwartz, M., 165
Seckler, A. B., 134
Seeman, T. E., 303
Sehgal, A., 103
Seicol, Rabbi S., 82
Seiden, R. H., 42
Selig, S., 206
Sengstock, M. C., 200, 211
Settles, B. H., 244
Shapiro, G., 95
Sharpe, A., 172
Shelp, F., 85
Sheps, S. B., 121
Sherman, E., 179, 180, 201
Showstack, J., 110
Shrager, D. S., 116, 117

Shue, H., 229
Sibert, T., 85
Siegel, B., 250
Siegler, M., 95
Sievertsen, D., 170–171, 172, 175
Silva, M. C., 213
Silverstein, M., 95, 243
Silverstein, S., 250
Simmons, J. L., 203
Simmons, G., 213
Simonsick, E. M., 303
Simpson, E. L., 33
Singer, P., 10, 13, 95
Skelly, J. R., 207, 314
Skogan, W. G., 201, 202
Smart, N., 71
Smith, B. K., 196
Smith, G. P., II, 1
Smith, J. L., 102
Smith, L., 217, 218
Smith, L. R., 120
Smith, P. K., 120
Solis, J. M., 45
Solomon, J. C., 251
Solomon, K., 212
Sorum, P. C., 109
Sowell, T., 264
Speare, A., 243
Speas, K., 206
Spector, M. I., 54
Spencer, C., 215, 218
Spiegel, D., 97
Spillman, B. C., 118
Sprafka, J. M., 212
Spring, J. C., 198, 199
Stacey-Konnert, C., 182
Stacks, J. F., 218
Stafford, R. S., 120
Stallard, E., 35
Stannard, C. I., 211
Starks, H. E., 101, 103, 107
Steering Committee for Physicians' Health Study Research Group, 294
Stein, K. F., 194
Steinmetz, S., 190
Stevens, J. A., 303
Stocking, C., 95
Stoeckle, J. D., 132

Stone, A., 128
Stone, D., 169
Stone, R., 206, 242
Strasser, D., 213
Strauss, M. A., 190
Strauss, W., 218
Strouse, T. B., 97
Sung, K. T., 15, 18
Swan, J., 170

Takeshita, J., 171, 174, 175, 176, 182
Tatai, K., 52
Tatara, T., 192, 193, 197
Taussig, H. B., 128
Taylor, A., 118
Taylor, C., 166, 168, 341
Teasdale, T. A., 207, 309, 313, 317
Teetzel, H., 103
Telfer, E., 144
ten Have, H.A.M.J., 117, 166
Tennstedt, S. L., 242, 243
Teno, J., 132
ter Meulen, R., 111, 348
Theilmann, J., 111
Thobaben, M., 192
Tilak, S., 76
Tilden, V. P., 141
Tillich, P., 59
Tinetti, M. E., 212
Tisdale, W. A., 198
Tobin, S. S., 173, 179, 182
Todd, S., 190
Toffler, A., 218
Toffler, H., 218
Tolle, S. W., 141
Tomita, S. K., 192, 194
Tomlinson, T., 206
Torres-Gil, F., 203
Toulmin, S., 12, 291
Townsend, C., 210
Traxler, A. J., 199
Tremblay, P. R., 264
Trials of War Criminals Before the Nuremberg Military Tribunals, 291
Truog, R., 96
Turner, H. B., 133, 135
Twycross, R. G., 146
Tyroler, H. A., 35

Urv-Wong, E. K., 214
U.S. Advisory Committee on Human Radiation Experiments, 290
U.S. Bureau of Census, 29, 34, 35, 38, 126, 243, 250
U.S. Bureau of Census Department of Housing and Urban Development, 38
U.S. Department of Health and Human Services, 25, 34, 35, 58, 211
U.S. General Accounting Office, 193, 214
U.S. House Select Committee on Aging, 29, 192, 193, 211
U.S. National Commission for the Protection of Human Subjects, 291
U.S. Preventive Services Task Force, 293
U.S. Senate Special Committee on Aging, 211, 216
United States vs. Karl Brandt, Trials of War Criminals, 291
Utech, M. R., 190

van Delden, J. J., 106
van der Maas, P. J., 106
Van Tassel, D., 343
Venesy, B. A., 151, 153, 161
Vinton, L., 196

Waite, L., 243
Walker, M., 257
Wallace, J. I., 107
Wanzer, S. H., 128
Ward, R. A., 39
Warwick, D. P., 56
Watson, M. M., 217
Waxman, H. A., 116, 117
Wear, S. S., 312
Weber, R., 197, 216
Weinstein, W. S., 215
Weisgraber, K. H., 111
Weld, T. D., 40
Welge, C., 212
Wennberg, J. E., 294
Westat, Inc., 29, 38
Wetle, T. T., 18, 85, 165, 192, 214, 313, 316, 317
Wexler, D. B., 269

Whalen, M. C., 197
Whitbeck, C., 208
Whitehouse, P. J., 208
Whitford, G., 260
Whittington, F., 213
Whyte, P., 111
Wiggins, O., 165
Wiggins, S., 111
Williams, G., 140
Wilson, E., 212
Wilson, N. L., 1, 14, 207, 307, 309, 313, 316, 317, 320, 330
Wing, S., 35
Winick, B. J., 269
Winkler, D., 153
Winkler, M. G., 80
Wolf, R. S., 216
Wood, E., 216
Wood, R. W., 141
Working Group on Client Capacity, 264

Working Group on Client Confidentiality, 264
Working Group on Divestment, 263
Working Group on Intergenerational Conflicts, 263
Working Group on Spousal Conflicts, 263
Wydra, H. A., 264
Wykle, M., 171, 173, 174, 175, 182

Yaffe, S., 201
Yamamoto, J., 47, 52
Yoshimura, S., 47
Young, P. A., 167, 206
Younger, S., 95, 96

Ziemba, S., 217
Zimmerman, J. McK., 142
Zoloth-Dorfman, L., 109
Zuckerman, C., 206, 207

Subject Index

Abandonment, 191, 199
Abstract ideals, 13
Abuse, 267–269
Access: to insurance, 170; to services, 172, 176
Accommodation, 208
Accountability, 19, 327–328
Acute care decisions, 311–312
Addiction, 146
Administration on Aging, 203
Adult protective services, 192, 193, 194–195, 196, 216; definition, 197; evolution of, 197–198; hierarchy of principles, 194; involuntary, 199; and self-neglect, 197
Advance care planning, 100
Advance directives, 87, 102, 123, 125, 129–132, 156–160, 163, 301; apppropriateness, 123; difficulties, 156, 159–160; performative, 160; planning 266–267; proxy directives, 157–159; for research, 301–302. *See also* Durable powers of attorney; Living wills
Advocacy, 87
Advocates, 263–264
African Americans, 39–42; attitudes, toward life, death and suicide, 40–41; funerals and the church, 42
Age, 64–68, 70–76

Ageism, 175, 192, 199, 201, 203, 206. *See also* Social attitudes
Aging, females, 283; losses, 282; nomenclature, 282; sex, 286
Aging of America, 150–153
Aging services, approach to home care, 223
Aging society, 342
Alcohol abuse, 176
Alcoholism, 247
Alzheimer's disease, 88, 152, 189, 208, 209, 246; special care units, 213. *See also* cognitive impairment
American Association of Retired Persons, 203, 206
American Bar Association, Commission on Legal Problems of the Elderly, 215
American College of Health Care Administrators, 214
American Psychiatric Association, 175
Americans with Disabilities Act, 262
Analgesics, 129, 146
Andrew House, 215
Animism, 13
Anxiety: as diagnosable disorder, 175; as symptom, 175
Applied ethics, 13–14
Aristotle, 340

Subject Index

Asset transfers, 261, 263, 270
Astronauts, 275–276
Attorneys, 262–264
Autism, 247
Autonomy, 16–17, 86, 129, 133, 147, 151–153, 187, 193, 195, 198, 199, 204, 205–208, 210, 212, 219, 327–328; dignity, 167–68; preserving at home, 206–209; preserving in institutions, 214–216; sense of self, 166–167

Baby boomers, 218
Balanced interest, 326–330, 332–333, 335
Belmont Report, 291
Beneficence, 17, 187, 195, 198, 204, 212, 290, 327–328
Benjamin Rose Institute, 215, 216
Best interests, 133–134, 154, 162–164
Bible, 61, 70
Bioethicists, 343
Biomedicine and mental illness, 175, 177, 178. *See also* Mental health care; Mental illness
Blinding (research), 293
Borowitz, Eugene, 65
Brave "old" world, 274
Buddhism, 48–49, 60–61

Canada National Workshop on Ethical Dilemmas in Abuse and Neglect Cases Involving Older Adults, 218
Cardiopulmonary resuscitation (CPR), 152, 157
Cardiovascular disease, 152
Care, home, 148; palliative, 142. *See also* Symptom care/control
Care (case) management, 221, 223
Caregiver burden, 255
Caregivers, 240–243, 246–247, 259; gender of, 243–244
Case analysis: Anna, 195–196, 198–199; Catherine, 204–205, 207; George, 200; Virginia, 209, 210; Wilma and Thomas, 188–199
Chardin, Teilhard de, 68
Choices, meaningfulness of, 166
Christianity, 60–61, 66

Cleveland Community Dialogue Series on Elder Abuse and Ethics, 218
Client's rights, 208, 215
Clinical practice guidelines, 116–118; Cookbook medicine, 117; Office for the Forum for Quality and Effectiveness in Health Care, 117
Coercion, 297
Cognitive development, 239
Cognitive impairment, 175, 189, 190, 204, 216. *See also* Alzheimer's disease; Mental health care; Mental illness; Mental impairment
Cohabiting, 241
Common law, 129
Communicative ethics, 204, 326, 346; assumptions, 336–337; implementing, 337–338
Community mental health movement, 170, 179, 184
Compassion, 74
Competency, 151–153, 157, 298–299
Complementary medical therapies, 97
Confidentiality, 189, 192, 193, 194, 264, 268
Confucianism, 49–50, 60, 61, 71
Confucius, 70, 72
Cookbook medicine, 117. *See also* Clinical practice guidelines
Crawford, S. C., 75
Crime, fear of, 200–204; against the elderly, 201–202; prevention, 202–203; reporting, 202
Criminal penalty, 192, 203, 216–217, 218
Cruzan v. Director, 119
Cruzan v. Harmon, 134
Cultural issues, 269; family care givers, 228; home care aides, shared culture, 227
Culture, 60

Davis, Prema Mathai, 59
De facto surrogates, 267
Death, 65, 74, 279; causes of, 126; place of, 126
Decalogue, 70
Decision makers, substitute, 155, 157, 161–163

Subject Index

Decision making, 20–21, 88
Decisions, capacity to make, 104, 151–153, 157, 263–264, 266–267
Deculturation, 181
Defensive medicine, 116
Degenerative diseases, 126
Demedicalization, 121–122; outcomes, 122
Dementia, 88–89, 175, 185, 246, 256; personhood, 167; sense of self, 166–167. *See also* Alzheimer's disease
Deontological theory, 253–254
Dependence, physical, 187, 190, 212; financial, 190, 195
Dependency, 276
Depression, 168, 175; preventable, 181–182; suicide, 176, 182
Developmental disabilities, 247–250, 253, 256. *See also* Autism
Dhammapada, 73–74
Dignity, 128, 136, 167, 168, 208. *See also* Autonomy
Disabilities, 189, 206, 210. *See also* Cognitive impairment; Dependence; Functional incapacity; Functional limitations; Mental impairment
Disabilities community, approach to home care, 223
Disability, 262
Discrimination, age, 262
Distributive justice, 27
Divorce, 279–280
DSM-IV: age-appropriateness of criteria, 176; mental illness, 175
Durable powers of attorney, 129, 131, 266; for health care, 156–159. *See also* Advance directives
Duty ethicist, 255
Dying, 136–138; needs of dying persons, 138–139, 142

Elder abuse, 188–195; intervention roles, 190–193; laws, 192, 193, 216, 218; other forms of family violence, in comparison with, 189–190; reports, 193, 194, 197; resident abuse, 210–212; self-neglect, 199
Elders, 68, 73, 76

Emotional support to homebound elderly, 221
Empathy, 74
Employment, 262
End-of-life decisions, 84, 119–10, 123, 125, 128–130, 135; medical decision making, 120, 123
Entitlements, 262
Environment, 148, 283; control, 277–278; restriction, 277–279; surveys, 281
Environmental hazards, 213–214
Epilepsy, 247
Equality, 62
Ethical decision making, protocols, 199, 218; guidelines, 207–208, 218; steps, 207
Ethical dilemmas, 21–22; environmental hazards, 213–214; paradigms for resolving, 193–195, 199, 203–204, 206, 208; regulations, 217; restraints, 212; risk in institutions, 209–210, 215; "value conflict: freedom versus safety," 198–199
Ethical egoism, 253–254
Ethical guidelines, 143–144
Ethical issues, 21; a case-based approach, 7–8
Ethical principles, 195, 204. *See also* Accountability; Autonomy; Beneficence; Fidelity; Justice; Nonmaleficence; Privacy
Ethical theory, 195
Ethical values, 56–57
Ethics, 60, 61, 64, 66; history of, 340–341; individual responsibility, 168; public policy, 168; situation, 342; social attitudes and values, 168, 170–172; social services, 168; "territory" of, 165–169
Ethics, aging as catalyst for growth of ethic, 2–3
Ethics, and politics, 331–332
Ethics, and power, 332
Ethics, concepts, 327
Ethics, decision-making process, 336
Ethics, doing, 14–15, 331, 336
Ethics, field of study, 11–14
Ethics, in aging, 1–9

Ethics, in relationships, 329
Ethics, multicultural, multidisciplinary setting, 333–334
Ethics, multiple perspectives, 8–9
Ethics, parameters of, 9–11
Ethics, personal, 328
Ethics, practice of, 14–15
Ethics Committee, Institutional, or Hospital Ethics Committee, 152, 154–156, 162
Ethics committees, 207, 208, 214, 218
Ethics in an Aging Society, 343
Ethics rounds, 214
Ethikos, 10
Ethnic cleansing, 341
Ethnic comparative life expectancy, 34
Ethnic ethics, 31–34
Ethnic-minority elderly, 25–28; data inadequacies, 35–36; death and dying, 39; living arrangements, 38; retirement, 36
Ethnicity, 243; death and dying, 54–55; modernization approach, 55–56
Ethnogenesis, 39
Ethos, 10
Euthanasia, 87, 90, 125, 127, 139–140
Everyday ethics, 168
Expertise, moral, medical, 155
Exploitation, 267
Extraordinary means, 127

Fairhill Center for Aging, 208
Families, 68, 72, 128–129, 133, 135–136, 139, 143, 147, 190, 191, 206, 263, 269; conflict, 247; distribution, 170, 172; justice, 167; of nonautonomous patients, 153, 157; role in mental health care, 170; stigma of mental illness, 170–171; violence, 189–190, 197
Feminist ethics, 247, 249, 257
Fidelity, 18, 195, 327–28
Fiduciary, 264, 268
Food and Drug Administration (FDA), 291
Four Quartets, 346
Freedom versus safety, 198–199
Functional incapacity, 189, 218. *See also* Functional limitations

Functional limitations, 196, 210. *See also* Dependence; Functional incapacity
Futility, 95
Future research, ethics of personal safety, 216

Gender, 348
General Accounting Office, 211
Generational-equity debate, 343
Generations, 165
Genetic screening 110
Gerontology, history of, 342; religious, 343
Government regulation, 210, 217
Grandchildren, 240–241, 243, 251
Grandparents, raising grandchildren, 251–252, 256–257; receiving care, 251
Great Britain, 265
Grief, 168
Group Randomized Study, 295–296
Guardian, 151, 162
Guardianship, 264–267, 270

H.R. 7551, 192
Handbooks, 340
Hastings Center, 344
Health care, 189, 193, 283
Health care costs, 115–116, 123; coronary artery bypass graft, 120; medical technology, 116, 121; resource allocation, 118, 121; withholding of benefits, 123
Health care delivery system, 114, 116
Health care reform, 114, 122, 124; attitudes toward, 122; health care costs, 118, 122; medical decision making, 122; politics, 124; rationing, 122–123
Helsinki Code, 291
High touch vs. high tech, 276
Hinduism, 60, 61
Hitler, Adolph, 341
Home, 64
Home care aide(s), 221, 223, 225
Home Care Aide Association of America, 221
Home Health Assembly of New Jersey, 207
Honor, 64, 70

Hospice, 142–43, 147
Hsuntzu, 71
Hydration and nutrition for incompetent patients, artificial tube feeding, 153, 157, 162

Ideology, 11–13; case-based, 12; casuistry, 12; character ethics, 12; common-morality theory, 12; communitarian, 12; community-based theory, 12; consequence theory, 11; duty theory, 11; ethics of care theory, 12; Kantianism, 12; liberal individualism, 12; obligation-based, 12; principle-based, 12; relationship-based, 12; rights theory, 12; social justice theory, 12; utilitarianism, 12
Imperfect duties, 255
In re Wanglie, 119
Incompetence, 153, 157, 163
Independence, 68
Independent providers, 224
Individual responsibility, 87
Industrial Revolution; First, 271; Second, 272
Infantilization, 189–190, 211, 217
In-home services, 193, 195
Inspection systems, 194
Institute for Bio-Ethics, Maastricht, Netherlands, 348
Institutional care, 188. *See also* Nursing homes
Institutional Review Boards (IRBs), 291–292, 297–299
Institutional structures and policies, 109
Intergenerational responsibility, 112
Interventional Research, 292
Invisibility of home care aides, 226
Islam, 60, 61, 69
Islamic view of aging and death, 79
Is–ought distinction, 314

Japanese Americans, 46; attitudes toward death, 50–52; ethical systems, 46–50; funerals, 52; suicide, 52
Jesus, 66, 68
Judaism, 61
Judgment impaired, 150–153, 163
Justice, 17, 63, 64, 165, 195, 203, 204, 269, 291, 327–328, 347. *See also* Families; Resource allocation

Kant, Immanuel, 340
Kethley House, 215
Kevorkian, Jack, 141, 344
Khrushchev, Nikita, 288
Koran, 69, 70

Labeling, 191, 192
Lake County, Ohio Ethics and Aging Committee, 207
Latino elderly, 29; health care delivery, 36–38
Law Enforcement Assistance Administration, 203
Least Restrictive Alternative (LRA) principle, 266
Legal realism, 270
Legal rights, 262
Legal services organizations, 264
Liberties, 262
Liberty limiting principles, 258
Life course perspective, 239
Life expectancy, 125
Life prolongation, 125, 127–128, 137
Life-sustaining treatment, 126–129, 137, 139; foregoing of, 127–128, 152, 155, 157, 158. *See also* Right to refuse medical treatment
Living Will Declaration, Society for the Right to Die, 152, 157–160
Living wills, 129–131, 266. *See also* Advance directives
Long Term Care Ombudsman Program, 209, 210, 214, 215, 216, 217
Long-term care, 285; definition of, 306; financing of, 309–10; international perspective on, 310–311
Long-term care decisions; control of resources in, 315–316, 318; distinct from acute-care decisions, 312, 318; elders with diminished decision-making capacity, 323; ethical decisions, 307; interpersonal stress in, 306; intrapsychic stress in, 306; management of ambiguity, 319; nondirective counseling in, 318, 322; obligation of elder in, 320,

322; obligations of family members in, 320; problem of competing realities in, 312–315, 318, 322; psychosocial decisions, 316–318; scope of, 306; self-identity and, 317; stepwise approach to, 321–324

Losses in old age, 282–283

Managed care, 108
Mandatory elder abuse reporting, 192–195, 217. *See also* Elder abuse
Marx, Karl, 340
Maslow's pyramid, 278
Mass media, 200, 217; journalism, 203
Maternalism and issues of control, 225, 226
Mediation, 215
Medicaid, 114, 262–263, 270; Fraud Control Units, 211; health care costs, 118
Medical decision making, 120; appropriateness, 123; health care reform, 122; idiosyncratic, 120, 121
Medical liability, 116; insurance premiums, 115, 120
Medical malpractice, 115–116; crisis, 115; medical liability, 115, 120
Medical technology, 114, 123; health care costs, 116; moral crisis, 123; rationing, 123
Medicalization of old age, 178. *See also* Biomedicine and mental illness
Medicare, 114, 262; health care costs, 118
Medications: effects on elders, 169–70; interactions as cause of mental symptoms, 174–175; self-medication, 175. *See also* Mental illness
Mental health: "adaptivity," 179; aging, 165–168; as by-product of way of life, 183–184; community, 180–181; concepts of, 178–181, 185–186; concepts of disease, 179; decline as "normal" with age, 169–170; "everyday" mental health, 180; gender, 173; as a goal to be pursued, 179; historical background of concept, 169–170; loss, 173, 180; mental illness, 173–174; poverty, 173; promotion of, 181–184; "psychological well-being," 173, 179; psychosocial and spiritual factors in, 179, 180–181; religious communities, 184; social roles of elders, 180–181, 183. *See also* Medications; Mental health care; Mental illness; Prevention, of mental illness; Promotion of mental health
Mental health care: and biomedical approach, 177–178; as enhancement, 177, 178; goals of, 177, 185–186; as "illness care," 178, 179; as prevention, 178, 181–182
Mental health professionals, role of, 168–169
Mental illness: and dementia, 175; *DSM-IV* criteria, 175; etiology, 185; factors contributing to, 173–174; physical ailments, 174; prevention, 181–184; recognition of, 174–176; reimbursement for, 174, 175–76, 182; stigma of, 170–171; symptoms, 175. *See also* Anxiety; Depression; Medications; Mental health; Problems in living; Research; Suicide
Mental impairment, 187, 196, 197. *See also* Alzheimer's disease; Cognitive impairment
Mental wellness, 178–181, 185–186. *See also* Mental health, concepts of
Metaethics, 11
Mexican Americans, 42–46; attitudes toward life and death, 43; death issues and suicide rate, 44; religion, family and acceptance of death, 44–46
Mind/body duality, 80
Minority elderly; barriers to health care, 58; health and health care delivery, 57–58; health problems, 34
Mistreatment by others. *See* Elder abuse
Moral crisis, 123; medical technology, 123; politics, 123–24
Moral pluralism, 26
Moral realism, 314–315
Moral relativism, 341
Mores, 10
Muhammad, 69
Muilenburg, James, 63

Nader, Ralph, 210
National Aging Resource Center on Elder Abuse, 193
National Institute on Aging, 151
National Values History Project, 206–207
Nation-states, variations in ethical styles of, 348
Native Americans, 53–54
Nazi Research, 289, 291
Need, definition of, 168–69, 171; Michael Ignatieff's view of, 169; theory of human good, 169
Neglect, 267–269
Negotiated consent, 208
Noncompliance, service receipt, 199–200
Nonethical issues, 22
Nonmaleficence, 18, 195, 204, 290, 327–328
Nontraditional relationships, 241
Normality, premises of, 169–71
Not clinically indicated, 122; resource allocation, 122
Nuremberg trials, 341
Nursing homes, 209, 210–215, 219, 262, 270. *See also* Institutional care

Observational research, 296–297
Office for the Forum for Quality and Effectiveness in Health Care and clinical practice guidelines, 117
Office of Protection from Research Risks (OPRR), 291
Old age, 64, 69; as a problem, 342
Old people's liberation movement, 210
Older adults, as consumers, 334; in the community, 5–7; differences, 4–5; subject of study, 3–4
Omissions, 127, 137
Omnibus Budget Reconciliation Act of 1987, 170, 215, 302
Open-label Studies, 295
Outcomes, 120, 122; demedicalization, 122; health care costs, 120; research, 116, 117

Pain, 141–143, 145–146; prevention/control, 145–146
Palliative care/treatment, 142–143

Papanicolaou Testing, 293
Paraprofessional, 327–330
Parens patriae, 264–265
Parents, 70, 72
Park Ridge Center, 344
Partnerships, professionals and clients, 339
Paternalism, 154–155, 160, 199, 246, 258
Patient Self-Determination Act, 131–134
Patient's best interests standard, 154
Perfect duties, 255
Perpetrator, 189, 190, 191. *See also* Elder abuse; Resident abuse
Personhood, 166–167. *See also* Autonomy
Philosophy and Public Affairs, 13
Physician, 85, 86, 89; assisted dying, 105; patient relationship, 98
Physicians Health Study, 294
Placebo, 293–294
Plato, 340
Political economy of aging, 342
Politics, 123–124; health care reform, 124; moral crisis, 123
Positive mental health, 178–181, 185–186. *See also* Mental health, concepts of
Poverty, 173. *See also* Mental health, poverty
Power, 244, 346–347
President's Commission for the Study of Ethical Problems in Medicine and Biomedical and Behavioral Research (President's Commission), 151, 153, 154, 155, 161–162, 163
Prevention, of mental illness, 181–184; need for research, 181–182; primary, 181; secondary, 181, 185. *See also* Mental health; Mental health care, as prevention
Preventive efforts, 118, 122; public health, 122; resource allocation, 122
Preventive ethics; implications for long-term care policy and planning, 324–325
Prima facie duty, 255–256
Primary caregiver, 242
Privacy, 17, 189, 191, 194, 215, 217, 327–328

Problems in living, 177, 178. *See also* Mental health; Mental illness
Professionals, 189, 191, 192, 193, 194, 206, 207; codes of ethics, 199, 207, 208
Promotion of mental health: and distribution, 181, 183, 185; as psychosocial, 182; reimbursement, 182
Propositions, 19
Prostate Specific Antigen, 293
Protective services, 268
Protocols, 19–20
Proxy health care, 131–132
Psychological well-being, 173. *See also* Mental health
Public good versus individual rights, 121
Public health, 122; preventive efforts, 122
Public Law 103-322, 203
Public policies, 269, 349

Quality Adjusted Life Years (QALYs), 171
Quality assurance, 114, 194; model, 115; tools, 115
Quality of care, 85
Quality of life, 128, 138, 144
Quality of life judgments, 157, 158
Quandary ethics, 166, 167; justice, 167. *See also* Ethics
Quinlan, Karen Ann, 114, 127, 162

Race, 243
Racial mortality crossover, 35
Randomized Control Trials, 292
Rationing, 122; health care reform, 122
Reciprocity, 70, 72
Regional differences, 347
Registries, abuse, 217
Reporting requirements, 268
Research, 181–182. *See also* Prevention, need for research
Resident abuse, 210–12
Resident councils, 215
Resource allocation, 118, 121, 171; availability and accessibility, 118; not clinically indicated, 122; rationing, 123. *See also* Families
Respect, 70

Restraints, 212–213, 219
Right of self-determination, 151–153
Right to die, 91
Right to refuse medical treatment, 157, 158, 159, 160
Rights, human, 256
Rights and responsibilities in the provision of home care, 229–234; particular rights, 234, 235; qualified, 234, 235; universal rights, 234
Risk, 187, 190, 191, 197, 216; at home, 204–208; greater risk, older people at, 187, 216; in institutions, 209–216; risk management, 209–210
Robots, 284
Rousseau, Jean-Jacques, 340

Saint Augustine, 340
Santayana, George, 340
Saunders, Cicely, 142
Self, sense of, 166–169. *See also* Autonomy; Dignity
Self-care, 196, 197
Self-determination, 86, 133, 144, 189, 194, 198, 206, 208, 212
Self-image, 137
Self-integrity, 144
Self-neglect, 195–200, 269
Sex, 348
Shintoism, 47–48
Shrinking environment for older adults, 277–280
Simple supernatural, 12
Social attitudes, 179, 182–183; liberal individualism, 184; worthiness, 185. *See also* Ageism
Social care relationships, 225
Social isolation, 196, 197, 198, 200, 202
Social roles: role equivalence, 282; role repetition, 22; role reversal, 283
Social Security, 262
Social support to homebound elderly, 221, 228, 230; personal emotional support, 222, 230–231; professional emotional support, 222, 232–234; social care relationship, 225
Spencer, Herbert, 340

Subject Index

Spiritual dimension, 78; maturity, 80, 82; needs, 82, 83, 84, 92; well-being, 81, 82; wellness, 81
Spirituality, 78–80, 81, 92
Spring Case, 163
Substituted judgment, 133–134
Suffering, 73, 76, 125. *See also* Pain
Suicide, 90, 139, 176, 182; physician assisted, 125, 139–142. *See also* Depression
Surrogate, 132–133
Surrogate families, 260. *See also* Nontraditional relationships
Symptom care/control, 142, 144–145

Technologies, 127; assessment, 117; biomedical, 126
Technology: advanced, 275–277; aging, 280–281; attitudes, 281; education, 281–282; fears, 272–74; future prospects, 286–287; health care, 283–85; long-term care, 285–286; objections to, 273; sex, 286
Teleological theory, 253
Theism, 12
Therapeutic jurisprudence, 269–270
Tillich, Paul, 59, 78–79
Title XX of Social Security Act, 198, 216
Torah, 61
Training, 208, 214, 215, 217
Trusts, 266; relationships, 264, 268

United Nations Charter, 341
Universal policies, 216–217
Universalistic morality, 26
U.S. Attorney General, 203
U.S. Senate Special Committee on Aging, 211
Utilitarianism, 253–254
Utility, 290–291

Value conflict, protective services and self-neglect, 198–200
Value systems, 118; resource allocation, 118
Values histories, 206–207
Values mapping, 207. *See also* Values histories
Victim, 189, 190, 193, 194, 200–202; 202; assistance programs, 202; compensation laws, 202. *See also* Crime; Elder abuse; Resident abuse
Virtue ethics, 41
Vital involvement, 178–181, 185–186. *See also* Mental health, concepts of
Voluntarism, 289–290
Voluntary passive euthanasia, 91

Wandering, 209, 213
Welfare services and mental illness, 171
Western tradition, 91
White House Conference on Aging, 200
Willowbrook Hepatitis Study, 290
Withholding of benefits, 123

Youth cult, 342

About the Editor and Contributors

W. ANDREW ACHENBAUM, Ph.D., teaches at the University of Michigan. He has published in the areas of the social history of aging and the history of gerontology. Dr. Achenbaum has participated in several international conferences in which ethics and aging were the focal issues. He becomes Chair of the National Council on Aging in 1999. His research interests include the development of the field of Gerontology, "wisdom" in the modern era, and policy issues in aging in a socioculturally diverse society.

GEORGIA J. ANETZBERGER, Ph.D., is Associate Director for Community Services at the Benjamin Rose Institute and Adjunct Assistant Professor of Medicine at Case Western Reserve University in Cleveland, Ohio. She is a Fellow of the Gerontological Society of America, is on the Board of Directors for the National Committee for the Prevention of Elder Abuse, and chairs its regional affiliate, the Western Reserve Consortium for the Prevention and Treatment of Elder Abuse.

ANTHONY BACK, M.D., is an Oncologist and Ethicist at the Veterans Administration Puget Sound Health Care System and an Assistant Professor at the University of Washington School of Medicine in Seattle, Washington. He is currently a Faculty Scholar for the Project on Death in America. His research interests include end-of-life suffering, and patient and family experiences with physician-assisted suicides.

ANTHONY J. CORTESE, Ph.D., is Associate Professor of Sociology at Southern Methodist University. His major area of research and teaching is Ethnic and Race Relations, and he has published in the area of Mexican American mental health. He currently serves on the American Sociological Association's Committee on Professional Ethics. Cortese has served as Director of Ethnic Studies and Director of Mexican American Studies at Southern Methodist University.

CROMWELL CRAWFORD, Ph.D., is a Professor of Religion at the University of Hawaii at Manoa. A specialist in Indian and Comparative Studies, he teaches courses in Ethics, Philosophy of Religion, and Medicine in World Religions. He has published widely in the areas of Comparative Bioethics, Religion and Medicine, and Environment, with a focus on Hinduism. He is active in the causes of South Asian Studies and is a member of the Inter-Religious Federation for World Peace.

CAROLEE A. DeVITO, Ph.D., M.PH., is a Professor in the Department of Psychiatry and Behavioral Sciences at the University of Miami Medical School and Director of the Health Services Research and Development Center at the Miami Veterans Affairs Medical Center. Research includes prevention of accidental injuries, particularly those associated with burns and falls. Dr. DeVito is principal investigator of a randomized study examining the benefits of physical restoration among elderly recently discharged from hospitals or deconditioned due to illness.

ARLENE GRUBER, M.SW., also has a Master's degree in Ethics. She has worked as a clinician at Loyola University Medical Center where she also has taught courses in Medical Ethics. In addition, she has taught Ethics at the Loyola Graduate School of Social Work and has served as an Ethics Consultant with the Loyola University Center for Ethics and the Inspector General's office of the Illinois Department of Children and Family Services. Related work has included home care, health care, and hospice for the elderly.

LAWRENCE HEINTZ, Ph.D., is a Professor of Philosophy at the University of Hawaii at Hilo. Since 1983 he has been a Medical Ethicist for the Hawaii Department of Health. He has taught at several British and American universities and was a member of the British National Working Party on Living Wills during 1986–1987. He is a member of Hawaii's Blue Ribbon Panel on Living and Dying with Dignity, and has published articles on ethics in philosophical and medical journals.

DALLAS M. HIGH, Ph.D., is Professor Emeritus of Philosophy and Senior Research Associate of the Sanders-Brown Center on Aging at the University of Kentucky. He has specialized in Aging and Ethics, Contemporary Philosophy, and Philosophy of Religion. He is a recipient of the Chancellor's Award for Outstanding Teaching at the University of Kentucky. His gerontological research interests include ethics and aging, family decision making in nursing home care, care of terminally ill persons, and the ethics of informed consent in Alzheimer's disease research.

MARTHA HOLSTEIN, Ph.D., is a Research Associate at the Park Ridge Center for the Study of Health, Faith, and Ethics. Her doctorate is in Medical Humanities. She has worked in the field of aging since 1973, focusing on ethics, public policy, social justice, dementia, and gender issues. Her writing covers a wide area including women, ethics, and home care, normative public policy, Alzheimer's disease, dying, and death.

BETTE A. IDE, Ph.D., R.N., is director of the Rural Health Nursing Specialization in the graduate program and Associate Professor in the College of Nursing, Department of Family and Community Nursing at the University of North Dakota in Grand Forks. She is currently involved in a study in collaboration with Montana State University on the use of complementary therapies by older rural adults. Her research interests include a spectrum of aging issues from health problems among the elderly to aging well.

TANYA FUSCO JOHNSON, M.Div., Ph.D., teaches Sociology at the University of Hawaii at Hilo. She is a Family Sociologist specializing in Gerontology. Dr. Johnson is a contributing editor of the *Journal of Elder Abuse and Neglect*, chairs the Aging Well Research Committee of the American Sociology Association, and is the Director of the Home Safety Monitoring Project for Frail Elderly at the University of Hawaii at Hilo. Her research in gerontology includes elder mistreatment, aging well, ethical practice in aging, and household safety for older adults.

MARSHALL B. KAPP, LL.B., is the Frederick A. White Distinguished Service Professor at Wright State University School of Medicine, where he teaches and conducts research in the area of legal and ethical aspects of health care, with particular emphasis on older patients. He serves as Director of Wright State University Office of Geriatric Medicine and Gerontology. He is a member of the adjunct faculty at the University of Dayton School of Law, where he teaches a seminar on Law and Aging. During 1998–1999, he will be the Dr. Arthur Grayson Memorial Distinguished Visiting Professor of Law and Medicine at Southern Illinois University.

GARI LESNOFF-CARAVAGLIA, Ph.D., is Professor in the School of Health Sciences at Ohio University. Prior to coming to Ohio University, she was Executive Director of the University Center on Aging at the University of Massachusetts Medical Center and Director of the Gerontology Institute and Program at the University of Illinois/Springfield. Research interests include technology and aging. Dr. Lesnoff-Caravaglia is the convener of the Formal Interest Group on Technology and Aging for the Gerontological Society of America.

LAURENCE B. McCULLOUGH, Ph.D., is a philosopher who teaches Medical Ethics at Baylor College of Medicine. He is Professor of Medicine and Medical Ethics in the Center for Medical Ethics and Health Policy. He teaches clinical ethics case conferences on Medicine, Geriatrics and Extended Care, Geropsychiatry, and Surgery services of the Houston Veterans Affairs Medical Center, where he is Staff Associate for Long-Term Care Research. Dr. McCullough has held fellowships at the Hastings Center and the American Council of Learned Societies. He is also a Faculty Associate of Baylor's Huffington Center on Aging and a Fellow of the Gerontological Society of America. Gerontological research interests include ethical issues in long-term care decision making, end-of-life decision making, and managed care for the elderly.

DAVID McCURDY, M.Div., is Co-Director of Clinical Healthcare Ethics Support Services, Park Ridge Center for the Study of Health, Faith, and Ethics. He has worked as a chaplain, clinical pastoral educator, and vice president of Religion and Health at Good Samaritan Hospital (Advocate Health Care), Downers Grove, Illinois. Previously, he served as a parish pastor and later, as a college chaplain at Elmhurst College. He continues as an adjunct faculty member in the Department of Theology and Religion of Elmhurst where he has taught courses in Health Care Ethics since 1985.

KATHY A. MARQUIS, J.D., FNP-L, is currently a member of the graduate faculty at Idaho State Department of Nursing in Pocatello, Idaho. She has been a faculty member as well as Family Nurse Practitioner preceptor in continuing education, undergraduate, and graduate Family Nurse Practitioner programs. She continues as a consultant on Medico-Legal and ethical issues relating to health care.

PHYLLIS B. MITZEN, M.A. in Social Service Administration, is the Director of Resources and Development at the Council for Jewish Elderly (CJE) in Chicago. She has developed programs for home community-based services. Ms. Mitzen founded and continues to serve as chair of CJE's Community Ethics Committee. Her research interests include ethics, aging, and long-term care.

ROBERT O. MORGAN, Ph.D., is a Psychometrician and Health Services researcher who studies predictors of health care use, with particular focus on elderly and disabled populations in Florida. He is an Associate Professor in the Department of Psychiatry and Behavioral Sciences at the University of Miami Medical School and Associate Director of the Health Services Research and Development Center at the Miami Veterans Affairs Medical Center.

ROBERT PEARLMAN, M.D., M.PH., is Associate Professor in the Department of Medicine, University of Washington and the Veterans Affairs Puget Sound Health Care System. He has served on Ethics Committees of the American Geriatric Society and Department of Veterans Affairs and has been an ethics consultant to the American Medical Association and the National Board of Medical Examiners. Dr. Pearlman directs his own research program in ethics at end-of-life care. His research interests include quality of life in medical decisions, medical futility, advance care planning, physician-assisted suicide, and patient suffering.

JILL A. RHYMES, M.D., is Director of the Geriatric Evaluation and Management Unit and the Geriatrics Consult Service at the Houston Veterans Affairs Medical Center and an Assistant Professor of Medicine at Baylor College of Medicine. She is also Faculty Associate of Baylor's Huffington Center on Aging. Her current research interests include values in long-term care decision making and the professional's role in long-term care decision making.

JENNIFER CREW SOLOMON, Ph.D., is Associate Professor of Sociology and Coordinator of the Gerontology Minor Program at Winthrop University where she teaches courses in Introductory Sociology, Social Theory, Social Psychology, Social Problems, Death and Grief, and Sociology of Aging. Her research includes grandparents raising grandchildren, gender and racial differences in retirement income, and humor and aging well.

PATRICIA SUGGS, M.Div., M.Ed., Ph.D., is a United Methodist minister of the Western North Carolina Conference and Director of the Appalachian Geriatric Education Center and of Aging Initiatives of the Northwest Area Health Education Center of the Wake Forest University School of Medicine. She is an Assistant Professor of Gerontology and Geriatrics at Wake Forest University School of Medicine and an instructor at Duke Divinity School. Her research includes gerontology/geriatric education, spirituality, health, and aging.

THOMAS A. TEASDALE, Dr.PH, teaches Research Methods, Educational Informatics, and Ethics at Baylor College of Medicine and the Veterans Affairs Medical Center at Houston, Texas. He has specialized in gerontology and is a founding faculty associate of Baylor's Huffington Center on Aging. His gerontological research interests include long-term care, medical decision making, and interdisciplinary training.

BETH A. VIRNIG, Ph.D., is an Assistant Professor in the Division of Health Management and Policy at the University of Minnesota's School of Public Health. She has served on the Research Ethics Committee for the Miami Veterans Affairs Medical Center where she has reviewed clinical research protocols and their corresponding consent forms. Her research includes medical care, epidemiology, use of medical claims data for research, research ethics, Medicare Hospice benefit in managed care and traditional fee-for-service populations, and Medicare data for cancer surveillance.

NANCY L. WILSON, Ph.D., is a social worker who has specialized in gerontology. She is an Assistant Professor in the Department of Medicine—Section of Geriatrics, Assistant Director of the Huffington Center on Aging, and Instructor at the Center for Medical Ethics and Health Policy at Baylor College of Medicine. Her research and practice interests are in the area of community long-term care, including ethical issues in long-term care, care management, and service delivery to elders with dementia and their families.

MANCHESTER COLLEGE LIBRARY

3 9315 01035756 1

174.2 H191j

Handbook on ethical issues in aging

DATE DUE

WITHDRAWN
from
Funderburg Library